GERIATRICS *At Your* FINGERTIPS®

2006-2007, 8th EDITION

AUTHORS

David B. Reuben, MD
Director, Multicampus Program in Geriatric Medicine and Gerontology
Chief, Division of Geriatrics
Archstone Foundation Chair
Professor of Medicine
David Geffen School of Medicine at UCLA
Los Angeles, CA

Keela A. Herr, PhD, RN
Professor
Chair, Adult and Gerontological Nursing
College of Nursing
The University of Iowa
Iowa City, IA

James T. Pacala, MD, MS
Associate Professor
Distinguished Teaching Professor
Department of Family Medicine and Community Health
University of Minnesota School of Medicine
Minneapolis, MN

Bruce G. Pollock, MD, PhD
Sandra A. Rotman Chair in Neuropsychiatry
Professor and Head, Division of Geriatric Psychiatry
The Rotman Research Institute
Baycrest Centre for Geriatric Care
University of Toronto
Toronto, Ontario, Canada

Jane F. Potter, MD
Chief, Section of Geriatrics and Gerontology
Harris Professor of Geriatric Medicine
University of Nebraska Medical Center
Omaha, NE

Todd P. Semla, MS, PharmD
Clinical Pharmacy Specialist
Department of Veterans Affairs
Pharmacy Benefits Management
Associate Professor
The Feinberg School of Medicine
Northwestern University
Chicago, IL

TABLE OF CONTENTS

Geriatrics At Your Fingertips® is published by the American Geriatrics Society as a service to health care providers involved in the care of older adults.

Although *Geriatrics At Your Fingertips*® is distributed by various companies in the health care field, it is independently prepared and published. All decisions regarding its content are solely the responsibility of the authors. Their decisions are not subject to any form of approval by other interests or organizations.

Some recommendations in this publication suggest the use of agents for purposes or in dosages other than those recommended in product labeling. Such recommendations are based on reports in peer-reviewed publications and are not based on or influenced by any material or advice from pharmaceutical or health care product manufacturers.

No responsibility is assumed by the authors or the American Geriatrics Society for any injury or damage to persons or property, as a matter of product liability, negligence, warranty, or otherwise, arising out of the use or application of any methods, products, instructions, or ideas contained herein. No guarantee, endorsement, or warranty of any kind, express or implied (including specifically no warrant of merchantability or of fitness for a particular purpose) is given by the Society in connection with any information contained herein. Independent verification of any diagnosis, treatment, or drug use or dosage should be obtained. No test or procedure should be performed unless, in the judgment of an independent, qualified physician, it is justified in the light of the risk involved.

Citation: Reuben DB, Herr KA, Pacala JT, *et al. Geriatrics At Your Fingertips: 2006-2007, 8th Edition.* New York: The American Geriatrics Society; 2006.

ISBN 1-886775-18-4
Library of Congress Control Number 2005933837

GERIATRICS *At Your* FINGERTIPS®

2006-2007, 8th EDITION

AUTHORS:

David B. Reuben, MD

Keela A. Herr, PhD, RN

James T. Pacala, MD, MS

Bruce G. Pollock, MD, PhD

Jane F. Potter, MD

Todd P. Semla, MS, PharmD

ABBREVIATIONS

ABG	arterial blood gas
ABI	ankle-brachial index
ACC	American College of Cardiology
ACE	angiotensin-converting enzyme
ACIP	Advisory Committee on Immunization Practices
ACOG	American College of Obstetrics and Gynecology
ACR	American College of Rheumatology
ACTH	adrenocorticotropic hormone
AD	Alzheimer's disease
ADA	American Diabetes Association
ADLs	activities of daily living
AFB	acid-fast bacillus
AGS	American Geriatrics Society
AHA	American Heart Association
AHRQ	Agency for Healthcare Research and Quality
AIDS	acquired immune deficiency syndrome
AIMS	Abnormal Involuntary Movement Scale
ALT	alanine aminotransferase
AMD	age-related macular degeneration
APAP	acetaminophen
ARB	angiotensin receptor blocker
AS	aortic stenosis
ASA	acetylsalicylic acid or aspirin
ASA class	American Society of Anesthesiologists grading scale for surgical patients
AST	aspartate amino transferase
ATA	American Thyroid Association
ATS	American Thoracic Society
AUA	American Urological Association
BMD	bone mineral density
BMI	body mass index
BP	blood pressure
BPH	benign prostatic hyperplasia
BUN	blood urea nitrogen
C&S	culture and sensitivity
CABG	coronary artery bypass graft
CAD	coronary artery disease
CBC	complete blood cell count
cfu	colony-forming unit
CHD	coronary heart disease
CI	confidence interval
CMS	Centers for Medicare and Medicaid Services
CNS	central nervous system
COPD	chronic obstructive pulmonary disease
CPAP	continuous positive airway pressure

CPK	creatine phosphokinase
CPR	cardiopulmonary resuscitation
Cr	creatinine
CrCl	creatinine clearance
CT	computed tomography
CXR	chest x-ray
CYP	cytochrome P-450
D&C	dilation and curettage
D5W	dextrose 5% in water
DBP	diastolic blood pressure
D/C	discontinue
DHIC	detrusor hyperactivity with impaired contractility
DMARD	disease-modifying anti-rheumatoid drug
DSM-IV	*Diagnostic and Statistical Manual of Mental Disorders*, 4th ed. (Washington, DC: American Psychiatric Association; 1994)
DVT	deep-vein thrombosis
ECF	extracellular fluid
ECG	electrocardiogram, electrocardiography
EEG	electroencephalogram
EF	ejection fraction
EPS	extrapyramidal symptoms
ESR	erythrocyte sedimentation rate
FDA	Food and Drug Administration
FEV_1	forced expiratory volume in 1 sec
FI	fecal incontinence
FOBT	fecal occult blood test
FVC	forced vital capacity
GAD	generalized anxiety disorder
GDS	Geriatric Depression Scale
GERD	gastroesophageal reflux disease
GFR	glomerular filtration rate
GI	gastrointestinal
GnRH	gonadotropin-releasing hormone
GU	genitourinary
Hb	hemoglobin
HbA_{1c}	glycosylated hemoglobin
HCTZ	hydrochlorothiazide
HDL	high-density lipoprotein
HF	heart failure
HR	heart rate
HT	hormone therapy
HTN	hypertension
hx	history
IADLs	instrumental activities of daily living
IBS	irritable bowel syndrome
IBW	ideal body weight
ICD	implantable cardiac defibrillator
INH	isoniazid

INR	international normalized ratio
IOP	intraocular pressure
iPTH	intact parathyroid hormone
JNC 7	Seventh Joint National Committee on Prevention, Detection, Evaluation, and Treatment of High Blood Pressure
K+	potassium ion
LBW	lean body weight
LDL	low-density lipoprotein
LFT	liver function test
LMWH	low-molecular-weight heparin
LVEF	left ventricular ejection fraction
LVH	left ventricular hypertrophy
MAOI	monoamine oxidase inhibitor
MCV	mean corpuscular volume
MDI	metered-dose inhaler
MI	myocardial infarction
MMA	methylmalonic acid
MMSE	Mini-Mental State Examination (Folstein's)
MRA	magnetic resonance angiography
MRI	magnetic resonance imaging
MSE	mental status examination
NG	nasogastric
NSAIDs	nonsteroidal anti-inflammatory drugs
NPH	neutral protamine Hagedorn (insulin)
OCD	obsessive-compulsive disorder
OGTT	oral glucose tolerance test
OT	occupational therapy
PAD	peripheral arterial disease
PCA	patient-controlled analgesia
PE	pulmonary embolism
PEF	peak expiratory flow
PNS	peripheral nervous system
POMA	Performance-Oriented Mobility Assessment
PPD	purified protein derivative (of tuberculin)
PPI	proton-pump inhibitor
PSA	prostate-specific antigen
PT	prothrombin time *or* physical therapy
PTCA	percutaneous transluminal coronary angioplasty
PTH	parathyroid hormone
PTT	partial thromboplastin time
PUVA	psoralen plus ultraviolet light of A wavelength
QT$_c$	QT (cardiac output) corrected for heart rate
RA	rheumatoid arthritis
RBC	red blood cells *or* ranitidine bismuth citrate
RF	rheumatoid factor
sats	saturations
SBP	systolic blood pressure
SD	standard deviation

SIADH	syndrome of inappropriate secretion of antidiuretic hormone
SPEP	serum protein electrophoresis
SSRIs	selective serotonin-reuptake inhibitors
sTfR	soluble transferrin receptor
TCA	tricyclic antidepressant
TD	tardive dyskinesia
TDD	telephone device for the deaf
TG	triglycerides
TIA	transient ischemic attack
TIBC	total iron-binding capacity
TSG	thyroid-stimulating globulin
TSH	thyroid-stimulating hormone
TTP	thrombotic thrombocytopenic purpura
TUIP	transurethral incision of the prostate
TURP	transurethral resection of the prostate
U	unit(s)
UA	urinalysis
UFH	unfractionated heparin
UI	urinary incontinence
UTI	urinary tract infection
UV	ultraviolet
VF	ventricular fibrillation
VIN	vulvar intraepithelial neoplasia
VT	ventricular tachycardia
WBC	white blood cell(s)
WHO	World Health Organization
wt	weight

Drug Prescribing and Elimination

Drugs are listed by generic names; trade names are in *italics*. Check marks (✔) indicate drugs preferred for treating older persons. Formulations in text are bracketed and expressed in milligrams (mg) unless otherwise specified. Abbreviations for dosing, formulations, and route of elimination are defined below.

ac	before meals	h	hour(s)
bid	twice a day	hs	at bedtime
C	capsule, caplet	IM	intramuscular(ly)
ChT	chewable tablet	Inj	injectable(s)
conc	concentrate	IT	intrathecal(ly)
CR	controlled release	IV	intravenous(ly)
crm	cream	K	renal elimination
d	day(s)	L	hepatic elimination
ER	extended release	lot	lotion
F	fecal elimination	max	maximum
fl	fluid	mcg	microgram(s)
g	gram(s)	MDI	metered-dose inhaler
gran	granules	min	minute(s)
gtt	drop(s)	mo	month(s)

npo	nothing by mouth
NS	normal saline
oint	ointment
OTC	over-the-counter
OU	both eyes
pc	after a meal
Pch	patch
pk	pack, packet
po	by mouth
pr	per rectum
prn	as needed
pwd	powder
qam	every morning
qd	every day
qhs	each bedtime
qid	four times a day
qod	every other day
S	liquid (includes concentrate, elixir, solution, suspension, syrup, tincture)
SC	subcutaneous(ly)
sec	second(s)
shp	shampoo
sl	sublingual
sol	solution
Sp	suppository
spr	spray(s)
SR	sustained release
sus	suspension
syr	syrup
T	tablet
tab(s)	tablet(s)
tbsp	tablespoon(s)
tinc	tincture
tid	three times a day
TR	timed release
tsp	teaspoon(s)
wk	week(s)
XR	extended release
yr	year(s)

INTRODUCTION

Providing high-quality medical care for older adults requires a special set of knowledge, clinical skills, and attitudes. Many resources contain current, accurate information on evaluation and management of the older patient. However, few are portable enough to be used in the examining room, on nursing home or hospital rounds, or when the clinician is on call outside the office.

In 1998, the American Geriatrics Society (AGS) first published *Geriatrics At Your Fingertips (GAYF)*, a pocket guide that provides immediate access to specific information needed to care for older adults in various health care settings. The response was extraordinary, and *GAYF* soon became the society's best-selling publication. As electronic media have increasingly expanded into clinical practice, the AGS has created new platforms for *GAYF* including an Internet edition (http://www.geriatricsatyourfingertips.org) and Palm and Windows CE operating systems versions (available for download at the Web site listed above).

In this 8th edition, we have added new sections on dysphagia, irritable bowel syndrome, myeloproliferative disorders, the metabolic syndrome, orthostatic hypotension, plantar fasciitis, rheumatoid arthritis, treatment of early prostate cancer, and Medicare Part D. Throughout the text and tables, we have updated information including recommended diagnostic tests, management strategies, and assessment instruments. Tables and lists of drugs are designed to facilitate appropriate prescribing. Generic and trade names are provided, as well as information on dosages, how the drugs are metabolized or excreted, and which formulations are available. Specific caveats and cautions to be observed when using the medication in older adults are also included.

The goal of *GAYF* is to reduce to a minimum the amount of time that a practicing clinician must spend searching for specific information that is needed immediately to make patient care decisions. Accordingly, *GAYF* does not attempt to explain in detail the rationale underlying the strategies presented. In many instances, these strategies have been derived from guidelines published by organizations such as the Agency for Healthcare Research and Quality, the American Geriatrics Society, the American Heart Association, and the American Diabetes Association. Many of the guidelines can be obtained from the National Guideline Clearinghouse (http://www.guidelines.gov). When no such guidelines exist, the strategies recommended herein represent the best opinions of the authors and the experts they have asked to review the chapters. In an effort to be comprehensive yet concise, references have been provided sparingly, but many others that are relevant are available from the organizations mentioned or in the most recent edition of the AGS *Geriatrics Review Syllabus*.

The authors welcome comments about the format and content of this edition of *GAYF* that may guide the preparation of future editions. All comments should be addressed to the American Geriatrics Society, Empire State Building, 350 Fifth Avenue, Suite 801, New York, NY 10118.

The authors are particularly grateful to Nancy Lundebjerg at the AGS, who has served a vital role in the development of this book and its readership. We are also grateful to the John A. Hartford Foundation for generously supporting the development and distribution of *GAYF* PDA versions.

We would also like to thank the following persons who have reviewed parts of this edition:

Catherine A. DuBeau, MD
Perry Fine, MD
Rita A. Frantz, PhD, RN
Gail Greendale, MD
Jerry C. Johnson, MD
James Judge, MD
Catherine MacLean, MD, PhD

Patrick E. McBride, MD, MPH
Elizabeth C. Reed, MD
Larissa Rodriguez, MD
Jules Rosen, MD
Ruth Wintz, MD
Thomas T. Yoshikawa, MD

Guidelines of the following organizations are the basis of parts of specific chapters:

Advisory Committee on Immunization Practices
Agency for Healthcare Research and Quality
Alzheimer's Association
American Academy of Neurology
American Association for Geriatric Psychiatry
American College of Cardiology
American College of Chest Physicians
American College of Gastroenterology
American College of Obstetrics and Gynecology
American College of Rheumatology
American Diabetes Association
American Geriatrics Society
American Heart Association
American Lung Association
American Pain Society
American Psychiatric Association
American Society of Anesthesiologists
American Thyroid Association
American Urological Association
Ethnogeriatrics Committee, American Geriatrics Society
National Cholesterol Education Program
National Heart, Lung, and Blood Institute
U.S. Preventive Services Task Force
World Health Organization

Staff
Managing Editor (all versions): Carol S. Goodwin
Medical Editor (print version): Susan E. Aiello, DVM, ELS
Medical Editor (PDA and Web versions): Barbara B. Reitt, PhD, ELS(D)
Medical Indexer (all versions): L. Pilar Wyman

Fry Communications, Inc.
Technical development and production of print and electronic versions:
Robyn Diven, Composition
Melissa Durborow, Group Manager
Gwen Eckenrode, Composition
Jason Hughes, Technical Services Manager
Julie Stevens, Account Administrator
Terry Plyler, Systems Architect/Engineer

Table 1. Conversions		
Temperature	**Liquid**	**Weight**
F = (1.8)C + 32	1 fl dram = 4 mL	1 lb = 0.453 kg
C = (F − 32) / (1.8)	1 fl oz = 30 mL	1 kg = 2.2 lb
	1 tsp = 5 mL	1 oz = 30 g
	1 tbsp = 15 mL	1 grain = 60 mg

Alveolar-Arterial Oxygen Gradient

$A - a = 148 - 1.2(Paco_2) - Pao_2$
[normal = 10−20 mm Hg, breathing room air at sea level]

Calculated Osmolality

2Na + glucose / 18 + BUN / 2.8 + ethanol / 4.6 + isopropanol / 6 + methanol / 3.2 + ethylene glycol / 6.2   [normal = 280–295]

Golden Rules of Arterial Blood Gases
- Pco_2 change of 10 corresponds to a pH change of 0.08.
- pH change of 0.15 corresponds to base excess change of 10 mEq/L.

Creatinine Clearance
See Appropriate Prescribing, p 9.
For renally eliminated drugs, dosage adjustments may be necessary if CrCl <60.
Cockcroft-Gault formula:

$$\frac{IBW(140 - age) (0.85 \text{ if female})}{(72) (\text{stable serum creatinine})}$$

Erythrocyte Sedimentation Rate
Westergren: women = (age + 10) / 2
men = age / 2

Ideal Body Weight
- Men = 50 kg + (2.3 kg) (each inch of height >5 feet)
- Women = 45.5 kg + (2.3 kg) (each inch of height >5 feet)

Lean Body Weight
IBW + 0.4 (actual body weight − IBW)

Body Mass Index

$$\frac{\text{weight in kg}}{(\text{height in meters})^2} \quad or \quad \frac{\text{weight in lb}}{(\text{height in inches})^2} \times 704.5$$

Partial Pressure of Oxygen, Arterial (Pao$_2$) While Breathing Room Air

100 − (age/3) estimates decline

Table 2. Motor Function by Nerve Roots

Level	Motor Function	Level	Motor Function
C4	Spontaneous breathing	L1–L2	Hip flexion
C5	Shoulder shrug	L3	Hip adduction
C6	Elbow flexion	L4	Hip abduction
C7	Elbow extension	L5	Great toe dorsiflexion
C8/T1	Finger flexion	S1–S2	Foot plantar flexion
T1–T12	Intercostal abdominal muscles	S2–S4	Rectal tone

Table 3. Lumbosacral Nerve Root Compression

Root	Motor	Sensory	Reflex
L4	Quadriceps	Medial foot	Knee jerk
L5	Dorsiflexors	Dorsum of foot	Medial hamstring
S1	Plantar flexors	Lateral foot	Ankle jerk

Figure 1. Dermatomes

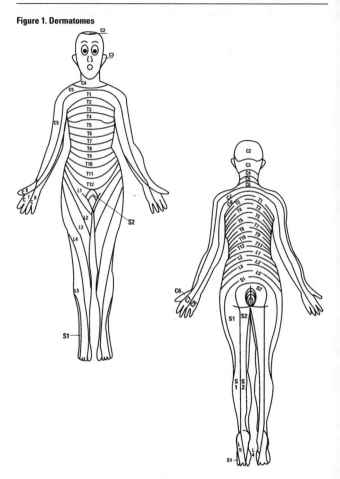

Source: *The Tarascon Pocket Pharmacopoeia*, 2006 classic shirt-pocket edition. Lompoc, CA: Tarascon Publishing, 2006:94. Reprinted with permission.

ASSESSMENT AND APPROACH

ASSESSMENT

Table 4. Assessing Older Adults*

Assessment Domain	Screening Methods	Further Assessment (if screen is positive)	See Page(s)
Medical			
Medical illnesses	Hx, screening physical examination	Additional targeted physical examination, laboratory and imaging tests	
Medications	Medications review	Pharmacy referral	9, 231
Nutrition	Inquire about weight loss (>10 lbs in past 6 mo), weigh patient	Dietary hx, malnutrition evaluation	118
Dentition	Oral examination	Dentistry referral	
Hearing	Handheld audioscope, Brief Hearing Loss Screener, whisper test	Ear examination, audiology referral	81, 220
Vision	Inquire about vision changes, Snellen chart testing	Eye examination, ophthalmology referral	203
Pain	Inquire about pain	Pain inventory	148, 225, 227
Urinary incontinence	Inquire if patient has lost urine >5 times in past year	UI evaluation	89
Mental			
Cognitive status	3-item recall, Mini-Cog, MMSE	Mental status examination, dementia evaluation	215
Emotional status	PHQ-9, GDS, or other depression screen, inquire "Do you ever feel sad or blue?"	In-depth interview	217, 219
Spiritual status	Spiritual hx	In-depth interview, chaplain or spiritual advisor referral	
Physical			
Functional status	ADLs, IADLs	PT/OT referral	215, 216
Balance and gait	Observe patient getting up and walking, orthostatic BP and HR	POMA scale	221
Falls	Inquire about falls in past year	Falls evaluation	66
Environmental			
Social, financial status	Social hx	In-depth interview, social work referral	
Environmental hazards	Inquire about living situation, home safety checklist	Home evaluation	**Table 37**

*See also Assessment Instruments, pp 215–231.

HOUSING ALTERNATIVES FOR OLDER ADULTS

Depending on need for assistance and financial resources, various options are available. Specific names may differ by region, and some may be combinations of various types (see also **Table 74**).

- **Home** with support, if necessary, including caregiver (private pay [PP] or limited hours if on Medicaid), home-delivered meals (usually PP with sliding scale), homemaker (usually PP with sliding scale)
- **Senior citizen housing** typically does not provide individual services although some may have a social worker available and may provide access to hiring help (PP, may be subsidized for older adults spending over one-third of income for rent)
- **Continuing care retirement communities** provide living arrangements ranging from independent to skilled (PP)
- **Assisted living facilities, residential care facilities, board-and-cares** provide meals, housekeeping services, and medication management (PP and Medicaid for some facilities)
- **Nursing homes** provide skilled and custodial care, some have separate units for residents with dementia and behavioral problems (PP, Medicaid, Medicare only if after a 3-day or longer hospital stay and only for a limited duration)

SCHEDULED NURSING-HOME VISIT CHECKLIST

1. Evaluate patient for interval functional change
2. Check vital signs, weight, laboratory tests, consultant reports since last visit
3. Review medications (correlate to active diagnoses)
4. Sign orders
5. Address nursing staff concerns
6. Write a SOAP note (subjective data, objective data, assessment, plan)
7. Revise problem list as needed
8. Update advance directives at least yearly
9. Update resident; update family member(s) as needed

INFORMED DECISION MAKING

Physicians have no ethical obligation to offer care that is judged to be futile.
Three elements are needed for a patient's choices to be legally and ethically valid:

- A capable decision maker: Capacity is for the decision being made; patient may be capable of making some but not all decisions. If a person is sufficiently impaired, a surrogate decision maker must be involved. (See also **Figure 2**.)
- Patient's voluntary participation in the decision-making process.
- Sufficient information: Patient must be sufficiently informed; items to disclose in informed consent include:
  ○ Diagnosis
  ○ Nature, risks, costs, and benefits of possible interventions
  ○ Alternative treatments; relative benefits, risks, and costs
  ○ Likely results of no treatment
  ○ Likelihood of success
  ○ Advice or recommendation of the clinician

Figure 2. Informed Decision Making

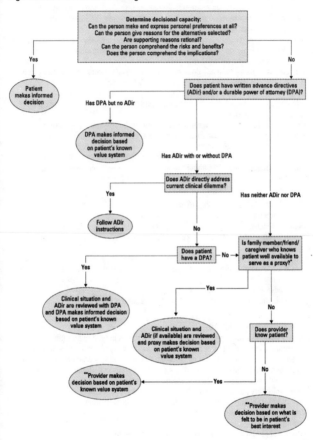

* Most states have laws specifying who should serve as proxy when no ADir or DPA exists. For most of these states, the specified hierarchy of decision makers is (in order): legal guardian, spouse or domestic partner, adult children, parents, adult siblings, closest living relative, close friend.

** Or court-appointed decision maker; laws vary by state.

ELDER MISTREATMENT
Risk Factors for Inadequate or Abusive Caregiving
- Cognitive impairment in patient, caregiver, or both
- Dependency (financial, psychological, etc) of caregiver on elderly patient, or vice versa
- Family conflict
- Family history of abusive behavior, alcohol or drug problems, mental illness, or mental retardation
- Financial stress
- Isolation of patient or caregiver, or both
- Depression or malnutrition in the patient
- Living arrangements inadequate for needs of the ill person
- Stressful events in the family, such as death of a loved one or loss of employment

Source: Adapted from: Fulmer T. Elder mistreatment. In: Pompei P, Murphy JB, eds. *Geriatrics Review Syllabus: A Core Curriculum in Geriatric Medicine*, 6*th* ed. New York, NY: American Geriatrics Society; 2006:87. Reprinted with permission.

Table 5. Signs that Raise Suspicion of Elder Mistreatment

Type of Mistreatment	Some Clinical Signs of Possible Mistreatment	Questions to Ask Patient to Gather more Hx
Abandonment	Evidence that patient is left alone unsafely Evidence of sudden withdrawal of care by caregiver Statements by patient about abandonment	Is there anyone you can call to come and take care of you?
Abuse	Anxiety, nervousness, especially toward caregiver Bruising, in various healing stages, especially bilateral or on inner arms or thighs Fractures, especially in various healing stages Lacerations Repeated emergency department visits Repeated falls Signs of sexual abuse Statements by patient about abuse	Has anyone at home ever hit you or hurt you?
Exploitation	Evidence of misuse of patient's assets Inability of patient to account for money and property or to pay for essential care Reports of demands for money or goods in exchange for caregiving or services Unexplained loss of Social Security or pension checks Statements about exploitation by patient	Has anyone taken your things?
Neglect	Contractures Dehydration Depression Diarrhea Failure to respond to warning of obvious disease Fecal impaction Inappropriate use of medications Malnutrition Poor hygiene Pressure ulcers Repeated falls Repeated hospital admissions Statements by patient about neglect Urine burns	Are you receiving enough care at home?

(cont.)

		Questions to Ask
Type of Mistreatment	Some Clinical Signs of Possible Mistreatment	Patient to Gather more Hx
Psychological abuse	Observed impatience, irritability, or demeaning behavior toward patient by caregiver Anxiety, fearfulness, ambivalence, or anger shown by patient about caregiver	Has anyone ever scolded or threatened you? Has anyone made fun of you?

Table 5. Signs that Raise Suspicion of Elder Mistreatment (cont.)

Source: Adapted from Fulmer T. Elder mistreatment. In: Pompei P, Murphy JB, eds. *Geriatrics Review Syllabus: A Core Curriculum in Geriatric Medicine, 6th ed.* New York, NY: American Geriatrics Society; 2006:88. Reprinted with permission.

Assessment and Management
- Interview patient and caregiver separately.
- Ask patient some general screening questions, such as, "Are there any problems with family or household members that you would like to tell me about?" Follow up a positive response with more direct questions such as those suggested in **Table 5**.
- On physical examination, look for any unusual marks, signs of injury, or conditions listed in **Table 5**.
- If mistreatment is suspected, report case to Adult Protective Services (most states have mandatory reporting laws).
- If patient is in immediate danger of harm, create and implement plan to remove patient from danger (hospital admission, court protective order, placement in safe environment, etc).

CROSS-CULTURAL GERIATRICS
Clinicians should remember that:
- Individuals within every ethnic group can differ widely.
- Familiarity with a patient's background is useful only if his or her preferences are linked to the cultural heritage.
- Ethnic groups differ widely in
  - approach to decision making (eg, involvement of family and friends),
  - disclosure of medical information (eg, cancer diagnosis),
  - end-of-life care (eg, advance directives and resuscitation preferences).

In caring for older adults of any ethnicity:
- Use the patient's preferred terminology for his or her cultural identity in conversation and in health records.
- Determine whether interpretation services are needed; if possible use professional interpreter rather than family member.
- Recognize that the patient may not conceive of illness in Western terms.
- Determine whether the patient is a refugee or survivor of violence or genocide.
- Explore early on the patient's preferences for disclosure of serious clinical findings and reconfirm at intervals.
- Ask if the patient prefers to involve or defer to others in the decision-making process.
- Follow the patient's preferences regarding gender roles.

APPROPRIATE PRESCRIBING, DRUG INTERACTIONS, AND ADVERSE EVENTS

HOW TO PRESCRIBE APPROPRIATELY

- **Obtain a complete drug history.** Ask about previous treatments and responses as well as about other prescribers. Ask about allergies, OTC drugs, nutritional supplements, alternative medications, alcohol, tobacco, caffeine, and recreational drugs.
- **Avoid prescribing before a diagnosis is made.** Consider nondrug therapy. Eliminate drugs for which no diagnosis can be identified.
- **Review medications regularly and before prescribing a new medication.** D/C medications that have not had the intended response or are no longer needed prescribed. Monitor the use of prn and OTC drugs.
- **Know the actions, adverse events, and toxicity profiles of prescribed medications.** Consider how new prescriptions might interact or complement existing drug therapy.
- **Start chronic drug therapy at a low dose and titrate dose on the basis of tolerability and response.** Use drug concentration monitoring when available.
- **Attempt to reach a therapeutic dose before switching to or adding another drug.**
- **Educate patient and/or caregiver about each medication.** Include the regimen, therapeutic goal, cost, and potential adverse events or drug interactions. Provide written instructions.
- **Avoid using one drug to treat the adverse events caused by another.**
- **Attempt to use one drug to treat two or more conditions.**
- **Use combination products cautiously.** Establish need for more than one drug. Titrate individual drugs to therapeutic doses and switch to combinations if appropriate.
- **Communicate with other prescribers.** Don't assume patients will—they assume you do!
- **Avoid using drugs from the same class or with similar actions** (eg, alprazolam and zolpidem).

See also Medication Appropriateness Assessment, p 231. For more on drugs that should be avoided in all older adults, see p 236.

WAYS TO REDUCE MEDICATION ERRORS

- Be knowledgeable about the medication's dose, adverse events, interactions, and monitoring.
- Write legibly to avoid misreading of the drug name (*Celexa* versus *Celebrex*).
- Write out the directions, strength, route, quantity, and number of refills.
- Always precede a decimal expression of <1 with a zero (0); never use a zero after a decimal.
- Avoid abbreviations, especially easily confused ones (qd and qid).
- Do not use ambiguous directions, eg, as directed (ud) or as needed.
- Include the medication's purpose in the directions (eg, for high blood pressure).
- Write dosages for thyroid replacement therapy in mcg not mg.
- Always re-read what you've written.

CRITERIA FOR DRUGS OF CHOICE FOR OLDER ADULTS

- Established efficacy
- Compatible safety and adverse-event profile

- Low risk of drug or nutrient interactions
- Half-life <24 h with no active metabolites
- Elimination does not change with age or known dose adjustments for renal or hepatic function
- Convenient dosing—once or twice daily
- Strength and dosage forms match recommended doses for older adults
- Affordable to the patient
- See also Medicare Part D Prescription Drug Plan, p 239.

PHARMACOLOGIC THERAPY AND AGE-ASSOCIATED CHANGES

Table 6. Age-associated Changes in Pharmacokinetics and Pharmacodynamics

Parameter	Age Effect	Disease, Factor Effect	Prescribing Implications
Absorption	Rate and extent are usually unaffected	Achlorhydria, concurrent medications, tube feedings	Drug-drug and drug-food interactions are more likely to alter absorption
Distribution	Increase in fat:water ratio; decreased plasma protein, particularly albumin	HF, ascites, and other conditions increase body water	Fat-soluble drugs have a larger volume of distribution; highly protein-bound drugs have a greater (active) free concentration
Metabolism	Decreases in liver mass and liver blood flow may decrease drug metabolism	Smoking, genotype, concurrent drug therapy, alcohol and caffeine intake may have more effect than aging	Lower doses may be therapeutic
Elimination	Primarily renal; age-related decrease in GFR*	Kidney impairment with acute and chronic diseases; decreased muscle mass results in less Cr production	Serum creatinine not a reliable measure of kidney function; best to estimate CrCl using formula (see p 1)
Pharmaco-dynamics	Less predictable and often altered drug response at usual or lower concentrations	Drug-drug and drug-disease interactions may alter responses	Prolonged pain relief with opioids at lower doses; increased sedation and postural instability to benzodiazepines; altered sensitivity to β-blockers

* Many laboratories are reporting an estimated GFR as a measure of renal function. GFR should not be equated to CrCl. Only CrCl should be used to adjust drug dosages and can be estimated using the equation on p 1.

COMPLICATING FACTORS
Drug-Food or -Nutrient Interactions
Physical Interactions: Mg^{++}, Ca^{++}, Fe^{++}, Al^{++}, or zinc can lower oral absorption of levothyroxine and some quinolone antibiotics. Tube feedings decrease absorption of oral phenytoin and levothyroxine.
Decreased Drug Effect: Warfarin and vitamin K-containing foods (eg, green leafy vegetables, broccoli, brussels sprouts, greens, cabbage).

Decreased Oral Intake or Appetite: Drugs can alter the taste of food (dysgeusia) or decrease saliva production (xerostomia), making mastication and swallowing difficult. Drugs associated with dysgeusia include captopril and clarithromycin. Drugs that can cause xerostomia include antihistamines, antidepressants, antipsychotics, clonidine, and diuretics.

Drug-Drug Interactions

A drug's effect can be increased or decreased by another drug because of impaired absorption (eg, sucralfate and ciprofloxacin), displacement from protein-binding sites (eg, warfarin and sulfonamides), inhibition or induction of metabolic enzymes (see **Table 7**), or because two or more drugs have a similar pharmacologic effect (eg, potassium-sparing diuretics, potassium supplements, and ACE inhibitors).

Top Ten Dangerous Drug Interactions in Long-Term Care: *

Warfarin — NSAIDs (excluding celecoxib)

Warfarin — sulfa drugs

Warfarin — macrolides

Warfarin — quinolones (eg, ciprofloxacin, levofloxacin, enoxacin, norfloxacin, ofloxacin)

Warfarin — phenytoin

ACE inhibitors — potassium supplements

ACE inhibitors — spironolactone

Digoxin — amiodarone

Digoxin — verapamil

Theophylline — quinolones (eg, ciprofloxacin, enoxacin, norfloxacin, ofloxacin)

* As determined by the American Society of Consultant Pharmacists Multidisciplinary Management Project (http://www.scoup.net/M3Project/topten/)

Digoxin: Digoxin levels must be monitored with concomitant administration of many other drugs.

The following **increase** digoxin concentration or effect, or both:

amiodarone	hydroxychloroquine	quinine
diltiazem	ibuprofen	spironolactone
erythromycin	indomethacin	tetracycline
esmolol	nifedipine	tolbutamide
flecainide	quinidine	verapamil

The following **decrease** digoxin concentration or effect, or both:

aminosalicylic acid	colestipol	psyllium
antacids	kaolin pectin	sulfasalazine
antineoplastics	metoclopramide	St. John's wort
cholestyramine		

Enzyme Inhibitors and Inducers: **Table 7** is a list of common drug-drug interactions via this mechanism.

Table 7. Selected CYP Isozyme Substrates, Inducers, and Inhibitors

Isozyme	Substrates*		Inducers**	Inhibitors†
CYP1A2				
	Amitriptyline	Naproxen	Carbamazepine	Amiodarone
	APAP	Nortriptyline	Cigarette smoke	Cimetidine
	Clozapine	Olanzapine	Omeprazole	Diltiazem
	Estradiol	Verapamil	Phenobarbital	Estradiol
	Imipramine	Warfarin-R‡	Phenytoin	Fluoroquinolones
			Rifampin	Fluvoxamine
				Isoniazid
				Ketoconazole
				Ticlopidine
CYP2C9				
	Celecoxib	Phenytoin	Carbamazepine	Amiodarone
	Diclofenac	Piroxicam	Phenobarbital	Cimetidine
	Fluvastatin	Sulfamethoxazole	Phenytoin	Fluconazole
	Glipizide	Tamoxifen	Rifampin	Fluvoxamine
	Ibuprofen	Tolbutamide		Isoniazid
	Irbesartan	Warfarin		Omeprazole
	Losartan			Propoxyphene
				Ticlopidine
				Valproic acid
CYP2B6				
	Bupropion		Phenobarbital	Thiotepa
	Cyclophosphamide		Rifampin	Ticlopidine
	Methadone			
CYP2C19				
	Amitriptyline	Pantoprazole	Fluoxetine	
	Cyclophosphamide	Phenobarbital	Fluvoxamine	
	Diazepam	Phenytoin	Ketoconazole	
	Lansoprazole	Progesterone	Lansoprazole	
	Omeprazole		Omeprazole	
			Ticlopidine	
CYP2D6				
	Amitriptyline	Imipramine		Amiodarone
	Aripiprazole	Metoprolol		Bupropion
	Codeine‡	Ondansetron		Celecoxib
	Clomipramine	Paroxetine		Chlorpheniramine
	Desipramine	Risperidone		Cimetidine
	Dextromethorphan	Tamoxifen		Clomipramine
	Donepezil	Thioridazone		Darifenacin
	Duloxetine	Timolol		Diltiazem
	Haloperidol	Tramadol§		Duloxetine
		Venlafaxine		Fluoxetine
				Haloperidol
				Methadone
				Paroxetine
				Propoxyphene
				Quinidine
				Valproic acid

(cont.)

Table 7. Selected CYP Isozyme Substrates, Inducers, and Inhibitors (cont.)

Isozyme	Substrates*		Inducers**	Inhibitors†
CYP3A4,5,7				
	Alprazolam	Ketoconazole	Carbamazepine	Amiodarone
	Amiodarone	Lovastatin	Glucocorticoids	Cimetidine
	Aripiprazole	Methadone	Griseofulvin	Ciprofloxacin
	Astemizole	Nefazodone	Oxcarbazepine	Clarithromycin
	Atorvastatin	Omeprazole	Phenobarbital	Cyclosporine
	Buspirone	Pioglitazone	Phenytoin	Diltiazem
	Carbamazepine	Quetiapine	Pioglitazone	Erythromycin
	Chlorpheniramine	Quinidine	Rifabutin	Fluconazole
	Clarithromycin	Risperidone	Rifampin	Fluoxetine
	Clozapine	Sildenafil	St. John's wort	Fluvoxamine
	Codeine	Simvastatin	Troglitazone	Grapefruit juice
	Cyclosporine	Solifenacin		Haloperidol
	Darifenacin	Tacrolimus		Isoniazid
	Diazepam	Tamoxifen		Itraconazole
	Dihydropyridine	Telithromycin		Ketoconazole
	calcium channel	Trazodone		Nefazodone
	blockers	Triazolam		Norfloxacin
	Diltiazem	Venlafaxine		Propoxyphene
	Donepezil	Verapamil		Quinidine
	Erythromycin	Vincristine		Star fruit
	Estradiol	Warfarin		Telithromycin
	Fluoxetine	Ziprasidone		Verapamil
	Haloperidol	Zolpidem		
	Itraconazole			

* Substrate: a drug metabolized by the isozyme.
** Inducer: a drug that increases the capacity of the isozyme to metabolize the substrate and potentially decreases the therapeutic effect of the substrate.
† Inhibitor: a drug that prevents the isozyme from metabolizing the substrate and increases the risk for toxicity of the substrate.
‡ R-isomer
§ Analgesic effect decreased because of inhibition of substrate metabolism to its active metabolite by an inhibitor.
Note: The list of medications is not comprehensive, but represents medications often prescribed for older adults or medications involved in serious drug interactions (eg, cyclosporine). Some interactions in vivo or in vitro have been documented, whereas others are theoretical. For more information, consult a drug-drug interaction text or Internet resource, eg, http://medicine.iupui.edu/flockhart/.

Table 8. Commonly Used Herbal and Alternative Medications

Product	Common Uses	Adverse Events	Drug Interactions	Cautions
Chondroitin	Osteoarthritis	Nausea, dyspepsia, changes in intraocular pressure		
Echinacea	Immune stimulant	Hepatotoxicity	Immuno-suppressants	D/C ≥2 wk before surgery; cross-sensitivity with chrysanthemum, ragweed, daisy, and aster allergies; kidney disease; immunosuppression

(cont.)

	Table 8. **Commonly Used Herbal and Alternative Medications (cont.)**			
Product	Common Uses	Adverse Events	Drug Interactions	Cautions
Feverfew	Anti-inflammatory, migraine prophylaxis	Platelet inhibition, bleeding, GI upset	NSAIDs, antiplatelet agents, anticoagulants	D/C 7 d before surgery, active bleeding; cross-sensitivity with crysanthemum and daisy
Garlic	Hypertension, hypercholesterolemia, platelet inhibitor	Bleeding, GI upset, hypoglycemia	NSAIDs, antiplatelet agents, anticoagulants	D/C 7 d before surgery
Ginger	Antiemetic, anti-inflammatory, dyspepsia	Bleeding	NSAIDs, antiplatelet agents, anticoagulants	D/C 7 d before surgery
Ginkgo	Alzheimer's disease, memory, intermittent claudication, macular degeneration	Bleeding, nausea, headache, GI upset, diarrhea, anxiety	MAOIs	D/C 36 h before surgery
Ginseng	Physical and mental performance enhancer	Hypertension, tachycardia	Antiplatelet agents, anticoagulants, NSAIDs, MAOIs	D/C 7 d before surgery, kidney failure
Glucosamine	Osteoarthritis, rheumatoid arthritis	GI distress, anorexia, insomnia, painful and itchy skin, peripheral edema, tachycardia		Allergy to shellfish
Kava kava	Anxiety, sedative	Sedation, hepatotoxicity	Anticonvulsants (increased effect)	D/C 24 h before surgery
SAMe (S-adenosyl-methionine)	Depression, fibromyalgia, insomnia, osteoarthritis, rheumatoid arthritis	GI distress, insomnia, dizziness, dry mouth, headache, restlessness	Antidepressants, St. John's wort, NSAIDs, antiplatelet agents, anticoagulants	Not effective for bipolar depression, hyperhomocysteinemia (theoretical), D/C at least 14 d before surgery
Saw palmetto	BPH	Headache, nausea, GI distress, erectile dysfunction	Finasteride, α_1-adrenergic agonist properties in vitro may decrease efficacy	
St. John's wort	Depression, anxiety	Photosensitivity, hypomania	Potent CYP3A4 inducer (see **Table 7**)	Wear sunscreen, avoid in fair-skinned patients, D/C 5 d before surgery
Valerian	Anxiety, insomnia	Sedation, benzodiazepine-like withdrawal		Taper dose several weeks before surgery

ALCOHOL ABUSE

Definition

Possible Alcohol Dependence—DSM-IV: Three or more of the following:
- Tolerance, requiring more alcohol to get "high"
- Withdrawal, or drinking to relieve, prevent withdrawal
- Drinking in larger amounts, or for a longer time than intended
- Persistent desire to drink, or unsuccessful efforts to control drinking
- Spending a lot of time obtaining, using alcohol, or recovering from effects
- Giving up important occupational, social, or recreational activities because of drinking
- Drinking despite persistent or recurrent physical or psychologic problems caused or worsened by alcohol

Possible Alcohol Abuse—DSM-IV: Recurring problems with one or more of the following:
- Drinking resulting in the failure to fulfill major obligations at work or in the home
- Drinking in situations where it is physically hazardous
- Alcohol-related legal problems
- Continued drinking despite social problems caused or worsened by alcohol

Hazardous Drinking: WHO definition—use of alcohol that places a person at risk of physical or psychologic complications. Increases risk of HTN, some cancers (eg, head and neck, esophagus, breast in women), and cirrhosis (higher in women). Possible increased risk of hip fracture and other injury.

Evaluation

Alcohol dependence or abuse is often missed in older adults because of reduced social and occupational functioning; signs more often are poor self-care, malnutrition, and medical illness.

Alcohol Misuse Screening: CAGE questionnaire has been validated in the older population.

   C Have you ever felt you should **C**ut down?
   A Does others' criticism of your drinking **A**nnoy you?
   G Have you ever felt **G**uilty about drinking?
   E Have you ever had an "**E**ye opener" to steady your nerves or get rid of a hangover?
   (*Positive response to any suggests problem drinking.*)

Detecting Harmful Drinking (*≥2 drinks/d for women, ≥3 drinks/d for men is potentially harmful*):
May be missed by CAGE; ask
- How many days per week?
- How many drinks on those days?
- Maximum intake on any one day?
- What type (ie, beer, wine, or liquor)?
- What is in "a drink"?

Aggravating Factors

Alcohol and Aging: Higher blood concentrations per amount consumed due to decreased lean body mass and total body water; concomitant medications may interact with alcohol.
Age-related Diseases: Cognitive impairment, HTN.
Medications: Many drug interactions, eg, APAP, antihypertensives, NSAIDs, sedatives, antidepressants.

Management

Alcohol Guidelines for Moderate Drinking: No more than 1 drink/d after age 65; 1 drink/d probably reduces cardiovascular and cerebrovascular risk.

Psychosocial Interventions:

• Problem drinking or alcohol misuse: Brief intervention; educate patient on effects of current drinking, point out current adverse events.

• Alcohol dependence or abuse: Self-help groups (eg, Alcoholics Anonymous); professional help (eg, psychodynamic, cognitive-behavioral, counseling, social support, family therapy, age-specific inpatient or outpatient).

Drug therapy: Is useful only when used as an adjunct to psychosocial therapy.

• Naltrexone *(Depade, REVIA, Trexan)* 25 mg × 2 d, then 50 mg qd [T: 50]; monitor liver enzymes, contraindicated in kidney failure; ~10% get nausea, headache (L, K).

• Acamprosate *(Campral)* 666 mg tid, reduce dosage to 333 mg tid if CrCl 30–50 mL/min [T: 333]; contraindicated in kidney failure, may be used in combination with naltrexone; diarrhea is most common adverse drug event (K).

Acute alcohol withdrawal: See p 44.

SMOKING CESSATION

Nonpharmacologic Therapy

What Health Providers Should Do:

• **Ask** about tobacco use at every visit

• **Advise** all users to quit

• **Assess** willingness to quit

• **Assist** the patient with a quit plan, education, pharmacotherapy

Making the Decision to Quit:

Patients are more likely to stop smoking if they:

• Believe they could get a smoking-related disease

• Believe they can make an honest attempt at quitting

• Believe the benefits of quitting outweigh the benefits of continued smoking

• Know someone who has had health problems as a result of smoking

Setting a Quit Date and Deciding on a Plan:

• Pick a specific day within the next month (gives time to develop a plan).

• Will nicotine replacement therapy be used?

• Will the patient attend a smoking cessation class?

• On quit day, get rid of all cigarettes and related items.

Managing Symptoms of Withdrawal:

• **Physical:** Pharmacotherapy (**Table 9**) helps physical symptoms.

• Who should or should not receive pharmacotherapy?

  ○ Nicotine replacement:

    ▪ Improves quit rates in most patients

    ▪ Is contraindicated with recent MI, uncontrolled high BP, arrhythmias, severe angina, gastric ulcer

    ▪ May not be needed if patient smokes fewer than 10 cigarettes/d; if used, recommend lower dosages

  ○ Other agents (bupropion, etc):

    ▪ May be used if nicotine contraindicated

    ▪ Use in combination with nicotine if prior failure using nicotine alone

- **Psychological:**
  ○ Smoking is linked with many activities, and the link must be unlearned.
  ○ Avoid people and places where tempted to smoke.
  ○ Alter habits: 1) switch to juices or water instead of alcohol or coffee, 2) take a brisk walk instead of a coffee break, and 3) use oral substitutions such as sugarless gum or hard candy.
  ○ Three types of counseling and behavioral therapies are effective: 1) problem solving or skills training, 2) social support as part of treatment, and 3) social support outside of treatment.

Maintaining Smoking Cessation: Use the same methods that helped during withdrawal.

Source: Adapted from *Global Strategy for the Diagnosis, Management, and Prevention of Chronic Obstructive Pulmonary Disease, Global Initiative for Chronic Obstructive Lung Disease (GOLD).* NHLBI/WHO Workshop Report, Executive Summary. National Institutes of Health, National Heart, Lung and Blood Institute. March 2001. NIH Publication No. 2701A (for full report, see http://www.goldcopd.com).

Table 9. Pharmacotherapy for Tobacco Abuse

Drug	Dosage	Formulations	Comments (Metabolism, Excretion)
Tobacco Abuse			
Bupropion* (*Wellbutrin SR, Zyban*)	150 mg bid × 7–12 wk	SR: 100, 150	Combined with nicotine replacement, doubles quit rate to 30% at 12 mo; contraindicated with seizure disorders (L)
Nicotine Replacement**			
Transdermal patches[†] (eg, *Habitrol, NicoDerm*)	21 mg/d × 4–8 wk[§] 14 mg/d × 2–4 wk 7 mg/d × 2–4 wk	7, 14, 21	Apply to clean, nonhairy skin on upper torso, rotate sites; start 14 mg/d with cardiovascular disease or body wt <100 lb or if smoking <10 cigarettes/d (L)
(*Nicotrol*)	15 mg/d × 8 wk[§] 10 mg/d × 4–6 wk 5 mg/d × 4–6 wk	5, 10, 15	Gradually released over 16 h (L)
(*ProStep*)	22 mg/d × 4–8 wk[§] 11 mg/d × 4–8 wk	11, 22	Persons <100 lb start lower dose; reduce or D/C after 4–8 wk (L)
Polacrilex gum (*Nicorette*)	9–12 pieces/d	2, 4	Chew 1 piece when urge to smoke; usual 10–12 pieces/d, max 30/d; 4 mg if smoking >21 cigarettes/d (L)
Nasal spray[‡] (*Nicotrol NS*)	1 spr each nostril q 30–60 min	0.5 mg/spr	Do not exceed 5 applications/h or 40 in 24 h (L)
Inhaler[‡] (*Nicotrol Inhaler*)	6–16 cartridges/d	4 mg delivered/ cartridge	Max 16 cartridges/d with gradual reduction after 6–12 wk if needed (L)
Lozenge	1 po prn	2, 4	Do not exceed 20/d; do not bite or chew; wean over 12 wk
Lollipop	1 po prn	1, 2, 3, 4	Place in mouth when urge to smoke; remove when craving passes; gradually reduce dose over 4–8 wk; do not exceed 7/d

* Bupropion is FDA approved. Nortriptyline is an effective alternative. Hughes JR, Stead LF, Lancaster T. Antidepressants for smoking cessation. *Cochrane Database Syst Rev* 2002; 1:000031.
** Best used in combination with smoking cessation program; dyspepsia is most common drug-related adverse event.
† In patients receiving >600 mg cimetidine, reduce to next lower patch dose.
§ The next lower dose is less toxic and probably equally effective.
‡ Available by prescription only.

WARFARIN THERAPY
Prescribing Warfarin
- For anticoagulation in nonacute conditions, initiate therapy by giving warfarin (*Coumadin, Carfin, Sofarin*) 2–5 mg/d as fixed dose [T: 1, 2, 2.5, 3, 4, 5, 6, 7.5, 10]; reduce dose if INR >2.5 on day 3.
- Half-life is 31–51 h; steady state is achieved on day 5–7 of fixed dose.
- Warfarin therapy is implicated in **many** adverse drug-drug interactions.
- Some drugs that **increase** INR in conjunction with warfarin:

  - alcohol (with concurrent liver disease)
  - amiodarone
  - androgens
  - antibiotics (many)
  - APAP (>1.3 g/d for >1 wk)
  - ASA (>3 g/d)
  - chloral hydrate
  - cimetidine
  - clofibrate
  - clotrimazole
  - fluconazole
  - flu vaccine
  - isoniazid
  - ketoprofen
  - metolazone
  - miconazole
  - piroxicam
  - propafenone
  - propranolol
  - sulindac
  - tolmetin
  - trimethoprim

- Some drugs that **decrease** INR in conjunction with warfarin:

  - barbiturates
  - carbamazepine
  - cholestyramine
  - cyclosporine
  - dicloxacillin
  - etretinate
  - griseofulvin
  - nafcillin
  - rifampin
  - sucralfate
  - trazodone
  - vitamin K

Table 10. Indications for Anticoagulation in the Absence of Active Bleeding or Severe Bleeding Risk

Condition	Target INR	Duration of Therapy
Hip or major knee surgery	2.0–3.0	At least 7–10 d
Idiopathic venous thromboembolism (includes PE)	2.0–3.0	At least 6–12 mo*
Atrial fibrillation	2.0–3.0	Indefinitely
Mitral valvular heart disease with hx of systemic embolization or left atrial diameter >5.5 cm	2.0–3.0	Indefinitely
Cardiomyopathy with EF <25%	2.0–3.0	Indefinitely
Mechanical aortic valve with normal left atrial size and sinus rhythm	2.0–3.0**	Indefinitely
Mechanical aortic valve with enlarged left atrium and/or atrial fibrillation	2.5–3.5**†	Indefinitely
Mechanical mitral valve	2.5–3.5**†	Indefinitely
Caged ball or caged disk valve	2.5–3.5‡	Indefinitely
Bioprosthetic heart valve	2.0–3.0	3 mo
Acute MI complicated by severe left ventricular dysfunction, HF, previous emboli, mural thrombus on echocardiography	2.0–3.0	1–3 mo

* For first event of idiopathic DVT or PE, consider indefinite anticoagulation, particularly after cases of life-threatening embolism or in patients with thrombophilia such as Factor V Leiden mutation.

** If additional risk factors are present or if there is systemic embolism despite anticoagulation treatment, target INR is 2.5–3.5 and ASA 80–100 mg/d should be added.

† Alternative target INR 2.0–3.0 with addition of ASA 80–100 mg/d.

‡ With addition of ASA 80–100 mg/d.

Cessation of Anticoagulation Before Surgery

• If INR is between 2.0 and 3.0, hold warfarin 4 doses before surgery; longer if INR >3.0.
• If patient has recurrent thromboembolic disease or a mechanical valve, unfractionated heparin or LMWH at DVT/PE treatment dosages (see **Table 12**) should be started when the INR falls after warfarin is discontinued.

Table 11. Treatment of Warfarin Overdose

INR	Clinical Situation	Action
≥3.5 and <5.0	No significant bleeding	Omit next warfarin dose and/or lower dose
≥5.0 and <9.0	No significant bleeding	Omit next 1–2 doses of warfarin and restart therapy at lower dose; alternatively, omit 1 dose and give VK 1.0–2.5 mg po
≥9.0	No significant bleeding	D/C warfarin and give VK 3.0–10.0 mg po; give additional VK po if INR is not substantially reduced in 24–48 h. Restart warfarin at lower dose when INR is therapeutic.
Any elevation	Serious bleeding	D/C warfarin; give VK 10.0 mg by slow IV infusion, supplemented with fresh frozen plasma or prothrombin complex concentrate depending on urgency of situation; check INR q 6 h; repeat VK q 12 h as needed
Any elevation	Life-threatening bleeding	D/C warfarin; give VK 10.0 mg by slow IV infusion, supplemented with prothrombin complex concentrate as needed; repeat this treatment as needed

Note: VK = vitamin K.
Source: American College of Chest Physicians Consensus Panel on Antithrombotic Therapy: Ansell J, Hirsch J, Pollar L, et al. The pharmacology and management of the vitamin K antagonists. In: Seventh ACCP Conference on Antithrombotic and Thrombolytic Therapy. *Chest.* 2004; 126:(204S–233S).

ACUTE ANTICOAGULATION

Table 12. Anticoagulants for DVT or PE Prophylaxis and Treatment

Class, Agent	DVT or PE Prophylaxis Dosage by Condition Type	DVT or PE Treatment Dosage	Comments
Heparin			
Unfractionated heparin (*Hep-Lock*)	General surgery: 5000 U SC 2 h before and q 12 h after surgery	5000 U/kg IV bolus followed by 15 mg/kg/h IV*	Bleeding, anemia, thrombocytopenia, hypertransaminase-mia, urticaria (L, K)
LMWH			
Enoxaparin (*Lovenox*)	THA, HFX: 30 mg SC q 12 h or 40 mg SC qd KR: 30 mg SC q 12 h; AS: 40 mg SC qd	Outpatient treatment of DVT: 1 mg/kg SC q 12 h; inpatient treatment of DVT ± PE: 1 mg/kg SC q 12 h or 1.5 mg/kg SC qd*	Bleeding, anemia, hyperkalemia, hyper-transaminasemia, thrombocytopenia, thrombocytosis, urticaria, angioedema (K)

(cont.)

Table 12. Anticoagulants for DVT or PE Prophylaxis and Treatment (cont.)

Class, Agent	DVT or PE Prophylaxis Dosage by Condition Type	DVT or PE Treatment Dosage	Comments
Dalteparin (*Fragmin*)	Low-risk THA: 2500–5000 U SC before surgery, 5000 U SC qd after surgery Abdominal surgery: 2500–5000 U SC before and after surgery	DVT: 100 U/kg SC q 12 h; also indicated for anticoagulation in acute coronary syndrome	Same (K)
Tinzaparin (*Innohep*)	NA	175 anti-Xa IU/kg SC qd*	Same (K)
Heparinoid			
Danaparoid (*Orgaran*)	THA, HFX, HIT: 750 anti-Xa U SC bid	NA	Same as LMWH (K)
Factor Xa Inhibitor			
Fondaparinux (*Arixtra*)	THA, HFX, KR: 2.5 mg SC qd beginning 6–8 h after surgery	Weight <50 kg: 5 mg SC qd; weight 50–100 kg: 7.5 mg SC qd; weight >100 kg: 10 mg SC qd	Contraindicated if CrCl <30 mL/min (K)
Direct Thrombin Inhibitors			
Argatroban	HIT: 2 mcg/kg/min IV infusion	HIT: 2 mcg/kg/min IV infusion	↓ Dosage if hepatic impairment (L)
Lepirudin (*Refludan*)	HIT: 4 mg/kg bolus, then 0.15 mg/kg/h	HIT: 4 mg/kg bolus, then 0.15 mg/kg/h	↓ Bolus to 0.2 mg/kg if CrCl <60
Thrombolytics			
Streptokinase (*Kabikinase, Streptase*)	NA	250,000 U IV over 30 min, then 100,000 U/h for 24 h†	Risk of hemorrhage ↑ with age and higher BMI; HTN, hallucination, agitation, confusion, serum sickness (L)

Note: THA = total hip arthroplasty (hip replacement); HFX = hip fracture surgery; KR = knee replacement; HIT = heparin-induced thrombocytopenia; NA = not applicable.
* Also indicated for anticoagulation in acute coronary syndrome (see **Table 14**).
† Dose in acute MI is 1.5 million U IV over 60 min.

ANXIETY

DIAGNOSIS

Anxiety disorders are less prevalent in older than in younger adults. New-onset anxiety in older adults is often secondary to physical illness, depression, medication adverse events, or withdrawal from drugs.

DSM-IV recognizes several anxiety disorders:
(*Italicized type indicates the most common anxiety disorders occurring in older adults.*)
- Acute stress disorder
- Agoraphobia without a history of panic
- *Generalized anxiety disorder (GAD)*
- *Anxiety disorder due to a general medical condition*
- Obsessive-compulsive disorder (OCD)
- Panic disorder, with or without agoraphobia
- Post-traumatic stress disorder
- Social phobia (social anxiety disorder)
- Specific phobia
- Substance-induced anxiety disorder

DSM-IV Criteria for GAD

- Excessive anxiety and worry on more days than not for ≥6 mo, about a number of events or activities
- Difficulty controlling the worry
- Anxiety and worry associated with ≥3 of 6 symptoms:
  - restlessness or feeling keyed up or on edge
  - being easily fatigued
  - difficulty concentrating or mind going blank
  - irritability
  - muscle tension
  - sleep disturbance (difficulty falling or staying asleep, or restless unsatisfying sleep)
- Focus of anxiety and worry not confined to features of an Axis I disorder (primary psychiatric disorder); often, about routine life circumstances; may shift from one concern to another
- Anxiety, worry, or physical symptoms cause clinically significant distress or impairment in social, occupational, or other important areas of functioning
- Disturbance not due to the direct physiologic effects of a drug of abuse or a medication or to a medical condition; does not occur exclusively during a mood disorder, psychotic disorder, or a pervasive development disorder

DSM-IV Criteria for Panic Attack

Discrete period of intense fear or discomfort with ≥4 of the following (also, must peak within 10 min):
- Palpitations, rapid HR
- Sweating
- Feeling dizzy, unsteady, lightheaded, or faint
- Trembling or shaking
- Sensations of shortness of breath or smothering
- Choking feeling
- Chest pain or discomfort
- Nausea or abdominal distress

- Feelings of unreality or being detached from self
- Fear of losing control or going crazy
- Fear of dying
- Paresthesias
- Chills or hot flushes

Differential Diagnosis
- Panic disorder: recurrent, unexpected panic attacks
- Physical conditions producing anxiety
  - Cardiovascular: Arrhythmias, angina, MI, HF
  - Endocrine: Hyperthyroidism, hypoglycemia, pheochromocytoma
  - Neurologic: Movement disorders, temporal lobe epilepsy, AD, stroke
  - Respiratory: COPD, asthma, pulmonary embolism
- Medications producing anxiety
  - Caffeine
  - Corticosteroids
  - Nicotine
  - Psychotropics: Antidepressants, antipsychotics, stimulants
  - Sympathomimetics: Pseudoephedrine, β-agonists
  - Thyroid hormones: Overreplacement
- Withdrawal states: alcohol, sedatives, hypnotics, benzodiazepines, SSRIs
- Depression

EVALUATION
- Past psychiatric hx
- Drug review: Prescribed, OTC, alcohol, caffeine
- Mental status evaluation
- Physical examination: Focus on signs and symptoms of anxiety (eg, tachycardia, hyperpnea, sweating, tremor)
- Laboratory tests: Consider CBC, blood glucose, TSH, B_{12}, ECG, oxygen saturation, drug and alcohol screening

MANAGEMENT
Nonpharmacologic
- Cognitive-behavior therapy may be useful for GAD, panic disorder, and OCD.
- May be effective alone but mostly used in conjunction with pharmacotherapy.
- Requires a cognitively intact, motivated patient.

Pharmacologic
Antidepressants Approved for Anxiety Disorders: See **Table 28** for dosing.
- Obsessive-compulsive: fluoxetine, fluvoxamine, paroxetine, sertraline; secondary choices include β-blockers and atypical antipsychotics
- Panic: sertraline, paroxetine; secondary choices include β-blockers and atypical antipsychotics
- Social phobia: paroxetine, sertraline, venlafaxine XR
- Generalized anxiety: escitalopram, paroxetine, sertraline, venlafaxine XR
- Post-traumatic stress: paroxetine, sertraline

Buspirone (BuSpar):
- Serotonin 1A partial agonist effective in GAD and anxiety symptoms accompanying general medical illness
- Not effective for acute anxiety, panic, or OCD
- May take 2–4 wk for therapeutic response
- Recommended geriatric dosage: 7.5–10 mg bid [T: 5, 10, 15, 30]
- No dependence, tolerance, withdrawal, CNS depression, or significant drug-drug interactions

Benzodiazepines:
- Most often used for acute anxiety, GAD, panic, OCD
- Preferred: Intermediate–half-life drugs inactivated by direct conjugation in liver and therefore less affected by aging
- Avoid long-acting benzodiazepines (eg, flurazepam, diazepam, chlordiazepoxide); linked to cognitive impairment, falls, sedation, psychomotor impairment
- Problems: Dependence, tolerance, withdrawal, more so with short-acting benzodiazepines; seizure risk with alprazolam withdrawal
- Potentially fatal if combined with alcohol or other CNS depressants
- Only short-term (60–90 d) use recommended
- Not covered by Medicare Part D

Table 13. Benzodiazepines for Anxiety Recommended for Older Adults

Drug	Dosage	Formulations
Lorazepam (Ativan)	0.5–2 mg in 2–3 divided doses	T: 0.5, 1, 2; S: 2 mg/mL; Inj: 2 mg/mL
Oxazepam (Serax)	10–15 mg bid–tid	T: 10, 15, 30

Nonbenzodiazepine Hypnotics:
Zoldipem (Ambien), zaleplon (Sonata), and eszopiclone (Lunesta) should not be used for treatment of anxiety disorders. See Sleep Disorders, **Table 94**.

CARDIOVASCULAR DISEASES

CORONARY ARTERY DISEASE
Diagnostic Cardiac Tests
- Cardiac catheterization is the gold standard.
- Stress testing: The heart is stressed either through exercise (treadmill, stationary bicycle) or, if the patient cannot exercise or the ECG is markedly abnormal, with pharmacologic agents (dipyridamole, adenosine, dobutamine). Exercise stress tests can be performed with or without cardiac imaging, while pharmacologic stress tests always include imaging. Imaging can be accomplished by echocardiography or single-photon-emission computed tomography (SPECT).

Acute Myocardial Infarction
Evaluation and Assessment
- Presentation frequently atypical—suspect MI with atypical chest pain; arm, jaw, or abdominal pain (with or without nausea); acute functional decline.
- As in younger persons, diagnosis is made by cardiac enzyme increases, with or without ECG changes. Serial enzyme measurements are necessary to exclude MI.
  - Both creatine kinase MB isoenzymes (CK-MB) and cardiac troponins T and I usually become elevated 4 h after myocardial injury.
  - CK-MB subforms are the most sensitive and specific test for detecting MI in the first 6 h, but troponin remains elevated longer.
  - Elevated troponin in the face of normal CK-MB can indicate increased risk of MI in the ensuing 6 mo.
  - Troponins are not useful for detecting reinfarction within first wk of an MI. CK-MB is the preferred marker for early reinfarction.
  - Both CK-MB and cardiac troponins can have false-positive results due to subclinical ischemic myocardial injury or nonischemic myocardial injury.
- Risk factors for acute MI in older adults:
  - Previous MI or angina
  - Age
  - Diabetes mellitus
  - Dyslipidemia
  - Family hx
  - Hypertension
  - Obesity
  - Sedentary life style
  - Severe coronary artery calcification
  - Smoking

Acute Management of MI
- At initial presentation of both ST segment elevation MI and acute coronary syndrome (unstable angina or non-ST segment elevation MI):
  - Bedrest with continuous ECG monitoring.
  - Oxygen to maintain saturation >90%.
  - ASA ± clopidogrel (*Plavix*) and an anticoagulant (see **Table 14**).
  - If catheterization with angioplasty or stent placement is planned, give a glycoprotein IIb/IIIa inhibitor (see **Table 14**).
  - β-Blockers given without delay and continued long term unless systolic failure or pronounced bradycardia is present. Acute phase: Atenolol (*Tenormin*) 5 mg IV over 5 min and repeat in 10 min, or metoprolol (*Lopressor*) 5 mg IV q 5 min up to a total of 15 mg. Begin chronic phase within 1–2 h: atenolol 25–100 mg po qd or metoprolol 50–200 mg po bid.

○ Nitroglycerin is indicated without delay for persistent ischemia, hypertension, large anterior infarction, or HF. Begin at 5–10 mcg/min IV and titrate to pain relief, SBP >90 mm Hg, or resolution of ECG abnormalities.

○ Morphine sulfate 1–5 mg IV if chest pain persists on nitroglycerin therapy.

Table 14. Antithrombotic Therapy in Acute Coronary Syndrome

Class, Agent	Dosage	Indications
Antiplatelet Agents		
ASA	162–325 mg po initially, followed by 75–160 mg po qd	PACS, DACS, PCI, CABG
Clopidogrel (*Plavix*)	300 mg po initially, followed by 75 mg po qd	DACS, PCI*
Anticoagulants		
Enoxaparin (*Lovenox*)	30 mg IV bolus, followed by 1 mg/kg SC q 12 h	DACS
Dalteparin (*Fragmin*)	120 IU/kg SC q 12 h	DACS
Heparin (*Hep-Lock*)	60–70 U/kg (max 5000 U) IV bolus followed by 12–15 U/kg/h IV	PCI, CABG
Glycoprotein IIb/IIIa Inhibitors		
Abciximab (*ReoPro*)	0.25 mg/kg IV bolus, followed by 0.125 mcg/kg/min (max 10 mcg/min)	PCI
Eptifibatide (*Integrilin*)	180 mcg/kg IV bolus, followed by 2.0 mcg/kg/min IV	PCI
Tirofiban (*Aggrastat*)	0.4 mcg/kg/min IV for 30 min, followed by 0.1 mcg/kg/min	PCI

Note: PACS = possible or suspected acute coronary syndrome; DACS = definite acute coronary syndrome; PCI = acute coronary syndrome with planned percutaneous cardiac intervention; CABG = acute coronary syndrome with emergent CABG a likely possibility

* Use clopidogrel in PACS if patient is allergic to ASA. In combination with ASA, clopidogrel causes increased risks of bleeding, so use carefully in older adults. After an episode of acute coronary syndrome, ASA therapy should be lifelong, while clopidogrel should be given for 9–12 mo. Do not use clopidogrel if there is a reasonable possibility that patient will be undergoing CABG within the next 5 d.

Acute Revascularization (Early Invasive Therapy)

• Re-establish blood flow via PTCA, preferably with stent placement, or perform thrombolytic therapy as soon as possible for the following indications:

○ Q-wave MI (chest pain <12 h, ≥1 mm ST-segment elevation)

○ Acute coronary syndrome with recurrent angina/ischemia at rest or with low-level activity, elevated troponins, new ST-segment depression, recurrent angina with HF, EF <40%, hemodynamic instability, sustained VT, PTCA in the previous 6 mo, or prior CABG

• Thrombolytic therapy for Q-wave MI is generally preferred over PTCA/stent if presentation is <3 h from symptom onset and PTCA/stent administration is delayed (eg, catheterization lab occupied or unavailable).

○ Age is not a contraindication.

○ Absolute contraindications (ACC/AHA):

- Prior hemorrhagic stroke
- Other stroke or intracerebral event in past yr

- Active internal bleeding
- Known malignant intracranial neoplasm
- Aortic dissection

- Structural cerebral vascular lesion (eg, arteriovenous malformation)
  - Relative contraindications:
    - BP >180/110 on presentation
    - Hx of prior stroke >3 mo, dementia or known intracerebral pathology not covered in absolute contraindications
    - Current therapeutic INR ≥3
    - Known bleeding diathesis
    - Recent (<3 wk) major surgery
    - Prolonged (>10 min) or traumatic CPR
- Significant closed head or facial trauma within 3 mo
- Recent (<2–4 wk) trauma or internal bleeding
- Noncompressible vascular puncture
- Active peptic ulcer
- Hx of severe, chronic HTN
- For streptokinase or anistreplase, prior exposure (5 d–2 yr) or prior allergic reactions

• Emergent CABG is an alternative to PTCA or thrombolytic therapy.

Subacute Management of MI

During hospitalization for both ST-segment elevation MI and acute coronary syndrome (unstable angina or non-Q-wave MI):

• Patients with hematocrit ≤30 and who are not in HF should be transfused to achieve hematocrit >33.
• ACE inhibitors should be started within first 24 h after MI with ST-segment elevation, particularly in cases with systolic dysfunction (see **Table 17**).
• Warfarin therapy is indicated in post-MI patients with atrial fibrillation, left ventricular thrombosis, or large anterior infarction (see **Table 10**).
• Lipid-lowering therapy (see Dyslipidemia, p 30) to achieve target levels (total cholesterol <160 mg/dL, LDL cholesterol <70–100 mg/dL, HDL cholesterol >45 mg/dL) should be initiated by the time of hospital discharge.
• At time of discharge, prescribe rapid-acting nitrates prn: Sublingual nitroglycerin or nitroglycerin spray every 5 min for max of 3 doses in 15 min. See **Table 15**.
• Longer-acting nitrates should be prescribed if symptomatic angina and treatment will be medical rather than surgical or angioplasty. May be combined with β-blockers or calcium channel blockers, or both. See **Table 15**.
• Calcium channel blockers should be used cautiously for management of angina only in non-Q-wave infarctions without systolic dysfunction and a contraindication to β-blockers.

Table 15. Nitrate Dosages and Formulations		
Drug	**Dosage**	**Formulations**
Oral		
Isosorbide dinitrate (*Isordil, Sorbitrate*)	10–40 mg tid (6 h apart)	T: 5, 10, 20, 30, 40; ChT: 5, 10
Isosorbide dinitrate SR (*Isordil Tembids, Dilatrate SR*)	40–80 mg bid–tid	T: 40
Isosorbide mononitrate (*ISMO, Monoket*)	20 mg bid (8 AM and 3 PM)	T: 10, 20
Isosorbide mononitrate SR (*Imdur*)	start 30–60 mg qd; max 240 mg/d	T: 30, 60, 120
Nitroglycerin (*Nitro-Bid*)	2.5–9 mg bid–tid	T: 2.5, 6.5, 9

(cont.)

Table 15. **Nitrate Dosages and Formulations (cont.)**		
Drug	**Dosage**	**Formulations**
Sublingual		
Isosorbide dinitrate (*Isordil, Sorbitrate*)	1 tab prn	T: 2.5, 5, 10
Nitroglycerin (*Nitrostat*)	0.4 mg prn	T: 0.15, 0.3, 0.4, 0.6
Oral spray		
Nitroglycerin (*Nitrolingual*)	1–2 spr prn; max 3/15 min	0.4 mg/spr
Ointment		
Nitroglycerin 2% (*Nitro-Bid, Nitrol*)	start 0.5–4 inches q 4–8 h	2%
Transdermal		
Nitroglycerin	1 Pch 12–14 h/d	(all in mg/h)
(*Deponit*)		0.2, 0.4
(*Minitran*)		0.1, 0.2, 0.4, 0.6
(*Nitrek*)		0.2, 0.4, 0.6
(*Nitro-Dur*)		0.1, 0.2, 0.3, 0.4, 0.6, 0.8
(*Nitrodisc*)		0.2, 0.3, 0.4
(*Transderm-Nitro*)		0.1, 0.2, 0.4, 0.6, 0.8

POST-MI AND CHRONIC STABLE ANGINA CARE
- Unless contraindicated, all patients should be on ASA, a β-blocker, and an ACE inhibitor.
- If β-blockers are contraindicated, use long-acting nitrates or long-acting calcium channel blockers for chronic angina.
- Use sublingual or spray nitroglycerin for acute angina.
- Treat hypertension (see p 31); goal of <140/90 or <130/80 if HF, diabetes mellitus, or kidney failure is present.
- Treat dyslipidemia (see p 30); goals of LDL <70–100 mg/dL and TG <150 mg/dL.
- Treat diabetes mellitus; see p 62 for target goals.
- Weight reduction in obese individuals; goal BMI (kg/m^2) <25.
- Aerobic exercise; goal 30 min at least 3 times/wk.
- Smoking cessation.
- Use folic acid 1 mg po qd to treat homocysteinemia; goal homocysteine <10 μmoles/L.
- Increase consumption of oily fish (eg, white canned or fresh tuna, salmon, mackerel, herring) and foods rich in α-linolenic acid (eg, flax-seed, canola, and soybean oils; flax seed; walnuts). Consider supplementation with fish oil capsules to achieve omega-3 fatty acid intake of 1 g/d.
- Strongly consider placement of implantable cardiac defibrillator (see p 42) in patients with LVEF ≤30% at least 1 mo after MI or 3 mo after CABG.

HEART FAILURE (HF)
Evaluation and Assessment
- All patients initially presenting with HF should have an echocardiogram to evaluate left ventricular function. An ejection fraction (EF) of <40% indicates systolic dysfunction. HF with an EF ≥40% indicates HF with preserved systolic function (diastolic dysfunction).

- Other routine assessment tests: ECG, CXR, CBC, electrolytes, creatinine, albumin, LFTs, TSH, UA
- Measurement of plasma brain natriuretic peptide (BNP) can be helpful in diagnosing acute HF. A BNP >100 pg/mL strongly suggests decreased left ventricular function or acute HF.
- Optional: Radionuclide ventriculography, which measures EF more precisely, provides a better evaluation of right ventricular function, and is more expensive than echocardiography.

Table 16. Heart Failure Staging

Clinical Profile	ACC/AHA Staging	New York Heart Association Staging
Asymptomatic but at high risk of developing HF (eg, HTN, diabetes mellitus, CAD present)	Stage A	—
Asymptomatic with structural disease: LVH, left ventricular dysfunction, prior MI, or valvular disease	Stage B	Class I
Structural disease; currently asymptomatic but with hx of symptoms	Stage C	Class I
Structural disease; patient comfortable at rest but symptomatic on normal physical activity	Stage C	Class II
Structural disease; patient comfortable at rest but symptomatic on slight physical activity	Stage C	Class III
Structural disease; patient symptomatic at rest	Stage C	Class IV
Refractory symptoms at rest in hospitalized patient requiring specialized interventions or hospice care	Stage D	Class IV

Management*
Nonpharmacologic:
- Exercise: Regular walking or cycling for NYHA Class I–III or AHA/ACC Stage A–C disability (see **Table 16**)
- Measure weight daily
- Salt restriction: 3 g sodium diet is reasonable goal; 2 g in severe HF

Pharmacologic: For information on drug dosages and adverse events not listed below, see **Table 20**. Efficacy of different medications may vary significantly across racial and ethnic groups; eg, blacks may require higher doses of ACE inhibitors and β-blockers and may benefit from isosorbide dinitrate/hydralazine therapy.
- Systolic dysfunction:
  ○ Diuretics if volume overload
  ○ ACE inhibitors to target levels (see **Table 17**)
  ○ Once volume status is stabilized, a β-blocker (metoprolol XL [*Toprol-XL*] 12.5–25 mg po qd initially, target 200 mg/d; or bisoprolol [*Zebeta*] 1.25 mg po qd initially, target 5 mg qd; or carvedilol [*Coreg*] 3.125 mg po bid initially, target 25 mg bid) should be added for long-term HF management if there is no contraindication to β-blockers (do not add β-blockers in acutely ill patients).
  ○ Add low-dose digoxin (*Lanoxin*) [T: 0.125, 0.25; S: 0.05 mg/mL]; (*Lanoxicaps*) [T: 0.05, 0.1, 0.2], 0.125–0.375 mg qd (target serum levels 0.5–0.8 mg/dL) if HF is not controlled

on diuretics and ACE inhibitors. Digoxin may be less effective and even harmful in women.

○ Adding an aldosterone antagonist can reduce mortality. Use either spironolactone (*Aldactone*) 25 mg qd [T: 25] in patients with NYHA Class III or IV failure or eplerenone (*Inspra*) 25–50 mg po qd [T: 25, 50, 100] in patients with LVEF <40% who have had MI in the previous 2 wk. Monitor serum potassium carefully and avoid these drugs if Cr ≥2.5 mg/dL.

○ An angiotensin II receptor blocker is indicated in patients being treated with a diuretic, a β-blocker, and digoxin and who cannot receive an ACE inhibitor secondary to cough or angioedema (see **Table 17**).

○ Some clinicians recommend anticoagulation in patients with EF <25% (see **Table 10**).

○ Adding a combination of isosorbide dinitrate and hydralazine (see **Table 15** and **Table 20**; also available as a single preparation: *BiDil* 1–2 tabs po tid [T: 20/37.5]) in blacks with advanced HF can lower risk of mortality from HF.

○ Calcium channel blockers and Class I antiarrhythmics are not indicated.

• HF with preserved systolic function (diastolic dysfunction):
  ○ Diuretics should be used judiciously and only if there is volume overload.
  ○ There is no agreed-upon primary treatment. β-Blockers, ACE inhibitors, and/or nondihydropyridine calcium channel blockers may be of benefit.

*Source: Hunt SA, Baker DW, Chin MH, et al. ACC/AHA guidelines for the evaluation and management of chronic heart failure in the adult: executive summary: a report of the American College of Cardiology/American Heart Association Task Force on Practice Guidelines (Committee to Revise the 1995 Guidelines for Evaluation and Management of Heart Failure). *Circulation* 2001;104:2996–3007.

Table 17. Target Doses of ACE Inhibitors and Angiotensin II Receptor Blockers in Patients with HF

Agent	Starting Dose	Target Dose
ACE Inhibitors		
Benazepril	2.5 mg qd	40 mg qd
Captopril	12.5 mg bid	50 mg tid
Enalapril	2.5 mg qd	10 mg bid
Fosinopril	5 mg qd	40 mg qd
Lisinopril	2.5 mg qd	20 mg qd
Moexipril	3.75 mg qd	15 mg qd
Perindopril	4 mg qd	8 mg qd
Quinapril	5 mg qd	40 mg qd
Ramipril	1.25 mg qd	10 mg qd
Trandolapril	1 mg qd	4 mg qd
Angiotensin Receptor Blockers		
Candesartan	4 mg qd	32 mg qd
Eprosartan	400 mg qd	400 mg bid
Irbesartan	75 mg qd	150 mg qd
Losartan	12.5 mg qd	50 mg bid
Olmesartan	20 mg qd	40 mg qd
Telmisartan	20 mg qd	80 mg qd
Valsartan	40 mg qd	320 mg bid

DYSLIPIDEMIA

Table 18. Treatment Indications for Dyslipidemia

Risk Category	Conditions	LDL-Cholesterol Goal	Initiate Nonpharmacologic Management	Consider Drug Therapy (see Table 19)
Low	0 or 1 risk factor*	<160 mg/dL	≥160 mg/dL	≥190 mg/dL; optional: 160–189 mg/dL
Moderate	≥2 risk factors; 10-yr CAD risk <10%[†]	<130 mg/dL	≥130 mg/dL	≥160 mg/dL
Moderately high	≥2 risk factors; 10-yr CAD risk 10–20%[†]	<130 mg/dL	≥130 mg/dL	≥130 mg/dL; optional: 100–129 mg/dL
High	CVD[‡], DM, or 10-yr CAD risk >20%[†]	<100 mg/dL	≥100 mg/dL	≥100 mg/dL
Very high	DM + CVD[‡]; acute coronary syndrome; multiple severe or poorly controlled risk factors	<70 mg/dL	≥100 mg/dL	≥100 mg/dL; optional: 70–99 mg/dL

Note: CVD = cardiovascular disease; DM = diabetes mellitus.
* Risk factors are cigarette smoking, HTN, HDL <40 mg/dL, family history of premature CAD, male age ≥45 yr, female age ≥55 yr.
† Calculation of 10-yr risk of CAD is available at http://www.nhlbi.nih.gov/guidelines/cholesterol/
‡ CVD refers to CAD, angina, PAD, TIA, stroke, abdominal aortic aneurysm, or 10-yr CAD risk >20%.

Management

Nonpharmacologic: A cholesterol-lowering diet should be considered initial therapy for dyslipidemia and should be used as follows:
• The patient should be at low risk of malnutrition.
• The diet should be nutritionally adequate, with sufficient total calories, protein, calcium, iron, and vitamins.
• The diet should be easily understood and affordable (a dietitian can be very helpful).
• Cholesterol-lowering margarines can lower LDL cholesterol by 10% to 15% (*Take Control* 1–2 tbsp/d; *Benecol* 3 servings of 1.5 tsp each/d).

Pharmacologic: Target drug treatment according to type of dyslipidemia.

Table 19. Drug Regimens for Dyslipidemia

Condition	Drug	Dosage	Formulations
Elevated LDL, normal TG	Statin (HMG-CoA reductase inhibitor)*		
	Atorvastatin (*Lipitor*)	10–80 mg qd	T: 10, 20, 40, 80
	Fluvastatin (*Lescol*)	20–80 mg qd in PM, max 80 mg	C: 20, 40; T: ER 80
	Lovastatin (*Mevacor, Altocor*)	10–40 mg qd in PM or bid	T: 10, 20, 40
	Pravastatin (*Pravachol*)	10–40 mg qd	T: 10, 20, 40, 80
	Rosuvastatin (*Crestor*)	10–40 mg qd	T: 5, 10, 20, 40
	Simvastatin (*Zocor*)	5–80 mg qd in PM	T: 5, 10, 20, 40, 80

(cont.)

Table 19. Drug Regimens for Dyslipidemia (cont.)

Condition	Drug	Dosage	Formulations
Elevated TG (>500 mg/dL)	Fenofibrate (*Tricor*)	54–160 mg qd	T: 54, 160
	Gemfibrozil (*Lopid*)	300–600 mg po bid	T: 600
	Omega-3-acid ethyl esters	4 g/d in single or divided doses	C: 1 g
Combined elevated LDL, low HDL, elevated TG	Fenofibrate, gemfibrozil, or HMG-CoA if TG <300 mg/dL	as above	as above
Alternative for any of above	Niacin†	100 mg tid to start; increase to 500–1000 mg tid; extended release 150 mg qhs to start, increase to 2000 mg qhs as needed	T: 25, 50, 100, 250, 500, ER 150, 250, 500, 750, 1000; C: TR 125, 250, 400, 500
Elevated LDL or combined with inadequate response to one agent	Lovastatin/niacin combination*† (*Advicor*)	20 mg/500 mg qhs to start; increase to 40 mg/2000 mg as needed	T: 20/500, 20/750, 20/1000
	Colesevelam (*WelChol*)	Monotherapy: 1850 mg po bid; combination therapy: 2500–3750 mg/d in single or divided doses	T: 625
	Ezetimibe (*Zetia*)	10 mg qd	T: 10
	Ezetimibe/simvastatin* combination (*Vytorin*)	1 tab qd	T: 10/10, 10/20, 10/40, 10/80

* Measure transaminases at baseline, at 3 mo, and then periodically. Watch for statin-induced myopathy, usually presenting as diffuse, symmetric myalgias. If myopathy is suspected (higher risk at higher statin doses or in combination with fenofibrate, gemfibrozil, or niacin), measure CPK and transaminases; CPK levels >10 times the upper limit of normal indicate serious myopathy/rhabdomyolysis. Even if CPK and transaminases are normal, myalgias still may be due to statin; if this is the case, myalgias should disappear within 1 wk of discontinuing statin.

† Monitor for flushing, pruritus, nausea, gastritis, ulcer. Dosage increases should be spaced 1 mo apart. ASA 325 mg po 30 min before first niacin dose of the day is effective in preventing adverse events.

HYPERTENSION (HTN)
Definition, Classification
JNC 7 defines HTN as SBP ≥140 or DBP ≥90. In older adults, base treatment decisions primarily on the SBP level.

Evaluation and Assessment
• Measure both standing and sitting BP after 5 min of rest.
• Base diagnosis on two or more readings at each of two or more visits. Once diagnosis is made, evaluation includes:
  ○ Assessment of cardiac risk factors: smoking, dyslipidemia, obesity, and diabetes mellitus are important in older adults.
  ○ Assessment of end-organ damage: LVH, angina, prior MI, prior coronary revascularization, HF, stroke or TIA, nephropathy, peripheral arterial disease, retinopathy.

○ Routine laboratory tests: CBC, UA, electrolytes, creatinine, fasting glucose, total cholesterol, HDL cholesterol, and ECG.
○ Consider renal artery stenosis if sudden onset of HTN, sudden rise in BP in previously well-controlled HTN, or HTN despite treatment with three antihypertensives.

Aggravating Factors
- Emotional stress
- Excessive alcohol intake
- Excessive salt intake
- Lack of aerobic exercise
- Low potassium intake
- Low calcium intake
- Nicotine
- Obesity

Management
JNC 7 recommendations: Target is <140/90 (130/80 in persons with diabetes or kidney disease). Lowering BP below 120/80 is not recommended. Particularly in patients with "white coat" HTN, home monitoring of BP with a properly calibrated machine can produce more reliable readings than office-based measurements.

Nonpharmacologic:
- Adequate calcium and magnesium intake as well as a low-fat diet for optimizing general health.
- Adequate dietary potassium intake; fruits and vegetables are the best sources.
- Aerobic exercise—30–45 min most days of the week.
- Moderation of alcohol intake—limit to 1 oz of ethanol/d.
- Moderation of dietary sodium: watch for volume depletion with diuretic use.
  Goal: ≤2.4 g Na^+/d.
- Smoking cessation
- Weight reduction if obese: even a 10-lb weight loss can significantly lower BP.
  Goal: BMI (kg/m^2) <25.

Pharmacologic: **Table 20** lists commonly used antihypertensives.
- Use antihypertensives carefully in patients with orthostatic BP drop.
- Base treatment decisions on standing BP.
- If no coexisting conditions, a thiazide diuretic, a β-blocker, or an ACE inhibitor can be used as a first-line drug.
- If coexisting conditions, therapy should be individualized (see **Table 21**).
- Combination drugs for hypertension are listed in **Table 22**.
- Available dose formulations of oral potassium supplements: [T: (mEq) 6, 7, 8, 10, 20; S: (mEq/15 mL) 20, 40; powders (mEq/pk) 15, 20, 25]
- Follow-up BP measurements monthly until target BP is attained; visits may be q 3–6 mo if BP is stable at target goal.

Hypertensive Emergencies and Urgencies:
- Elevated BP alone without symptoms or target end-organ damage rarely requires emergent BP lowering.
- Conditions requiring emergent BP lowering include hypertensive encephalopathy, intracranial hemorrhage, unstable angina, acute MI, acute left ventricular failure with pulmonary edema, dissecting aortic aneurysm.
- Most common initial treatment for emergent BP lowering is sodium nitroprusside (*Nipride*) 0.25–10 mg/kg/min as IV infusion.
- For nonemergent (ie, urgent) BP lowering, give a standard dose of a recommended antihypertensive orally (see **Table 20**) or an extra dose of the patient's usual oral antihypertensive.

Table 20. Oral Antihypertensive Agents

Class, Drug	Geriatric Dosage Range, Total mg/d (times/d)	Formulations	Comments (Metabolism, Excretion)
Diuretics			↓ Potassium, Na, magnesium levels; ↑ uric acid, calcium, cholesterol (mild), and glucose (mild) levels
Thiazides			
✔ Chlorothiazide (*Diuril*)	125–500 (1)	T: 250, 500	
✔ Chlorthalidone (*Hygroton*)	12.5–25 (1)	T: 15, 25, 50, 100	↑ Adverse events at >25 mg/d (L)
✔ HCTZ (*Esidrix, HydroDIURIL, Oretic*)	12.5–25 (1)	T: 25, 50, 100; S: 50 mg/mL; C: 12.5	↑ Adverse events at >25 mg/d (L)
✔ Indapamide (*Lozol*)	0.625–2.5 (1)	T: 1.25, 2.5	Less or no hypercholesterolemia (L)
✔ Metolazone (*Mykrox*)	0.25–0.5 (1)	T rapid: 0.5	Monitor electrolytes carefully (L)
✔ Metolazone (*Zaroxolyn*)	2.5–5 (1)	T: 2.5, 5, 10	Monitor electrolytes carefully (L)
✔ Polythiazide (*Renese*)	1–4 (1)	T: 1, 2, 4	
Loop diuretics			
♥ Bumetanide (*Bumex*)	0.5–4 (1–3)	T: 0.5, 1, 2	Short duration of action, no hypercalcemia (K)
♥ Furosemide (*Lasix*)	20–160 (1–2)	T: 20, 40, 80; S: 10, 40 mg/5 mL	Short duration of action, no hypercalcemia (K)
♥ Torsemide (*Demadex*)	2.5–50 (1–2)	T: 5, 10, 20, 100	Short duration of action, no hypercalcemia (K)
Potassium-sparing drugs			
Amiloride (*Midamor*)	2.5–10 (1)	T: 5	(L, K)
Triamterene (*Dyrenium*)	25–100 (1–2)	T: 50, 100	(L, K)
Aldosterone receptor-blockers			
♥ Eplerenone (*Inspra*)	25–100 (1)	T: 25, 50, 100	(L, K)
♥ Spironolactone (*Aldactone*)	12.5–50 (1–2)	T: 25, 50, 100	Gynecomastia (L, K)
Adrenergic Inhibitors			
α_1-Blockers			Avoid as primary therapy for HTN unless patient has BPH
Doxazosin (*Cardura*)	1–16 (1)	T: 1, 2, 4, 8	(L)
Prazosin (*Minipress*)	1–20 (2–3)	T: 1, 2, 5	(L)
Terazosin (*Hytrin*)	1–20 (1–2)	T: 1, 2, 5, 10; C: 1, 2, 5, 10	(L, K)

(cont.)

Note: Listing of adverse events is not exhaustive, and adverse events are for the class of drugs except where noted for individual drugs. ✔ = preferred for treating older adults; ♥ = useful in treating HF.

Table 20. Oral Antihypertensive Agents (cont.)

Class, Drug	Geriatric Dosage Range, Total mg/d (times/d)	Formulations	Comments (Metabolism, Excretion)
Central α_2-agonists and other centrally acting drugs			Sedation, dry mouth, bradycardia, withdrawal hypertension
Clonidine (*Catapres, Catapres-TTS*)	0.1–1.2 (2–3) *or* 1 Pch/wk	T: 0.1, 0.2, 0.3; Pch: 0.1, 0.2, 0.3 mg/d	Continue oral for 1–2 d when converting to patch (L, K)
Guanfacine (*Tenex*)	0.5–2 (1)	T: 1, 2	(K)
Methyldopa (*Aldomet*)	250–2500 (2)	T: 125, 250, 500; S: 250 mg/5 mL	(L, K)
Reserpine (*Serpasil*)	0.05–0.25 (1)	T: 0.1, 0.25	Depression, nasal congestion, activation of peptic ulcer (L, K)
β-Blockers			Bronchospasm, bradycardia, acute HF, may mask insulin-induced hypoglycemia; lipid solubility is a risk factor for delirium
✔ Acebutolol (*Sectral*)	200–800 (1)	C: 200, 400	β_1, low lipid solubility, intrinsic sympathomimetic activity (L, K)
✔ Atenolol (*Tenormin*)	12.5–100 (1)	T: 25, 50, 100	β_1, low lipid solubility (K)
✔ Betaxolol (*Kerlone*)	5–20 (1)	T: 10, 20	β_1, low lipid solubility (L, K)
✔♥ Bisoprolol (*Zebeta*)	2.5–10 (1)	T: 5, 10	β_1, low lipid solubility (L, K)
✔ Carteolol (*Cartrol*)	1.25–10 (1)	T: 2.5, 5	β_1, low lipid solubility, intrinsic sympathomimetic activity (K)
✔ Metoprolol (*Lopressor*)	25–400 (2)	T: 25, 50, 100	β_1, moderate lipid solubility (L)
✔♥ Long-acting (*Toprol XL*)	50–400 (1)	T: 25, 50, 100, 200	(L)
Nadolol (*Corgard*)	20–160 (1)	T: 20, 40, 80, 120, 160	β_1, β_2, low lipid solubility (K)
Penbutolol (*Levatol*)	10–40 (1)	T: 20	β_1, β_2, high lipid solubility, intrinsic sympathomimetic activity (L, K)
Pindolol (*Visken*)	5–40 (2)	T: 5, 10	β_1, β_2, moderate lipid solubility, intrinsic sympathomimetic activity (K)
Propranolol (*Inderal*)	20–160 (2)	T: 10, 20, 40, 60, 80, 90; S: 4 mg/mL, 8 mg/mL, 80 mg/mL	β_1, β_2, high lipid solubility (L)
Long-acting (*Inderal LA, InnoPran XL*)	60–180 (1)	C: 60, 80, 120, 160	β_1, β_2, high lipid solubility (L)
Timolol (*Blocadren*)	10–40 (2)	T: 5, 10, 20	β_1, β_2, low to moderate lipid solubility (L, K)

(cont.)

Note: Listing of adverse events is not exhaustive, and adverse events are for the class of drugs except where noted for individual drugs. ✔ = preferred for treating older adults; ♥ = useful in treating HF.

Table 20. Oral Antihypertensive Agents (cont.)

Class, Drug	Geriatric Dosage Range, Total mg/d (times/d)	Formulations	Comments (Metabolism, Excretion)
Combined α- and β-blockers			Postural hypotension, bronchospasm
✔♥ Carvedilol (Coreg)	3.125–25 (2)	T: 3.125, 6.25, 12.5, 25	β_1, β_2, high lipid solubility (L)
✔ Labetalol (Normodyne, Trandate)	100–600 (2)	T: 100, 200, 300	β_1, β_2, moderate lipid solubility (L, K)
Direct Vasodilators			Headaches, fluid retention, tachycardia
♥ Hydralazine (Apresoline)	25–100 (2–4)	T: 10, 25, 50, 100	Lupus syndrome; used in combination with isosorbide dinitrate for HF in blacks (L, K)
Minoxidil (Loniten)	2.5–50 (1)	T: 2.5, 10	Hirsutism (K)
Calcium Antagonists			
Nondihydropyridines			Conduction defects, worsening of systolic dysfunction, gingival hyperplasia
✔ Diltiazem SR (Cardizem CD, Cardizem SR, Dilacor XR, Tiazac)	120–360 (1–2) max 480	C: 1/d: 120, 180, 240, 300, 360, 420; 2/d: 60, 90, 120; T: 30, 60, 90, 120, ER: 120, 180, 240	Nausea, headache (L)
✔ Verapamil SR (Calan SR, Covera-HS, Isoptin SR, Verelan)	120–360 (1–2)	T: SR 120, 180, 240; C: SR 100, 120, 180, 200, 240, 300, 360; T: 40, 80, 120	Constipation, bradycardia (L)
Dihydropyridines			Ankle edema, flushing, headache, gingival hypertrophy
✔ Amlodipine (Norvasc)	2.5–10 (1)	T: 2.5, 5, 10	(L)
✔ Felodipine (Plendil)	2.5–20 (1)	T: 2.5, 5, 10	(L)
✔ Isradipine (DynaCirc)	2.5–20 (2)	T: 2.5, 5	(L)
✔ Sustained release (DynaCirc CR)	2.5–10 (1)	T: 5, 10	
✔ Nicardipine (Cardene)	60–120 (3)	C: 20, 30	(L)
✔ Sustained release (Cardene SR)	60–120 (2)	T: 30, 45, 60	(L)
✔ Nifedipine SR (Adalat CC, Procardia XL)	30–60 (1)	T: 30, 60, 90	(L)
✔ Nisoldipine (Sular)	10–40 (1)	T: ER 10, 20, 30, 40	(L)
ACE Inhibitors*			Cough (common), angioedema (rare), hyperkalemia, rash, loss of taste, leukopenia
✔♥ Benazepril (Lotensin)	2.5–40 (1–2)	T: 5, 10, 20, 40	(L, K)

(cont.)

Note: Listing of adverse events is not exhaustive, and adverse events are for the class of drugs except where noted for individual drugs. ✔ = preferred for treating older adults; ♥ = useful in treating HF.
* See **Table 17** for target doses in treating HF.

Table 20. Oral Antihypertensive Agents (cont.)

Class, Drug	Geriatric Dosage Range, Total mg/d (times/d)	Formulations	Comments (Metabolism, Excretion)
✔ ♥ Captopril (Capoten)	12.5–150 (2–3)	T: 12.5, 25, 50, 100	(L, K)
✔ ♥ Enalapril (Vasotec)	2.5–40 (1–2)	T: 2.5, 5, 10, 20	(L, K)
✔ ♥ Fosinopril (Monopril)	5–40 (1–2)	T: 10, 20, 40	(L, K)
✔ ♥ Lisinopril (Prinivil, Zestril)	2.5–40 (1)	T: 2.5, 5, 10, 20, 30, 40	(K)
✔ ♥ Moexipril (Univasc)	3.75–30 (1)	T: 7.5, 15	(L, K)
✔ ♥ Perindopril (Aceon)	4–8 (1–2)	T: 2, 4, 8	(L, K)
✔ ♥ Quinapril (Accupril)	5–40 (1)	T: 5, 10, 20, 40	(L, K)
✔ ♥ Ramipril (Altace)	1.25–20 (1)	T: 1.25, 2.5, 5, 10	(L, K)
✔ ♥ Trandolapril (Mavik)	1–4 (1)	T: 1, 2, 4	(L, K)
Angiotensin II Receptor Blockers (ARBs)*			Angioedema (very rare), hyperkalemia
✔ ♥ Candesartan (Atacand)	4–32 (1)	T: 4, 8, 16, 32	(K)
✔ ♥ Eprosartan (Teveten)	400–800 (1–2)	T: 400, 600	(biliary, K)
✔ ♥ Irbesartan (Avapro)	75–300 (1)	T: 75, 150, 300	(L)
✔ ♥ Losartan (Cozaar)	12.5–100 (1–2)	T: 25, 50, 100	(L, K)
✔ ♥ Olmesartan (Benicar)	20–40 (1)	T: 5, 20, 40	(F, K)
✔ ♥ Telmisartan (Micardis)	20–80 (1)	T: 20, 40, 80	(L)
✔ ♥ Valsartan (Diovan)	40–320 (1)	T: 80, 160, 320; C: 80, 160	(L, K)

Note: Listing of adverse events is not exhaustive, and adverse events are for the class of drugs except where noted for individual drugs. ✔ = preferred for treating older adults; ♥ = useful in treating HF.
* See **Table 17** for target doses in treating HF.
Source: Data in part from The seventh report of the Joint National Committee on Prevention, Detection, Evaluation, and Treatment of High Blood Pressure: The JNC 7 report. JAMA. 2003;289:2560–2572.

Table 21. Choosing Antihypertensive Therapy on the Basis of Coexisting Conditions

Condition	Appropriate for Use	Avoid or Contraindicated
Angina	β, D, non-D	
Atrial tachycardia and fibrillation	β, non-D	
Bronchospasm		β, αβ
Diabetes mellitus	ACEI, ARB, β, T*	T*
Dyslipidemia		β, T†
Essential tremor	β	
HF	AA, ACEI, ARB, β, αβ, L	D, non-D‡
Hyperthyroidism	β	
MI	β, AA, ACEI	non-D
Osteoporosis	T	
Prostatism (BPH)	α	

(cont.)

Table 21. Choosing Antihypertensive Therapy on the Basis of Coexisting Conditions (cont.)

Condition	Appropriate for Use	Avoid or Contraindicated
Renal insufficiency	AA, ACEI[§]	
Urge UI	D, non-D	L, T

Note: AA = aldosterone antagonist; α = α-blocker; β = β-blocker; $\alpha\beta$ = combined α- and β-blocker; ACEI = ACE inhibitor; ARB = angiotensin receptor blocker; D = dihydropyridine calcium antagonist; non-D = nondihydropyridine calcium antagonist; L = loop diuretic; T = thiazide diuretic.

* Low-dose diuretics probably beneficial in type 2 diabetes; high-dose diuretics relatively contraindicated in types 1 and 2.
† Low-dose diuretics have a minimal effect on lipids.
‡ May be beneficial in HF caused by diastolic dysfunction.
§ Use with great caution in renovascular disease.

Table 22. Combination Drugs for Hypertension

Combination Type	Fixed-dose Combination, mg*	Trade Name
ACE inhibitors and calcium channel blockers	Amlodipine/benazepril hydrochloride (2.5/10, 5/10, 5/20, 10/20)	Lotrel
	Enalapril maleate/felodipine (5/5)	Lexxel
	Trandolapril/verapamil (2/180, 1/240, 2/240, 4/240)	Tarka
ACE inhibitors and diuretics	Benazepril/HCTZ (5/6.25, 10/12.5, 20/12.5, 20/25)	Lotensin HCT
	Captopril/HCTZ (25/15, 25/25, 50/15, 50/25)	Capozide
	Enalapril maleate/HCTZ (5/12.5, 10/25)	Vaseretic
	Lisinopril/HCTZ (10/12.5, 20/25)	Prinzide
	Moexipril hydrochloride/HCTZ (7.5/12.5, 15/25)	Uniretic
	Quinapril hydrochloride/HCTZ (10/12.5, 20/12.5, 20/25)	Accuretic
Angiotensin-receptor blockers and diuretics	Candesartan cilexetil/HCTZ (16/12.5, 32/12.5)	Atacand HCT
	Eprosartan mesylate/HCTZ (600/12.5, 600/25)	Teveten HCT
	Irbesartan/HCTZ (75/12.5, 150/12.5, 300/12.5)	Avalide
	Losartan potassium/HCTZ (50/12.5, 100/25)	Hyzaar
	Telmisartan/HCTZ (40/12.5, 80/12.5)	Micardis HCT
	Valsartan/HCTZ (80/12.5, 160/12.5)	Diovan HCT
β-Blockers and diuretics	Atenolol/chlorthalidone (50/25, 100/25)	Tenoretic
	Bisoprolol fumarate/HCTZ (2.5/6.25, 5/6.25, 10/6.25)	Ziac
	Propranolol LA/HCTZ (40/25, 80/25)	Inderide
	Metoprolol tartrate/HCTZ (50/25, 100/25)	Lopressor HCT
	Nadolol/bendroflumethiazide (40/5, 80/5)	Corzide
	Timolol maleate/HCTZ (10/25)	Timolide
Centrally acting drug and diuretic	Methyldopa/HCTZ (250/15, 250/25, 500/30, 500/50)	Aldoril
	Reserpine/chlorothiazide (0.125/250, 0.25/500)	Diupres
	Reserpine/HCTZ (0.125/25, 0.125/50)	Hydropres
Diuretic and diuretic	Amiloride hydrochloride/HCTZ (5/50)	Moduretic
	Spironolactone/HCTZ (25/25, 50/50)	Aldactazide
	Triamterene/HCTZ (37.5/25, 50/25, 75/50)	Dyazide, Maxzide

*Some drug combinations are available in multiple fixed doses. Each drug dose is reported in mg.
Source: The seventh report of the Joint National Committee on Prevention, Detection, Evaluation, and Treatment of High Blood Pressure: The JNC 7 report. *JAMA*. 2003;289:2560–2572.

ATRIAL FIBRILLATION (AF)
Evaluation and Assessment
Causes:
- Cardiac disease: Cardiac surgery, cardiomyopathy, HF, hypertensive heart disease, ischemic disease, pericarditis, valvular disease
- Noncardiac disease: Alcoholism, chronic pulmonary disease, infections, pulmonary emboli, thyrotoxicosis

Standard testing: ECG, CXR, CBC, electrolytes, creatinine, BUN, TSH, echocardiogram

Management
- Correct precipitating cause.
- For both acute and chronic AF, the preferred management for most patients is rate control and anticoagulation rather than rhythm control.
  - Rate control (target <80 beats/min) can be achieved with atenolol, metoprolol, diltiazem, or verapamil, given IV (in cases of acute hemodynamic instability) or po.
  - Digoxin can be used as a second-line agent for rate control.
  - Anticoagulation to INR 2.0–3.0 should be achieved with oral warfarin (see p 18) and continued indefinitely.
  - If anticoagulation is contraindicated, use ASA 325 mg po qd and continue indefinitely.
- Rhythm control via direct current or pharmacologic cardioversion is an alternative treatment option in patients with unpleasant symptoms or decreased exercise tolerance on rate control therapy.
  - For direct-current cardioversion, two methods may be used:
    - Early cardioversion: perform transesophageal echocardiography to exclude intracardiac thrombus; if no thrombus, begin anticoagulation and cardiovert with 4 wk of post-cardioversion anticoagulation.
    - Delayed cardioversion: anticoagulate for 3 wk before cardioversion, followed by 4 wk of post-cardioversion anticoagulation.
  - For pharmacologic cardioversion and rhythm maintenance (recommended only if AF produces symptoms significantly impairing quality of life), rhythm control drugs may be tried (see **Table 23**).
- Direct-current cardioversion should be attempted in acute-onset AF with compromised cardiac output or angina.

Table 23. **Selected Rhythm Control Drugs for AF**

Drug	Dosage	Formulations	Comments (Metabolism)
Amiodarone *(Cordarone, Pacerone)*	100–400 qd	T: 200, 400	Most effective antifibrillatory agent but numerous adverse events, including pulmonary and hepatic toxic effects, hypothyroidism, corneal deposits, warfarin interaction (L)
Propafenone *(Rythmol)*	150–300 tid	T: 150, 225, 300	Contraindicated in patients with ischemic and structural heart disease; adverse events include VT and HF (L)
Sotalol *(Betapace, Betapace AF, Sorine)*	80–160 bid	T: 80, 120, 160, 240	Prolongs QT interval; adverse events include torsades de pointes, HF, exacerbation of COPD/bronchospasm (K)

AORTIC STENOSIS (AS)
Evaluation and Assessment
• Presence of symptoms—angina, syncope, HF (frequently diastolic dysfunction)—indicates severe disease and a life expectancy without surgery of <2 yr.
• Echocardiography is essential to measure aortic jet velocity (AJV) and aortic valve area (AVA).
  ○ Moderate AS is indicated by an AJV of 3.0–4.0 meters/sec and by an AVA of 1.0–1.5 cm².
  ○ Severe AS is indicated by an AJV >4.0 meters/sec and by an AVA <1.0 cm².
• For asymptomatic cases, echocardiography should be repeated annually for moderate AS and every 6–12 mo for severe AS.
• ECG and CXR should be obtained initially to look for conduction defects, LVH, and pulmonary congestion.

Treatment
• Aortic valve replacement (AVR) surgery
  ○ Alleviates symptoms and improves ventricular functioning.
  ○ In most cases, perform AVR promptly *after* symptoms have appeared.
  ○ Consider risks and benefits of AVR on individual basis (see pp 164–166).
• Avoid vasodilators if possible.

PERIPHERAL ARTERIAL DISEASE (PAD)

Table 24. Classes of Peripheral Arterial Disease

Class	ABI	Symptoms	Treatment
Normal	>0.9	None	RFM
Mild	0.8–0.9	No limitation in walking distance	RFM, AT
Moderate to severe	0.4–0.8	Walking limited by claudication	RFM, AT, CRx
Severe to critical	<0.4	Pain at rest; ischemia on exam	RFM, AT, CRx, LS

Note: ABI = ankle-brachial BP index; AT = antiplatelet therapy; CRx = claudication therapy; LS = limb salvage; RFM = risk factor modification.

Treatment
Risk Factor Modification:
• Low-fat diet
• Exercise: walking program
• Smoking cessation
• Lipid-lowering therapy
• BP control
• Glycemic control in diabetic patients

Antiplatelet Therapy:
• ASA 325 mg qd
• Clopidogrel (*Plavix*) 75 mg qd [T: 75] if no response to or intolerant to ASA

Claudication Treatment:
- Walking program
- Drug therapy: cilostazol (*Pletal*) 100 mg bid (contraindicated in patients with HF) 1 h before or 2 h after meals [T: 50, 100]; pentoxifylline (*Trental*) 400 mg tid [T: 400]; conventional analgesics

Limb Salvage:
- Percutaneous angioplasty
- Bypass surgery

SYNCOPE

Table 25. Classification of Syncope

Cause	Frequency (%)	Features	Increased Risk of Death
Vasovagal	21	Preceded by lightheadedness, nausea, diaphoresis; recovery gradual, frequently with fatigue	No
Cardiac	10	Little or no warning before blackout, rapid and complete recovery	Yes
Orthostatic	9	Lightheaded prodrome after standing, recovery gradual	No
Medication-induced	7	Lightheaded prodrome, recovery gradual	No
Seizure	5	No warning, may have neurologic deficits, slow recovery	Yes
Stroke, TIA	4	Little or no warning, neurologic deficits	Yes
Other causes	8	Preceded by cough, micturition, or specific situation	No
Unknown	37	Any of the above	Yes

Source: Adapted from Soteriades ES, Evans JC, Larson MG, et al. Incidence and prognosis of syncope. *N Engl J Med* 2002;347:878–885.

Evaluation
- Focus hx on events before, during, and after loss of consciousness; hx of cardiac disease (significantly worsens prognosis of syncope of all causes); careful medication review.
- Focus on cardiovascular and neurologic systems in physical examination.
- ECG and orthostatic BP or pulse check for all patients.
- Additional testing as suggested by initial evaluation:
  - Ambulatory ECG monitoring for further evaluation of arrhythmia
  - Stress testing to investigate ischemic heart disease
  - Echocardiography to investigate structural heart disease
  - Electrophysiologic studies in patients with prior MI or structural heart disease
  - Tilt-table testing for suspected vasovagal cause
  - Head imaging, electroencephalogram for suspected neurologic cause
  - If suspected orthostatic cause, evaluation for Parkinson's disease, autonomic neuropathy, diabetes mellitus, hypovolemia

Management
- Patients with cardiac syncope require immediate hospitalization on telemetry; exclude MI and PE.
- Strongly consider hospital admission for patients with syncope due to neurologic or unknown causes, particularly if concurrent heart disease.
- Patients with syncope due to vasovagal, orthostatic, medication-induced, or other causes can usually be managed as outpatients, particularly if there is no hx of heart disease.
- Treatment is correction of underlying cause.

ORTHOSTATIC (POSTURAL) HYPOTENSION
See also **Table 37**.
Evaluation and Assessment
- Associated with following symptoms usually after standing: lightheadedness, dizziness, syncope, blurred vision, diaphoresis, head or neck pain, decreased hearing
- Diagnosis: ≥20 mm Hg drop in SBP or ≥10 mm Hg in DBP within 3 min of rising to more upright position
- Causes
  - Medications, including antihypertensives, phenothiazines, tricyclic antidepressants, monoamine oxidase inhibitors, anti-Parkinsonian drugs, PDE5 inhibitors (for erectile dysfunction)
  - Autonomic dysregulation (suggested by lack of compensatory rise in heart rate with postural hypotension): age-related decreased baroreceptor sensitivity, Parkinson's disease and related disorders, peripheral neuropathy, prolonged bed rest
  - Hypovolemia
  - Anemia

Management
- Correct underlying disorder, particularly by discontinuing medications that could exacerbate hypotension
- Alter movement behavior: educate patients to rise slowly, flex calf and forearm muscles when standing, stand with one foot in front of other, avoid straining, and elevate head of the bed
- Dietary changes: avoid alcohol, maintain adequate fluid intake, increase salt and caffeine intake
- Above-the-knee compression stockings (at least medium strength, eg, Jobst)
- Pharmacologic interventions:
  - Fludrocortisone *(Florinef)*: 0.1 mg qd–tid [T: 0.1]; use with caution in patients with HF, cardiac disease, hypertension, renal disease, esophagitis, peptic ulcer disease, or ulcerative colitis
  - Midodrine *(ProAmantine)*: 2.5–5 mg qd–tid [T: 2.5, 5]; use with caution in patients with hypertension, diabetes, urinary retention, renal disease, hepatic disease, glaucoma
  - Caffeine: 1 cup of caffeinated coffee bid–tid; alternatively, caffeine tabs 100–200 mg bid–tid; useful for postprandial hypotension when taken with meals
  - Erythropoietin (see **Table 44**) can be useful for hypotension secondary to anemia

IMPLANTABLE CARDIAC DEFIBRILLATOR (ICD) PLACEMENT
Indications (consider life expectancy and comorbidities)
- Established:
  - Cardiac arrest due to ventricular fibrillation (VF) or ventricular tachycardia (VT)
  - Spontaneous sustained VT with structural heart disease
  - Spontaneous sustained VT without structural heart disease not alleviated by other treatments
  - Unexplained syncope with hemodynamically significant VF or VT inducible by electrophysiologic study when drug therapy is ineffective, not tolerated, or not preferred
  - Nonsustained VT, CAD, and inducible VF by electrophysiologic study that is not suppressed by Class I antiarrhythmic
  - LVEF ≤30% and CAD
  - ICD + biventricular pacing for advanced HF (NYHA Class III or IV) and QRS interval ≥120 millisec
- Less established: Nonischemic cardiomyopathy with LVEF ≤35% and either premature ventricular complexes or nonsustained VT

Contraindications
- Terminal illness with life expectancy <6 mo
- Unexplained syncope without inducible VT or VF and without structural heart disease
- VT or VF due to transient or easily reversible disorder
- End-stage HF (ACC/AHA Stage D) not awaiting cardiac transplant

Complications
- Surgical: infection (1%–2%), hematoma, pneumothorax
- Device-related: lead dislodgement or malfunction, connection problems, inadequate defibrillation threshold
- Therapy-related: frequent shocks (appropriate or inappropriate), acceleration of VT, anxiety and other psychological stress

DELIRIUM

DIAGNOSIS

Diagnostic Criteria—Adapted from *DSM-IV*
- Disturbed consciousness (ie, decreased attention, environmental awareness)
- Cognitive change (eg, memory deficit, disorientation, language disturbance) or perceptual disturbance (eg, visual illusions, hallucinations)
- Rapid onset (hours to days) and fluctuating daily course
- Evidence of a causal physical condition

Risk Factors
- Dementia greatly increases risk of delirium.
- Advanced age, comorbid physical problems (especially sleep deprivation, immobility, dehydration, pain, sensory impairment).

Evaluation
- Assume reversibility unless proven otherwise.
- Thoroughly review prescription and OTC medications.
- Exclude infection and other medical causes.
- Laboratory studies may include CBC, electrolytes, LFTs, renal function tests, serum albumin, serum calcium, serum glucose, UA, oxygen saturation, CXR, and ECG.
- Confusion Assessment Method (CAM): BOTH acute onset and fluctuating course AND inattention AND EITHER disorganized thinking OR altered level of consciousness (Inouye S, *Ann Intern Med.* 1990;113:941–948).

CAUSES

(Italicized type indicates the most common causes in older adults.)

Drugs
- *Anticholinergics* (eg, diphenhydramine), TCAs (eg, amitriptyline, imipramine), antipsychotics (eg, chlorpromazine, thioridazine)
- Anti-inflammatory agents, including prednisone
- Benzodiazepines or alcohol—acute toxicity or withdrawal
- Cardiovascular (eg, digitalis, antihypertensives)
- Diuretics
- Lithium
- GI (eg, cimetidine, ranitidine)
- Opioid analgesics (especially meperidine)

Infections
Respiratory, *skin*, *urinary tract*, and others

Metabolic Disorders
Acute blood loss, *dehydration*, *electrolyte imbalance*, end-organ failure (hepatic, renal), hyperglycemia, *hypoglycemia*, *hypoxia*

Cardiovascular
Arrhythmia, *HF*, *MI*, shock

Neurologic
CNS infections, head trauma, seizures, stroke, subdural hematoma, TIAs, tumors

Miscellaneous
Fecal impaction, *postoperative state*, sleep deprivation, urinary retention

MANAGEMENT

Nonpharmacologic

- Identify and remove or treat underlying cause(s)
- Provide general supportive measures:
  - Modify environment
    - communication to reorient to new surroundings
    - objects that provide orientation (eg, calendar, clock)
    - quiet, well-lit surroundings
    - familiar faces (eg, family members) at bedside for reassurance
    - sitters
  - Engage in stimulating activities during daytime
    - cognitive activities (eg, current events discussion, word games)
    - ambulation, active range-of-motion exercises
  - Correct sensory deficits
    - eyeglasses
    - adequate lighting
    - magnifying lenses
    - cerumen removal
    - hearing aids
    - portable amplification device
  - Promote normal sleep
    - warm milk at bedtime
    - relaxation tapes
    - back massage
    - nighttime noise reduction
  - Prevent dehydration: oral or parenteral supplementation if BUN/creatinine ratio >18
  - Use physical restraints only as last resort to maintain patient safety (eg, preventing patient from pulling out tubes or catheters)

Pharmacologic

- For acute agitation or aggression accompanying delirium, use a high-potency antipsychotic such as haloperidol (*Haldol*) 0.5–2 mg po [T: 0.5, 1, 2, 5, 10, 20; S: 2 mg/mL] or IV or IM (twice as potent as po). May also be given as slow IV push; titrate upward as needed. Reevaluate every 30 min. Observe for development of EPS.
- Other IM antipsychotics are less valuable because of the following concerns:
  - Ziprasidone (*Geodon*): cardiac conduction delays
  - Risperidone IM (*Risperdal Consta*): not appropriate for acute treatment, because only a small amount of drug is initially released from IM formulation.
  - Olanzapine IM (*Zyprexa IntraMuscular*): anticholinergic and hypotensive effects
- Avoid low-potency antipsychotics such as chlorpromazine (*Thorazine*) or thioridazine (*Mellaril*) because of their anticholinergic and arrythmogenic properties (torsades de pointes). If patient is able to take drugs po, consider low dose of atypical antipsychotic (see **Table 78**).
- If delirium is secondary to alcohol or benzodiazepine withdrawal, use a benzodiazepine such as lorazepam (*Ativan*) in doses of 0.5–2 mg every 4–6 h. Because these agents themselves may cause delirium, gradual withdrawal and discontinuation are desirable. If delirium is secondary to alcohol, also use thiamine 100 mg qd (po, IM, or IV).

DEMENTIA

DEMENTIA SYNDROME
Definition
Chronic acquired decline in memory and in at least one other cognitive function (eg, language, visual-spatial, executive) sufficient to affect daily life.

Estimated Frequencies of Causes of Dementia
- AD: 60% to 70%
- Other progressive disorders: 15% to 30% (eg, vascular, Lewy body, frontal temporal)
- Completely reversible dementia (eg, drug toxicity, metabolic changes, thyroid disease, subdural hematoma, normal-pressure hydrocephalus): 2% to 5%

DIAGNOSIS OF AD
- Dementia syndrome
- Gradual onset and continuing decline
- Not due to another physical, neurologic, or psychiatric condition or to medications
- Deficits not seen exclusively during delirium

PROGRESSION OF AD
Mild Cognitive Impairment (preclinical)   MMSE: 26–30
- Report by patient or caregiver of memory loss
- Delayed paragraph recall
- Cognition otherwise intact
- No functional impairment, normal ADL
- Mild construction, language, or executive dysfunction
- Some cases of mild cognitive impairment may not progress to AD

Early, Mild Impairment (yr 1–3 from onset of symptoms)   MMSE: 22–28
- Disoriented to date
- Naming difficulties (anomia)
- Recent recall problems
- Mild difficulty copying figures
- Decreased insight
- Social withdrawal
- Irritability, mood change
- Problems managing finances

Middle, Moderate Impairment (yr 2–8)   MMSE: 10–21
- Disoriented to date, place
- Comprehension difficulties (aphasia)
- Impaired new learning
- Getting lost in familiar areas
- Impaired calculating skills
- Delusions, agitation, aggression
- Not cooking, shopping, banking
- Restless, anxious, depressed
- Problems with dressing, grooming

Late, Severe Impairment (yr 6–12)   MMSE: 0–9
- Nearly unintelligible verbal output
- Remote memory gone
- Unable to copy or write
- No longer grooming or dressing
- Incontinent
- Motor or verbal agitation

NONCOGNITIVE SYMPTOMS
Psychotic Symptoms (eg, Delusions, Hallucinations)
• Seen in about 20% of AD patients
• Delusions may be paranoid (eg, people stealing things, spouse unfaithful)
• Hallucinations (approximately 11% of patients) are more commonly visual

Depressive Symptoms
• Seen in up to 40% of AD patients; may herald onset of AD
• May cause acceleration of decline if untreated
• Suspect if patient stops eating or withdraws

Agitation or Aggression
• Seen in up to 80% of patients with AD
• A leading cause of nursing-home admission
• Consider superimposed delirium or pain as a trigger

RISK AND PROTECTIVE FACTORS FOR AD

Definite Risks	Possible Risks	Possible Protections
Age	Other genes	Antioxidants (eg, vitamin E,
Family history	Head trauma	beta carotene)
Down syndrome	Hypercholesterolemia	
APOE-E4 (Caucasians)	Hypertension	
	Lower educational level	
	Depression	

Clinical Features Distinguishing AD and Other Types of Dementia
• AD: Memory, language, visual-spatial disturbances, indifference, delusions, agitation
• Frontotemporal dementia: Personality change, executive dysfunction, hyperorality, relative preservation of visual-spatial skills
• Lewy body dementia: visual hallucinations, delusions, EPS, fluctuating mental status, sensitivity to antipsychotic medications
• Vascular dementia: abrupt onset, stepwise deterioration, prominent aphasia, motor signs

EVALUATION
Although completely reversible dementia (eg, drug toxicity) is rare, identifying and treating secondary physical conditions may improve function.

• Hx: Obtain from family or other caregiver
• Physical and neurologic examination
• Assess functional status
• Evaluate mental status for attention, immediate and delayed recall, remote memory, executive function, and depression. Screening tests may include Mini-Cog (p 215), number of animals named in 1 min, MMSE, PHQ-9 (p 217), GDS (p 219)

Laboratory Testing
CBC, TSH, B_{12}, folate, serum calcium, liver and kidney function tests, electrolytes, serologic test for syphilis (selectively); at this time genetic testing and commercial "Alzheimer blood tests" are not recommended for clinical use.

Neuroimaging
The likelihood of detecting structural lesions is increased with:
• Onset age <60 yr
• Focal (unexplained) neurologic signs or symptoms
• Abrupt onset or rapid decline (weeks to months)
• Predisposing conditions (eg, metastatic cancer or anticoagulants)
Neuroimaging may detect the 5% of patients with clinically significant structural lesions that would otherwise be missed.
FDG-PET scans approved by Medicare for atypical presentation or course of AD in which frontal temporal dementia diagnosis is suspected. See www.petscaninfo.com/portals/pat/medicare_guidelines_alzheimers.

TREATMENT
Primary goals of treatment are to improve quality of life and maximize functional performance by enhancing cognition, mood, and behavior.

General Treatment Principles
• Identify and treat comorbid physical illnesses (eg, HTN, diabetes mellitus)
• Avoid anticholinergic medications, eg, benztropine, diphenhydramine, hydroxyzine, oxybutynin, TCAs, clozapine, thioridazine
• Set realistic goals
• Limit prn psychotropic medication use
• Specify and quantify target behaviors
• Maximize and maintain functioning

Nonpharmacologic Approaches
To improve function:
• Behavior modification, scheduled toileting, and prompted toileting (see p 90) for UI
• Graded assistance (as little help as possible to perform ADLs), practice, and positive reinforcement to increase independence
For problem behaviors:
• Music during meals, bathing
• Walking or light exercise
• Simulate family presence with video or audio tapes
• Pet therapy
• Speak at patient's comprehension level
• Bright light, "white" noise (ie, low-level, background noise)

Pharmacologic Treatment of Cognitive Dysfunction
• Patients with a diagnosis of mild or moderate AD should receive a cholinesterase inhibitor that will increase level of acetylcholine in brain (**Table 26**).

- ○ Controlled data show modest symptomatic benefit for cognition, mood, behavioral symptoms, and daily function of cholinergic drugs compared with placebo for 1 yr, and open trials demonstrate benefit for 3 yr.
- ○ Only 10%–25% of patients taking cholinesterase inhibitors show clinical improvement, but 80% have less rapid decline.
- ○ Initial studies show benefits of these drugs for patients with dementia associated with Parkinson's disease, Lewy body dementia, and vascular dementia.
- ○ Cholinesterase inhibitors have not been convincingly demonstrated to slow progression of mild cognitive impairment to dementia.
- ○ Cholinesterase inhibitors may attenuate noncognitive symptoms and delay nursing-home placement.
- ○ To evaluate response:
  - ▪ Elicit caregiver observations of patient's behavior (alertness, initiative) and follow functional status (ADLs [p 215] and IADLs [p 216]).
  - ▪ Follow cognitive status (eg, improved or stabilized) by caregiver's report or serial ratings of cognition (eg, Mini-Cog, see p 215; MMSE).
- Memantine (*Namenda*) demonstrated modest efficacy compared with placebo in moderate to severe AD as monotherapy and when combined with donepezil (*Aricept*).
- Vitamin E at 1000 IU bid found to delay functional decline in AD (caution in those with cardiovascular disease because ≥400 IU may increase mortality).
- *Ginkgo biloba* is not generally recommended because clinical trial results are not yet definitive, and preparations vary because such nutriceuticals are not regulated by the FDA (see **Table 8**).
- Postmenopausal hormone therapy in older women may increase risk of developing AD.

Table 26. Cognitive Enhancers

Drug	Formulations	Dosing (Metabolism)
Donepezil (*Aricept*)*	T: 5, 10; ODT: 5, 10;** S: 5 mg/mL	Start at 5 mg qd, increase to 10 mg qd after 1 mo (CYP2D6, 3A4) (L)
Galantamine (*Razadyne* [formerly *Reminyl*])***	T: 4, 8, 12; S: 4 mg/mL	Start at 4 mg bid, increase to 8 mg bid after 4 wk; recommended dosage 8 or 12 mg bid (CYP2D6, 3A4) (L)
Extended release (*Razadyne ER*)	C: 8, 16, 24	Start at 1 capsule daily, preferably with food; titrate as above
Rivastigmine (*Exelon*)*	T: 1.5, 3, 4.5, 6	Start at 1.5 mg bid and gradually titrate up to 6 mg bid as tolerated; retitrate if drug is stopped (K)
Memantine (*Namenda* [NMDA antagonist])	T: 5, 10	Start at 5 mg qd, increase by 5 mg at weekly intervals to max of 10 mg bid; reduce dose if kidney function impaired (K)

* Cholinesterase inhibitors. Continue if improvement or stabilization occurs; stopping drugs can lead to rapid decline. Adverse events increase with higher dosing. Possible adverse events include nausea, vomiting, diarrhea, dyspepsia, anorexia, weight loss, leg cramps, bradycardia, insomnia, and agitation.

** ODT = oral disintegrating tablet.

*** Increased mortality found in controlled studies of mild cognitive impairment.

Treatment of Agitation

First, identify and examine context of behavior (is it harmful to patient or others), environmental triggers (eg, overstimulation, unfamiliar surroundings, frustrating interactions); exclude underlying physical discomfort (eg, illnesses or medication); consider nonpharmacologic strategies (see p 47). See also **Table 78**, Antipsychotic Medications.

Table 27. Agitation Treatment Guidelines

Symptom	Drug	Dosage	Formulations
Agitation in context of nonacute psychosis	Risperidone* (*Risperdal*)	0.25–1.5 mg/d	T: 0.25, 0.5, 1, 2, 3, 4; S: 1 mg/mL
	Olanzapine* (*Zyprexa*) (*Zydis*)	2.5–10 mg/d	T: 2.5, 5, 7.5, 10, 15, 20 T: oral disintegrating 5, 10, 15, 20
	Quetiapine* (*Seroquel*)	25–400 mg/d	T: 25, 100, 200, 300
	Aripiprazole* (*Abilify*)	5–10 mg/d	T: 5, 10, 15, 20, 30
Acute psychosis agitation if IM or IV is needed	Haloperidol* (*Haldol*)	0.5–2 mg/d**	T: 0.5, 1, 2, 5, 10, 20; S: 2 mg/mL; Inj
Agitation in context of depression	SSRI, eg, citalopram (*Celexa*)	10–30 mg/d	T: 20, 40; S: 2 mg/mL
Anxiety, mild to moderate irritability	Trazodone (*Desyrel*) Buspirone (*BuSpar*)	50–100 mg/d† 30–60 mg/d‡	T: 50, 100, 150, 300 T: 5, 7.5, 10, 15, 30
As a possible second-line treatment for significant agitation or aggression	Divalproex sodium (*Depakote, Epival*)	500–1500 mg/d§	T: 125, 250, 500; S: syr 250 mg/mL; sprinkle capsule: 125
	Carbamazepine (*Tegretol*)	300–600 mg/d§§	T: 200; ChT: 100; S: sus 100/5 mL
	Olanzapine (*Zyprexa IntraMuscular*)	2.5–5 mg IM	Inj
Sexual aggression, impulse-control symptoms in men	Atypical antipsychotic or divalproex	See dosages above	
	If no response, estrogen (*Premarin*) or	0.625–1.25 mg/d	T: 0.3, 0.625, 0.9, 1.25, 2.5
	medroxyprogesterone (*Depo-Provera*)	100 mg IM/wk	Inj

* Increased risk of mortality and cerebrovascular events compared with placebo; use with particular caution in patients with cerebrovascular disease or hypovolemia.

** May need to give higher dosages in emergency situations; should be used for only short periods of time.

† Small divided daytime dosage and larger bedtime dosage; watch for sedation and orthostasis.

‡ Can be given bid; allow 2–4 wk for adequate trial.

§ Can monitor serum levels; usually well tolerated; check CBC, platelets for agranulocytosis, thrombocytopenia risk in older adults.

§§ Monitor serum levels; periodic CBCs, platelet counts secondary to agranulocytosis risk. Beware of drug-drug interactions.

CAREGIVER ISSUES
• Over 50% develop depression.
• Physical illness, isolation, anxiety, and burnout are common.
• Intensive education and support of caregivers may delay institutionalization.
• Adult day care for patients and respite services may help.
• Alzheimer's Association offers support, education; chapters are located in major cities throughout US (see p 240 for telephone, Web site).
• Family Caregiver Alliance offers support, education, information for caregivers (see p 240 for telephone, Web site).

ADDITIONAL REFERENCES
Doody RS, Stevens JC, Beck C, et al. Practice parameter: management of dementia (an evidence-based review): report of the Quality Standards Subcommittee of the American Academy of Neurology. *Neurology* 2001; 56(9):1154–1166.

Palmer K, Fratiglioni L, Winblad B. What is mild cognitive impairment? Variations in definitions and evolution of nondemented persons with cognitive impairment. *Acta Neuro Scand.* 2003;107(Suppl 179):14–20.

DEPRESSION

EVALUATION AND ASSESSMENT

Recognizing and diagnosing late-life depression can be difficult. Older adults may complain of lack of energy or other somatic symptoms, attribute symptoms to old age or other physical conditions, or neglect to mention them to a health care professional. Consider evaluation and follow-up with structured self-assessment scale such as PHQ-9 (see p 217).

Medical Evaluation

TSH, B_{12}, calcium, LFTs, kidney function tests, electrolytes, UA, CBC

DSM-IV Criteria for Major Depressive Episode (Abbreviated)

Five or more of the following symptoms have been present during the same 2-wk period and represent a change from previous functioning; at least one of the symptoms is either (1) depressed mood or (2) loss of interest or pleasure.

- Depressed mood
- Loss of interest or pleasure in activities
- Significant weight loss or gain (not intentional), or decrease or increase in appetite
- Insomnia or hypersomnia
- Psychomotor agitation or retardation
- Fatigue or loss of energy
- Feelings of worthlessness or excessive or inappropriate guilt
- Diminished ability to think or concentrate, or indecisiveness
- Recurrent thoughts of death; suicidal ideation, attempt, or plan

The *DSM-IV* criteria are not specific for older adults; cognitive symptoms may be more prominent. The GDS, PHQ-9, and other instruments are useful for screening and monitoring (see p 217, 219).

MANAGEMENT

Treatment should be individualized on the basis of hx, past response, and severity of illness as well as concurrent illnesses. Treatments may be combined.

Nonpharmacologic

For mild to moderate depression or in combination with pharmacotherapy: cognitive-behavioral therapy, interpersonal therapy, problem-solving therapy.
For severe or psychotic depression, consider ECT (see p 53).

Pharmacologic

For mild, moderate, or severe depression: the duration of therapy should be at least 6–12 mo after remission for patients experiencing their first depressive episode. Most older adults with major depression require maintenance antidepressant therapy.

Choosing an Antidepressant (see Table 28 and list on p 53)

First-line Therapy: Consider an SSRI for most older adults, especially those with:
- Heart conduction defects or ischemic heart disease
- Prostatic hyperplasia
- Uncontrolled glaucoma

Second-line Therapy: Consider venlafaxine, mirtazapine, or bupropion.
Third-line Therapy: Consider nortriptyline or desipramine for patients with severe melancholic depression.

Table 28. Antidepressants Used for Older Adults

Class, Drug	Initial Dosage	Usual Dosage	Formulations	Comments (Metabolism, Excretion)
Selective Serotonin-Reuptake Inhibitors				Class adverse events (EPS, hyponatremia) (L, K [10%])
Citalopram (*Celexa*)	10–20 mg qam	20–30 mg/d	T: 20, 40, 60; S: 5 mg/10 mL	
Escitalopram (*Lexapro*)	10 mg/d	10 mg/d	T: 10, 20	
Fluoxetine (*Prozac*)	5 mg qam	5–60 mg/d	T: 10; C: 10, 20, 40; S: 20 mg/5 mL; C: SR 90 (weekly dose)	Long half-lives of parent and active metabolite may allow for less frequent dosing; may cause more insomnia than other SSRIs; CYP2D6, -2C9, -3A4 inhibitor (L)
Fluvoxamine (*Luvox*)	25 mg qhs	100–300 mg/d	T: 25, 50, 100	Not approved as an antidepressant in US; CYP1A2, -3A4 inhibitor (L)
Paroxetine (*Paxil*)	5 mg	10–40 mg/d	T: 10, 20, 30, 40	Helpful if anxiety symptoms are prominent; increased risk of withdrawal symptoms (dizziness); CYP2D6 inhibitor (L)
(*Paxil CR*)	12.5 mg/d	—	T: ER 12.5, 25, 37.5; S: 10 mg/5 mL	Increase by 12.5 mg/d no faster than 1/wk (L)
Sertraline (*Zoloft*)	25 mg qam	50–200 mg/d	T: 25, 50, 100; S: 20 mg/mL	(L)
Additional Medications				
Bupropion (*Wellbutrin, Zyban*)	37.5–50 mg bid 100 mg (SR) qd or bid	75–150 mg bid 100–150 mg (SR) bid	T: 75, 100, SR 100, 150	Consider for SSRI, TCA nonresponders; safe in HF; may be stimulating; can lower seizure threshold (L)
Duloxetine (*Cymbalta*)	20 mg qd	20–30 mg bid	C: 20, 30, 60	Most common side effects: nausea, dry mouth, constipation, diarrhea, urinary hesitancy (L)
Methylphenidate (*Ritalin*)	2.5–5 mg at 7 AM and noon	5–10 mg at 7 AM and noon	T: 5, 10, 20	Short-term treatment of depression or apathy in physically ill older adults; used as an adjunct (L)
Mirtazapine (*Remeron*)	15 mg qhs	15–45 mg/d	T: 15, 30, 45	May increase appetite; sedating; oral disintegrating tab (SolTab) available (L)
Trazodone (*Desyrel*)	25 mg qhs	75–600 mg/d	T: 50, 100, 150, 300	Sedation may limit dose; may be used as a hypnotic; ventricular irritability; priapism in men (L)

(cont.)

Table 28. **Antidepressants Used for Older Adults** (cont.)

Class, Drug	Initial Dosage	Usual Dosage	Formulations	Comments (Metabolism, Excretion)
Venlafaxine (*Effexor*)	25–50 mg bid	75–225 mg/d	T: 25, 37.5, 50, 75, 100	Low anticholinergic activity; minimal sedation and hypotension; may increase BP and QT_c; may be useful when somatic pain present; EPS, withdrawal symptoms, hyponatremia (L)
(*Effexor XR*)	75 mg qam	75–225 mg/d	C: 37.5, 75, 150	Same as above
Tricyclic Antidepressants				
Desipramine (*Norpramin*)	10–25 mg qhs	50–150 mg/d	T: 10, 25, 50, 75, 100, 150	Therapeutic serum level >115 ng/mL (L)
Nortriptyline (*Aventyl, Pamelor*)	10–25 mg qhs	75–150 mg/d	C: 10, 25, 50, 75; S: 10 mg/5 mL	Therapeutic window (50–150 ng/mL) (L)
Monoamine Oxidase Inhibitors				Hypotension; drug, food interactions (K, L)
Isocarboxazid (*Marplan*)	10 mg bid–tid	10 mg tid	T: 10	
Phenelzine (*Nardil*)	15 mg qd	15–60 mg/d	T: 15	
Tranylcypromine (*Parnate*)	10 mg bid	20–40 mg/d	T: 10	

Antidepressants to Avoid in Older Adults

- Amitriptyline (eg, *Elavil*): anticholinergic, sedating, hypotensive
- Amoxapine (*Asendin*): anticholinergic, sedating, hypotensive; also associated with EPS, tardive dyskinesia, and neuroleptic malignant syndrome
- Doxepin (eg, *Sinequan*): anticholinergic, sedating, hypotensive
- Imipramine (*Tofranil*): anticholinergic, sedating, hypotensive
- Maprotiline (*Ludiomil*): seizures, rashes
- Protriptyline (*Vivactil*): very anticholinergic; can be stimulating
- St. John's wort: decreases effects of digoxin and CYP3A4 substrates; efficacy questioned
- Trimipramine (*Surmontil*): anticholinergic, sedating, hypotensive

Electroconvulsive Therapy (ECT)

Generally safe and very effective. Potential complications include temporary confusion, arrhythmias, aspiration, falls.

Indications: Severe depression when a rapid onset of response is necessary; when depression is resistant to drug therapy; for patients who are unable to tolerate antidepressants, have previous response to ECT, have psychotic depression, severe catatonia, or depression with Parkinson's disease.

Evaluation: Before ECT, perform CXR, ECG, serum electrolytes, and cardiac examination. Additional tests (eg, stress test, neuroimaging, EEG) are used selectively.

Contraindications:
- Increased intracranial pressure
- Intracranial tumor
- MI within 3 mo (relative)
- Stroke within 1 mo (relative)

BIPOLAR DISORDER
- 5%–19% of mood disorders in older adults.
- Usually begins in early adulthood, family hx.
- 10% may develop after age 50.
- Distinct period of abnormally and persistently elevated, expansive, or irritable mood for longer than 1 wk.
- Symptoms may include racing thoughts, pressured speech, decreased need for sleep, distractibility, grandiose delusions.
- A single manic episode is sufficient for a diagnosis if secondary causes are excluded.
- Late-onset mania may be secondary to head trauma, stroke, delirium, other neurologic disorders, alcohol abuse, or medications (eg, corticosteroids, L-dopa, thyroxine).
- Use aripiprazole, olanzapine, quetiapine, risperidone, or ziprasidone for acute mania (see **Table 78**) and D/C antidepressants if taking.
- Initiate long-term treatment (**Table 29**) as soon as patient is able to comply with oral therapy.

Table 29. Long-term Treatment of Bipolar Disorders*

Drug	Initial Dosage	Usual Dosage	Formulation	Comments
Lithium (*Eskalith, Eskalith CR, Lithobid*)	150 mg/d	300–900 mg/d Levels 0.4–0.8 mEq/L	C, T, XR	Risk of CNS toxicity; cognitive impairment; hypothyroidism; interactions with diuretics, ACE inhibitors, calcium channel blockers, NSAIDs
Carbamazepine (*Tegretol, Tegretol XR*)	100 mg bid	800–1200 mg/d Levels 4–12 mcg/L	T	Many drug interactions; may cause SIADH; risk of leukopenia, neutropenia, agranulocytosis, thrombocytopenia; monitor CBC; drowsiness, dizziness
Valproic acid (*Depacon, Depakene, Depakote*)	125 mg bid	750 mg/d divided doses Levels 50–125 mcg/L	T	Can cause weight gain, tremor, several drug interactions; risk of hepatotoxicity, pancreatitis, neutropenia, thrombocytopenia; monitor LFTs and platelets
Lamotrigine (*Lamictal*)	25 mg/d	100–200 mg/d	T	D/C if rash; interaction with valproate (when used together, begin at 25 mg qod, titrate to 25–100 mg bid); prolongs PR interval; somnolence, headache common

* Limited evidence base in older adults. See www.dshs.state.tx.us/mhprograms/TIMABDman.pdf. (See also **Table 63**.)

DERMATOLOGIC CONDITIONS

COMMON DERMATOLOGIC CONDITIONS

Table 30. Dermatologic Conditions Common in Older Adults

Condition	Areas Affected	Description
Candidiasis	Body folds	Erythema, pustules, or cheesy, whitish matter, satellite lesions

Treatment: See intertrigo, next; antifungal powders, p 57.

Intertrigo	Any place two skin surfaces rest against one another (eg, under the breasts)	Moist, erythematous with local superficial skin loss; satellite lesions due to *Candida*

Treatment: Keep area dry; topical antifungals, absorbent pwd, 1% hydrocortisone or 0.1% triamcinolone crm bid × 1 or 2 d if inflamed.

Neurodermatitis	Any skin surface	Generalized, localized itching

Treatment: Mid- to higher-potency topical corticosteroids (**Table 33**); exclude other causes.

Onychomycosis	Nails (*Tinea unguium*)	Thickening and discoloration

Treatment: Itraconazole (*Sporanox*), contraindicated in HF—Toenails: 200 mg po qd × 3 mo, or 200 mg po bid × 1 wk/mo × 3 mo, or pulse 400 mg/d × 7 d of each of 4 mo; Fingernails: 200 mg po bid × 1 wk/mo × 2 mo (L); fluconazole (*Diflucan*)—Toenails: 150 or 300 mg po/wk × 6–12 mo; Fingernails: 150 or 300 mg po/wk × 3–6 mo (L); terbinafine (*Lamisil*), avoid if CrCl <50 mL/min—Toenails: 250 mg po qd × 12 wk; Fingernails: 250 mg qd × 6 wk. Obtain nail specimens for laboratory culturing to confirm diagnosis before prescribing itraconazole or terbinafine.

Psoriasis	All skin areas, nails (pitting)	Well-defined, erythematous plaques covered with silver scales; severity varies

Treatment: Topical corticosteroids, UV light, PUVA, methotrexate, cyclosporine, etretinate, sulfasalazine; anthralin preparations and tar + 1%–4% salicylic acid; calcipotriene for nonfacial areas.

Rosacea	Face (nose, chin, cheeks, forehead); ocular (dryness, blepharitis, conjunctivitis)	Vascular and follicular dilation; mild to moderate; may accompany seborrhea

Treatment: Avoid triggers (stress, prolonged sun exposure and exercise, hot and humid environment, alcohol, hot drinks, spicy foods). Wear sun screen (SPF ≥15) or sunblock with titanium and zinc oxide. See www.rosacea.org or www.aad.org.

Topical: Azelaic acid 15% gel bid (*Finacea*) or 20% crm bid (*Azelex, Finevin*); metronidazole 0.75% crm or gel bid (*MetroCream, MetroGel*) or 1% crm qd (*Noritate*); sodium sulfacetamide 10% + sulfa 5% qd (*Rosula* aqueous gel, *Clenia* crm, foaming wash), avoid if sulfa allergy or kidney disease (K); erythromycin 2% sol bid; tretinoin 0.025% crm or liq, 0.01% gel qhs.

Oral: Tetracycline 500 mg bid–tid × 6–12 wk, doxycycline 50–100 mg qd–bid × 6–12 wk, minocycline 50–100 mg bid × 6–12 wk, clarithromycin 250–500 mg bid × 6–12 wk, metronidazole 200 mg qd–bid × 4–6 wk, erythromycin 250–500 mg qd–bid × 6–12 wk.

Scabies	Interdigital webs, flexor aspects of wrists, axillae, umbilicus, nipples, genitals	Burrows, erythematous papules or rash, dry or scaly skin, pruritus (worse at night); spread by close, skin-to-skin or sexual contact

Treatment: Infestation can result in epidemics; treat all contacts and treat environment. Apply topical products from head to toe: Permethrin (*Elimite*) 5% crm, wash off after 8–14 h repeat in 7–10 d if symptomatic or if live mites were found; 1% lindane (*K-well, Scabene*) crm, wash off after 8–12 h; crotamiton (*Eurax*) 10% crm, less effective, leave on 48 h, repeat in 7–10 d if necessary; oatmeal baths, topical corticosteroids, or emollient creams for symptom relief; ivermectin (*Stromectol*) 200 mcg/kg po, may repeat once in 1 or 2 wk [T: 3, 6].

(cont.)

Table 30. Dermatologic Conditions Common in Older Adults (cont.)

Condition	Areas Affected	Description
Seborrheic dermatitis	Nasal labial folds, eyebrows, hairline, sideburns, posterior auriculare and midchest	Greasy, yellow scales with or without erythematous base; common in Parkinson's disease and in debilitated patients

Treatment: Hydrocortisone 1% crm bid or triamcinolone 0.1% oint bid × 2 wk; scalp: shp (selenium sulfide, zinc, or tar); ketoconazole 2% crm for severe conditions when *Pityrosporum orbiculare* infection is suspected.

Condition	Areas Affected	Description
Skin maceration	Any area constantly in contact with moisture, covered with occlusive dressing or bandage; skin folds, groin, buttocks	Erythema; abraded, excoriated skin; blisters; white and silver patches

Treatment: Eliminate cause of moisture: toileting program for incontinence; condom catheter; indwelling catheter (reserve for most intractable conditions); fecal incontinence collector. Protect skin from moisture: clean gently with mild soap after each incontinent episode; apply moisture barrier (eg, *Vaseline, Proshield, Smooth and Cool, Calmoseptine*) to repel moisture; use disposable briefs that wick moisture from the skin; use linen incontinence pads when disposable briefs accentuate perineal dermatitis.

Condition	Areas Affected	Description
Urticaria		
Hives	Skin surface	Uniform, red edematous plaques surrounded by white halos

Treatment: Identify cause, oral H$_1$ antihistamines (see **Table 81**), oral glucocorticoids (eg, prednisone 40 mg qd), oral H$_2$ antihistamines, or doxepin (po or topical *Zonalon 5%*) for refractory cases.

Angioedema	Lips, eyelids, tongue, larynx, GI tract	Larger, deeper than hives

Treatment: Oral H$_1$ antihistamines (see **Table 81**), oral glucocorticoids. Severe reactions: SC epinephrine 0.3 mL of a 1:1000 dilution (*EpiPen*).

Cholinergic	Skin surface	Round, red papular wheals

Treatment: Oral H$_1$ antihistamines (see **Table 81**) 1 h before exercise. Hot shower may relieve itching.

Xerosis	All skin surfaces	Dull, rough, flaky, cracked; nummular

Treatment: ↑ Humidity, apply emollient oint (eg, *Aquaphor*) or crm (eg, *Eucerin*) immediately after bathing; oatmeal baths; hydrocortisone 1% oint; avoid excess bathing and use of bath oils, which can lead to falls from slippery feet.

Table 31. Skin and Soft-tissue Infections

Condition	Areas Affected	Description
Erysipelas	Lower dermis and subcutaneous tissue, face and legs	Bright red, edematous, tender; unilateral distribution; orange peel appearance; well-demarcated border with vesicles and bullae

Treatment: Penicillin; erythromycin or cephalosporin if penicillin allergy.

Condition	Areas Affected	Description
Cellulitis	Lower dermis and subcutaneous soft tissue, commonly on the legs	Ill-defined erythema, pain, blisters and exudates; group A streptococci and *Staphylococcus aureus* most frequent

Treatment: Antistaphylococcal penicillin, amoxicillin-clavulanate × 10 d; macrolide (eg, erythromycin), 1st-generation cephalosporin (eg, cephalexin), or tetracycline if penicillin allergy.

(cont.)

Table 31. Skin and Soft-tissue Infections (cont.)		
Condition	**Areas Affected**	**Description**
Impetigo	Face around the nose and mouth	Very contagious; nonbullous and bullous variant; honey-colored crusts
Treatment: Small, localized lesions; topical mupirocin 2% (*Bactroban*) × 7–10 d; widespread: oral antistaphylococcal penicillin, erythromycin, or a cephalosporin × 10 d.		
Folliculitis	Areas with coarse, short hair, ie, neck, beard, buttocks, thighs	Multiple small erythematous papules and pustules surrounding a hair
Treatment: Mild localized cases can be treated with topical antibiotic: mupirocin 2%, erythromycin, or clindamycin; extensive or severe cases: oral antistaphylococcal penicillin, amoxicillin-clavulanate, or erythromycin.		

DERMATOLOGIC MEDICATIONS

Table 32. Antifungal Medications			
Agent	**Formulation**	**Dermatologic Indications**	**Dosing Frequency**
Topical Antifungals			
Amphotericin B (*Fungizone*)	3% crm, lot, oint	Candidiasis	2–4 times/d
Ciclopirox (*Loprox, Penlac*)	0.77% crm, gel, lot, sus; 1% shp; 8% lacquer	*Tinea pedis, T cruris, T corpis, T versicolor;* candidiasis; scalp seborrhea; onychomycosis	2 times/d; shp 3 times/wk; lacquer qhs
Clotrimazole* (*Cruex, Mycelex,* others)	1% crm, sol	Candidiasis, dermatophytoses; superficial mycoses	2 times/d
Econazole nitrate (*Spectazole*)	1% crm		
Ketoconazole (*Nizoral, Nizoral A-D**)	2% crm, 1% shp	Candidiasis; *Tinea cruris, T corpis, T versicolor*	1 or 2 times/d; shp 2 times/wk
Miconazole* (eg, *Micatin, Monistat-Derm*)	2% crm, lot, pwd, spr, tinc	*Tinea cruris, T corpis, T pedis*	2 times/d
Naftifine (*Naftin*)	1% crm, gel	*Tinea cruris, T corpis, T pedis*	2 times/d
Nystatin (*Mycostatin, Nilstat, Nystex*)	100,000 units/g crm, oint, pwd	Mucocutaneous candidiasis	2–3 times/d
Terbinafine (*Lamisil, LamisilAT**)	1% crm, sol	*Tinea cruris, T corpis, T pedis, T versicolor*	2 times/d
Tolnaftate* (*Absorbine Jr. Antifungal, Tinactin,* others)	1% crm, gel, S, pwd, spr	*Tinea cruris, T corpis, T pedis*	2 times/d

(cont.)

Table 32. Antifungal Medications (cont.)

Agent	Formulation	Dermatologic Indications	Dosing Frequency
Oral Antifungals			
Fluconazole (*Diflucan*)	T: 50, 100, 150, 200 S: 10, 40 mg/mL		
Itraconazole (*Sporonax*)	C: 100 S: 100 mg/mL		
Ketoconazole (*Nizoral*)	T: 200		
Terbinafine (*Lamisil*)	T: 250		

*OTC

Table 33. Topical Corticosteroids

Name	Strength and Formulations	Frequency of Application
Lowest Potency		
Dexamethasone phosphate (*Decadern*)	0.1% crm	qd–qid
Hydrocortisone acetate (*Hytone*)	0.25%, 0.5%, 1%, 2.5% crm, oint	tid–qid
Low Potency		
Alclometasone dipropionate (*Aclovate*)	0.05% crm, oint	bid–tid
Betamethasone valerate (*Valisone*)	0.1% lot	bid–qid
Desonide (*DesOwen, Tridesilon*)	0.05% crm, lot, oint	bid–qid
Fluocinolone acetonide (*Synalar*)	0.01% crm, sol	bid–qid
Triamcinolone acetonide (*Aristocort, Kenalog*)	0.1% crm, 0.025% crm, lot, oint	bid–tid
Mid-potency		
Betamethasone dipropionate (*Diprosone*)	0.05% lot	bid–qid
Betamethasone valerate (*Valisone*)	0.1% crm	bid–qid
Clocortolone pivalate (*Cloderm*)	0.1% crm	qd–qid
Desoximetasone (*Topicort*)	0.05% crm	bid
Fluocinolone acetonide (*Synalar*)	0.025% crm, oint	bid–qid
Flurandrenolide (*Cordran*)	0.05% crm, oint, lot	qd–bid
Fluticasone propionate (*Cutivate*)	0.05% crm	bid
Hydrocortisone butyrate (*Locoid*)	0.1% crm	qd–bid
Hydrocortisone valerate (*Westcort*)	0.2% crm, oint	tid–qid
Mometasone furoate (*Elocon*)	0.1% crm, lot	qd
Prednicarbate (*Dermatop*)	0.1% crm, lot	bid
Triamcinolone acetonide (*Aristocort, Kenalog*)	0.1% lot, oint	bid–tid

(cont.)

Table 33. **Topical Corticosteroids (cont.)**

Name	Strength and Formulations	Frequency of Application
High Potency		
Amcinonide (*Cyclocort*)	0.1% crm, lot	bid–tid
Betamethasone dipropionate (*Diprosone*)	0.05% crm	bid–qid
Betamethasone valerate (*Valisone*)	0.1% oint	bid–qid
Diflorasone diacetate (*Florone, Maxiflor*)	0.05% crm	bid–qid
Fluocinonide (*Lidex-E*)	0.05% crm	bid–qid
Triamcinolone acetonide (*Aristocort, Kenalog*)	0.5% crm, oint	bid–tid
Higher Potency		
Amcinonide (*Cyclocort*)	0.1% oint	bid–tid
Betamethasone dipropionate (*Diprolene AF*)	0.05% augmented crm	bid–qid
Betamethasone dipropionate (*Diprosone*)	0.05% oint	bid–qid
Desoximetasone (*Topicort*)	0.25% crm, oint; 0.05% gel	bid
Diflorasone diacetate (*Florone, Maxiflor*)	0.05% oint	bid–qid
Fluocinonide (*Lidex*)	0.05% crm, oint, gel	bid–qid
Halcinonide (*Halog*)	0.1% crm, oint, sol	qd–tid
Mometasone furoate (*Elocon*)	0.1% oint	qd
Super Potency		
Betamethasone dipropionate (*Diprolene*)	0.05% oint	bid–qid
Clobetasol propionate (*Temovate*)	0.05% crm, oint, sol, gel	bid
Diflorasone diacetate (*Psorcon*)	0.05% optimized oint	qd–tid
Halobetasol propionate (*Ultravate*)	0.05% crm, oint	bid

ADRENAL INSUFFICIENCY

Common Causes
- Chronic glucocorticoid administration
- Pituitary tumors
- Tuberculosis
- Autoimmune

Evaluation
- Basal plasma cortisol >15 mcg/dL excludes adrenal insufficiency.
- ACTH stimulation test: tetracosactin (*Synacthen Depot*) 250 mcg IM or IV; peak value >19 mcg/dL is normal.

Pharmacologic Therapy
For corticosteroid dose equivalencies, see **Table 34**.

Management
Stress doses of corticosteroids for patients with severe illness, injury, or undergoing surgery: In emergency situations, do not wait for test results. Give hydrocortisone 100 mg IV q 8 h. For less severe stress, double or triple usual oral replacement dose and taper back to baseline as quickly as possible.

Table 34. Corticosteroids

Drug	Approx Equivalent Dose (mg)	Relative Anti-Inflammatory Potency	Relative Mineralo-corticoid Potency	Biologic Half-life (h)	Formulations
Betamethasone (*Celestone*)	0.6–0.75	20–30	0	36–54	T: 0.6; S: 0.6 mg/5 mL
Cortisone (*Cortone*)	25	0.8	2	8–12	T: 5; S: 50 mg/mL
Dexamethasone (*Decadron, Dexone, Hexadrol*)	0.75	20–30	0	36–54	T: 0.25, 0.5, 0.75, 1, 1.5, 2, 4; S: elixir 0.5 mg/5 mL; Inj
Fludrocortisone (*Florinef*)*	NA	10	4	12–36	T: 0.1
Hydrocortisone (*Cortef, Hydrocortone*)	20	1	2	8–12	T: 5, 10, 20; S: 10 mg/5 mL; Inj
Methylprednisolone (eg, *Medrol, Solu-Medrol, Depo-Medrol*)	4	5	0	18–36	T: 2, 4, 8, 16, 24, 32; Inj
Prednisolone (eg, *Delta-Cortef, Prelone Syrup, Pediapred*)	5	4	1	18–36	S: 5 mg/5 mL; syr 5, 15 mg/5 mL
Prednisone (*Deltasone, Liquid Pred, Meticorten, Orasone*)	5	4	1	18–36	T: 1, 2.5, 5, 10, 20, 50; S: 5 mg/5 mL
Triamcinolone (eg, *Aristocort, Kenacort, Kenalog*)	4	5	0	18–36	T: 1, 2, 4, 8; S: syr 4 mg/5 mL

Note: NA = not available.
* Usually given for orthostatic hypotension at 0.1 mg qd–tid.

HYPOTHYROIDISM
Common Causes
- Autoimmune (primary thyroid failure)
- Following therapy for hyperthyroidism
- Pituitary or hypothalmic disorders (secondary thyroid failure)
- Medications, especially amiodarone (rare after first 18 mo of therapy) and lithium

Evaluation
TSH, free T_4

Pharmacologic Therapy
- Thyroxine (T_4, levothyroxine [*Eltroxin, Levo-T, Levothroid, Levoxyl, Synthroid*]). Start at 25 mcg and increase by 25-mcg intervals q 3–6 wk [T: 25, 50, 75, 88, 100, 112, 125, 137, 150, 175, 200, 300 mcg].
- Thyroxine and liothyronine (T_3) (*Thyrolar*). Start ¼ strength and increase [T: 12.5/3.1 (¼ strength), 25/6.25 (½ strength), 50/12.5, 100/25, 150/37.5 mcg].
- For myxedema coma: Load 400 mcg IV or 100 mcg q 6–8 h for 1 d, then 100 mcg/d for 4 d; then start usual replacement regimen.
- To convert thyroid USP to thyroxine: 60 mg USP = 50 mcg thyroxine.
- If patients are npo and must receive IV thyroxine, dose should be half usual po dose.

Monitoring
In primary hypothyroidism, the goal of therapy is to maintain plasma TSH within the normal range. Further adjustments are made q 3–6 wk (12- to 25-mcg increments) on basis of TSH levels until TSH is in normal range. Monitor TSH level at least q 12 mo (ATA) in patients on chronic thyroid replacement therapy. After dose adjustment, recheck TSH in 3–6 wk.

HYPERTHYROIDISM
Common Causes
- Graves' disease
- Toxic nodule
- Toxic multinodular goiter
- Medications, especially amiodarone (can occur any time during therapy) and lithium

Evaluation
TSH, free T_4; when indicated, T_3, thyroid autoantibodies, radioactive iodine uptake.

Pharmacologic Therapy
- Radioactive iodine ablation is usual treatment of choice, but surgery or medical therapy (see Monitoring above) are options.
- Propylthiouracil (PTU): Start 100 po tid, then adjust up to 200 po tid as needed [T: 50].
- Methimazole (*Tapazole*): Start 5–20 mg po tid, then adjust [T: 5, 10].
- Adjunctive therapy with β-blockers (see **Table 20**) or calcium antagonists (see **Table 20**) may improve symptoms.

METABOLIC SYNDROME
Definition (Adult Treatment Panel III)
Increased risk of CAD, PAD, and type 2 diabetes
Presence of 3 or more of the following:
- Central obesity as measured by waist circumference: men >40 inches, women >35 inches
- Fasting blood triglycerides ≥150 mg/dL
- Blood HDL cholesterol: men <40 mg/dL, women <50 mg/dL
- BP ≥130/85 mm Hg
- Fasting glucose ≥110 mg/dL

Management
- Weight loss if overweight
- Exercise
- Monitor and treat individual risk factors

DIABETES MELLITUS
Definition and Classification (ADA)
Diabetes mellitus is a group of metabolic diseases characterized by hyperglycemia resulting from defects in insulin secretion, insulin action, or both.
Type 1: Caused by an absolute deficiency of insulin secretion.
Type 2: Caused by a combination of resistance to insulin action and an inadequate compensatory insulin secretory response.
Criteria for Diagnosis: One or more of the following:
- Symptoms of diabetes (eg, polyuria, polydipsia, unexplained weight loss) plus casual plasma glucose concentration ≥200 mg/dL
- Fasting (no caloric intake for ≥8 h) plasma glucose ≥126 mg/dL
- 2 h Plasma glucose ≥200 mg/dL during an OGTT
Diagnosis should be confirmed by reevaluating on a subsequent day.
Pre-diabetes: Either of the following:
- Impaired fasting glucose: Defined as fasting plasma glucose ≥100 and <126 mg/dL
- Impaired glucose tolerance: Abnormal casual plasma glucose concentration or response to OGTT but not meeting diagnostic criteria for diabetes

Management
Prevention/Delay of Type 2 Diabetes in Patients with Impaired Glucose Tolerance
- Weight loss (5%–10%) if overweight
- Exercise (30 min daily)
Evaluate for Comorbid Conditions (AGS, ADA): Depression (see p 51), polypharmacy (see p 9), cognitive impairment (see p 215), urinary incontinence (see p 89), falls (see p 66), pain (see p 148) (AGS), PAD (claudication history and assessment of pedal pulses) (see p 39) (ADA), stress test if ≥2 additional CAD risk factors (see p 24).
Goals of Treatment (ADA, AGS):
- Outpatient: Average preprandial capillary blood glucose 80–120 mg/dL, average bedtime capillary blood glucose 100–140 mg/dL, and HbA_{1c} <7% (ADA) (<8% if frail; life expectancy <5 yr; or high risk of hypoglycemia, polypharmacy, or drug interaction) (AGS).

- Inpatient: ≤110 mg/dL in intensive-care units and preprandial in noncritical-care units; ≤180 mg/dL postprandial in noncritically ill patients.

Nonpharmacologic Interventions:

- Individualized nutrition therapy (see p 118)
- Lifestyle (eg, regular exercise, alcohol and smoking cessation)
- Patient and family education for self-management
- Self-monitoring of blood glucose
- High-fiber diet (25 g insoluble and 25 g soluble/d)

Pharmacologic Interventions for Type 2: Stepped therapy:

1. Monotherapy with a 2nd-generation sulfonylurea agent, metformin, α-glucosidase inhibitor, or thiazolidinedione (see **Table 35**)
2. Combination therapy with 2 or more agents with different actions
3. Add insulin hs or switch to insulin bid (see **Table 36**)
4. Switch insulin to long-acting insulin daily plus meal-time insulin
5. Add pramlintide *(Symlin)*, a synthetic analog of amylin, beginning at 60 mcg SC immediately before meals; side effects include hypoglycemia and nausea

- Manage HTN (BP goal <130/80 mm Hg; also see HTN, p 31).
- Treat lipid disorders (see p 30) as CHD risk equivalent with target LDL <70 mg/dL if other risk factors are present (NHLBI), HDL >40 mg/dL, TG <150 mg/dL, as appropriate. If total cholesterol ≥135 mg/dL and no overt heart disease, statin therapy to reduce LDL by 30%–40% regardless of baseline LDL (ADA) with goal of LDL <100 mg/dL; if overt heart disease, LDL goal of <70 mg/dL, using a high-dose statin, is an option. Statins should be used as primary prevention against macrovascular complications in patients with type 2 diabetes and other cardiovascular risk factors (ACP).
- ACE inhibitor or angiotensin II receptor blocker (ARB) if albuminuria, HTN, or another cardiovascular risk factor. Check kidney function within 1–2 wk of initiation of therapy, with each dose increase, and at least yearly.
- Daily ASA 75–162 mg.

Table 35. **Non-insulin Agents for Treating Diabetes Mellitus**			
Drug	**Dosage**	**Formulations**	**Comments (Metabolism)**
Oral Agents			
2nd-Generation Sulfonylureas			Increase insulin secretion; lower HbA$_{1c}$ by 1.0%–2.0%
Glimepiride *(Amaryl)*	4–8 mg once, begin 1–2 mg	T: 1, 2, 4	Numerous drug interactions, long-acting (L, K)
Glipizide (generic or *Glucotrol)*	2.5–40 mg once or divided	T: 5, 10	Short-acting (L, K)
(Glucotrol XL)	5–20 mg once	T: ER 2.5, 5, 10	Long-acting (L, K)
Glyburide (generic or *DiaBeta, Micronase)*	1.25–20 mg once or divided	T: 1.25, 2.5, 5	Long-acting, risk of hypoglycemia (L, K)
Micronized glyburide *(Glynase)*	1.5–12 mg once	T: 1.5, 3, 4.5, 6	(L, K)

(cont.)

Table 35. **Non-insulin Agents for Treating Diabetes Mellitus** (cont.)

Drug	Dosage	Formulations	Comments (Metabolism)
α-Glucosidase Inhibitors			Delay glucose absorption; lower HbA_{1c} by 0.5%–1.0%
Acarbose (*Precose*)	50–100 mg tid, just before meals, start with 25 mg	T: 25, 50, 100	GI adverse events common, avoid if Cr >2 mg/dL, monitor LFTs (gut, K)
Miglitol (*Glyset*)	25–100 mg tid, with 1st bite of meal; start with 25 mg qd	T: 25, 50, 100	Same as acarbose but no need to monitor LFTs (L, K)
Biguanides			Decrease hepatic glucose production; lower HbA_{1c} by 1.0%–2.0%
Metformin (*Glucophage*)	500–2550 mg divided	T: 500, 850, 1000	Avoid in patients >80 yr, Cr >1.5 in men, Cr >1.4 in women, HF, COPD, ↑ LFTs; hold before contrast radiologic studies; may cause weight loss (K)
(*Glucophage XR*)	1500–2000 mg qd	T: ER 500	
Meglitinides			Increase insulin secretion; lower HbA_{1c} by 1.0%–2.0%
Nateglinide (*Starlix*)	60–120 mg tid	T: 60, 120	Give 30 min before meals
Repaglinide (*Prandin*)	0.5 mg bid–qid if HbA_{1c} <8% or previously untreated; 1–2 mg bid–qid if HbA_{1c} ≥8% or previously treated	T: 0.5, 1, 2	Give 30 min before meals, adjust dose at wkly intervals; potential for drug interactions, caution in hepatic, renal insufficiency (L)
Thiazolidinediones			Insulin resistance reducers; lower HbA_{1c} by 0.5%–1.0%; ↑ risk of HF; avoid if NYHA Class III or IV cardiac status; D/C if any decline in cardiac status
Pioglitazone (*Actos*)	15 or 30 mg qd; max 45 mg/d as monotherapy, 30 mg/d in combination therapy	T: 15, 30, 45	Check LFTs at start, q 2 mo during 1st yr, then periodically; avoid if clinical evidence of liver disease or if serum ALT levels >2.5 times upper limit of normal (L, K)
Rosiglitazone (*Avandia*)	4 mg qd–bid	T: 2, 4, 8	Check LFTs at start, q 2 mo during 1st yr, then periodically; avoid if clinical evidence of liver disease or if serum ALT levels >2.5 times upper limit of normal (L, K)
Combinations			
Glipizide and metformin (*METAGLIP*)	2.5/250 once; 20/2000 in 2 divided doses	T: 2.5/250, 2.5/500, 5/500	Avoid in patients >80 yr, Cr >1.5 in men, Cr >1.4 in women; see individual drugs (L, K)

(cont.)

Table 35. Non-insulin Agents for Treating Diabetes Mellitus (cont.)			
Drug	**Dosage**	**Formulations**	**Comments (Metabolism)**
Glyburide and metformin (*Glucovance*)	1.25/250 mg initially if previously untreated; 2.5/500 mg or 5/500 mg bid with meals; max 20/2000/d	T: 1.25/250, 2.5/500, 5/500	Starting dose should not exceed total daily dose of either drug; see individual drugs (L, K)
Rosiglitazone and metformin (*Avandamet*)	4/1000– 8/2000 in 2 divided doses	T: 1/500, 2/500, 4/500, 2/1000, 4/1000	Avoid in patients >80 yr, Cr >1.5 in men, Cr >1.4 in women; see individual drugs (L, K)
Injectable Agents			
Exenatide (*Byetta*)	5–10 mcg SC bid	1.2-, 2.4-mL pre-filled syringes	Incretin mimetic; lowers HbA$_{1c}$ by 0.4%–0.9%; nausea and hypoglycemia common; less weight gain than insulin; avoid if CrCl <30 mL/min (K)
Pramlintide (*Symlin*)	60 mcg SC immediately before meals	0.6 mg/mL in 5-mL vial	Amylin analog; lowers HbA$_{1c}$ by 0.4%–0.7%; nausea and hypoglycemia common; reduce pre-meal dose of short-acting insulin by 50% (K)

Table 36. Insulin Preparations			
Preparations	**Onset**	**Peak**	**Duration**
Insulin glulisine (*Apidra*)	20 min	0.5–1.5 h	3–4 h
Insulin lispro (*Humalog*)	15 min	0.5–1.5 h	3–4 h
Insulin (eg, *Humulin, Novolin*)*			
Regular	0.5–1 h	2–3 h	8–12 h
NPH	1–1.5 h	4–12 h	24 h
Insulin aspart (*NovoLog*)	0.5 h	1–3 h	3–5 h
Long-acting (*Ultralente*)	4–8 h	16–18 h	>36 h
Insulin glargine (*Lantus*)**	1–2 h	—	24 h
Insulin, zinc (*Lente*)	1–2.5 h	8–12 h	18–24 h
Isophane insulin and regular insulin inj. (*Novolin 70/30*)	0.5 h	2–12 h	24 h

* Also available as mixtures of NPH and regular in 50:50 proportions.

** To convert from NPH dosing, give same number of units once a day. For patients taking NPH bid, decrease the total daily units by 20%, and titrate on basis of response. Starting dose in insulin-naive patients is 10 U once daily hs.

Monitoring (ADA)

- Weight, BP, and foot examination, including monofilament testing at 4 plantar sites (great toe and base of first, third, and fifth metatarsals), palpation, and inspection, each visit
- HbA$_{1c}$ twice/yr in patients with stable glycemic control; quarterly, if poor control
- Annual comprehensive dilated eye and visual examinations by an ophthalmologist or optometrist who is experienced in management of diabetic retinopathy
- Lipid profiles q 1–2 yr depending on whether values are in normal range
- Annual (unless microalbuminuria has previously been demonstrated) test for microalbuminuria by measuring albumin:creatinine ratio in a random spot collection

FALLS

DEFINITION
An event that results in a person's inadvertently coming to rest on the ground or lower level with or without loss of consciousness or injury. Excludes falls from major intrinsic event (eg, seizure, stroke, syncope) or overwhelming environmental hazard.

ETIOLOGY
Typically multifactorial. Composed of intrinsic (eg, poor balance, weakness, chronic illness, visual or cognitive impairment), extrinsic (eg, polypharmacy), and environmental (eg, poor lighting, no safety equipment, loose carpets) factors. Commonly a nonspecific sign for one of many acute illnesses in older adults.

EVALUATION
Exclude acute illness or underlying systemic or metabolic process (eg, infection, electrolyte imbalance as indicated by hx, examination, and laboratory studies). See **Figure 3** for recommended assessment and management. See also p 145.
- Laboratory tests for persons at risk: CBC, serum electrolytes, BUN, Cr, glucose, B_{12}, thyroid function
- Bone densitometry in women with additional risk factors for osteoporotic fracture (see p 145)
- Imaging: neuroimaging if head injury or new, focal neurologic findings on examination or if a CNS process is suspected
- Ambulatory cardiac monitoring rarely helpful
- Arrhythmic evaluation only if clinical evidence of this diagnosis (eg, hx of cardiac events or abnormal ECG)
- Drug concentrations for anticonvulsants, antiarrhythmics, TCAs, and high-dose aspirin

History
- Circumstances of fall (eg, activity at time of fall, location, time)
- Associated symptoms (eg, lightheadedness, vertigo, syncope, weakness, confusion, palpitations)
- Relevant comorbid conditions (eg, prior stroke, parkinsonism, cardiac disease, diabetes mellitus, seizure disorder, depression, anxiety, anemia, sensory deficit, glaucoma, cataracts, osteoporosis, cognitive impairment)
- Previous falls
- Medication review, including OTC medications and alcohol use; note recent changes in medications; note drugs that have hypotensive or psychoactive effects (see p 68)
- Ask about person's ability to complete ADLs: bathing, dressing, transferring, continence

Physical
Look for:
- Vital signs: postural pulse and BP changes at 1 and 2 min, fever, hypothermia
- Head and neck: visual impairment (especially poor acuity, reduced contrast sensitivity, decreased visual fields, cataracts), motion-induced imbalance (Dix-Hallpike test), bruit, nystagmus
- Musculoskeletal: arthritic changes, motion or joint limitations (especially lower extremity joint function), postural instability, skeletal deformities, podiatric problems

Figure 3. Assessment and Management of Falls

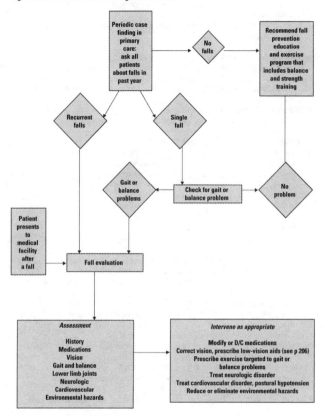

Sources: Adapted from American Geriatrics Society, British Geriatrics Society, and American Academy of Orthopaedic Surgeons Panel on Falls Prevention. Guideline for the prevention of falls in older persons. *J Amer Geriatr Soc.* 2001; 49(5):666, and Tinetti M. Preventing falls in elderly persons. *N Engl J Med* 2003;348(1):42–49.

- Neurologic: slower reflexes, altered proprioception, altered mental status, focal deficits, peripheral neuropathy, gait or balance disorders, muscle weakness (especially leg), instability, tremor, rigidity
- Cardiovascular: heart arrhythmias, cardiac valve dysfunction
- Other: fever; hypothermia

Gait, Balance, and Mobility Assessment
- Functional gait: observe patient rising from chair, walking (stride, length, velocity, symmetry), turning, sitting (Timed Get Up and Go test; see also POMA, p 221)
- Balance: Side-by-side, semi-tandem, and full tandem stance; Functional Reach test (see also POMA, p 221)
- Mobility: observe patient's use of assistive device (eg, cane, walker) or personal assistance, extent of ambulation, restraint use, footwear evaluation

Medications Associated with Increased Fall Risk
- Antipsychotics (especially phenothiazines)
- Sedatives, hypnotics (including benzodiazepines)
- Antidepressants (including MAOIs, SSRIs, TCAs)
- Antiarrhythmics (Class 1A)
- Anticonvulsants
- Anxiolytics
- Antihypertensives
- Diuretics

PREVENTION
Goal is to minimize risk of falling without compromising mobility and functional independence.
- Assess fall risk as part of routine primary health care visit (at least annually). Risk of falling significantly increases as number of risk factors increases.
- Assess for risk factors using a multidisciplinary approach, including physical and occupational therapy if appropriate.
- Diagnose and treat underlying cause.
- Focus on most common risk factors, which include muscle weakness, hx of falls, gait deficit, balance deficit, use of assistive devices, visual deficit, arthritis, impaired ADLs, depression, cognitive impairment, age >80 yr old.
- Begin fall prevention program targeting interventions for risk factors (see **Table 37**). A structured, interdisciplinary approach should be used.
  ○ Offer hip protectors to non-bedbound residents of nursing homes and others at high risk—available via http://www.hipprotector.com, http://www.hipsaver.com, or http://www.fallgard.com/index.asp.
  ○ Recommend daily supplementation of calcium (1200 mg) and vitamin D (800 IU).

Table 37. Preventing Falls: Selected Risk Factors and Suggested Interventions

Factors	Suggested Interventions
Medication-related Factors	
Use of benzodiazepines, sedative-hypnotics, or antipsychotic	Consider agents with less risk of falls (eg, atypical antipsychotics such as olanzapine, risperidone, or quetiapine)
	Taper and D/C medications, as possible
	Address sleep problems with nonpharmacologic interventions (see p 199)
	Educate regarding appropriate use of medications and monitoring for adverse events
Recent change in dosage or number of prescription medications *or* use of ≥4 prescription medications *or* use of other medications associated with fall risk	Review medication profile and modify, as possible Monitor response to medications and to dosage changes
Mobility-related Factors	
Presence of environmental hazards (eg, improper bed height, cluttered walking surfaces, lack of railings, poor lighting)	Improve lighting, especially at night
	Remove floor barriers (eg, loose carpeting)
	Replace existing furniture with safer furniture (eg, correct height, more stable)
	Install support structures (eg, railings and grab bars, especially in bathroom)
	Use nonslip bathmats
Impaired gait, balance, or transfer skills	Refer to PT for comprehensive evaluation and rehabilitation
	Gait training
	Balance or strengthening exercises (see also p 170)
	If able to perform tandem stance, refer for Tai Chi, dance, yoga, or postural awareness
	Provide training in transfer skills
	Prescribe appropriate assistive devices
	Recommend protective hip padding
	Environmental changes (eg, grab bars, raised toilet seats)
	Recommend appropriate footwear (eg, good fit, non-slip)
Impaired leg or arm strength or range of motion, or proprioception	Strengthening exercises (eg, use of resistive rubber bands, putty)
	Resistance training 2–3 times/wk to 10 repetitions with full range of motion, then increase resistance
	Tai Chi
	Physical therapy

(cont.)

Table 37. Preventing Falls: Selected Risk Factors and Suggested Interventions (cont.)

Factors	Suggested Interventions
Medical Factors	
Parkinson's disease, osteoarthritis, depressive symptoms, impaired cognition, other conditions associated with increased falls	Optimize medical therapy
	Monitor for disease progression and impact on mobility and impairments
	Determine need for assistive devices
	Use bedside commode if frequent nighttime urination
Postural hypotension: drop in SBP ≥20 mm Hg (or ≥20%) with or without symptoms, either immediately or within 3 min of standing (see also orthostatic postural hypotension, p 41)	Review medications potentially contributing and adjust dosing or switch to less hypotensive agents; avoid vasodilators and diuretics if possible
	Educate on activities to decrease effect (eg, slow rising, ankle pumps, hand clenching, elevation of head of bed) and to slow rising from recumbent or seated position, grab bars by toilet and bath
	Prescribe pressure stockings (eg, Jobst)
	Liberalize salt intake
	Caffeinated coffee (1 cup) or caffeine 100 mg with meals for postprandial hypotension
	Consider medication to increase pressure (if HTN, HF, and hypokalemia not serious [for fludrocortisone]): -midodrine (*ProAmatine*) 2.5–5 mg tid [T: 2.5, 5] -fludrocortisone (*Florinef*) 0.1 mg qd–tid [T: 0.1]
Vision or hearing impairment (see Hearing Impairment, p 81; Visual Impairment, p 203)	Refraction
	Cataract extraction
	Good lighting
	Home safety evaluation
	Mobility training for visually impaired
	Cerumen removal
	Audiological evaluation with hearing aid, if appropriate

GASTROINTESTINAL DISEASES

DYSPHAGIA

See also p 161.

Definition
- Inability to initiate a swallow, or a sensation that solids or liquids do not pass easily from the mouth into the stomach.
- Classified as oropharyngeal or esophageal dysphagia.

Presentation/Patient Complaints

Structural:
- Pocketing of food in cheeks, on hard palate, or under tongue
- Food gets stuck after swallowing
- Speech abnormalities: slurring, gurgly voice
- Orofacial changes: facial weakness, abnormal tongue movements

Functional:
- Inability to initiate a swallow
- Impaired ability to transfer food from mouth to esophagus
- Nasal regurgitation
- Coughing
- Drooling or excessive secretions
- Reluctance to eat specific foods or foods of certain consistency, or to eat at all

Common Causes
- Cerebrovascular accident/stroke
- Parkinson's disease
- Oropharyngeal tumors
- Zenker's diverticulum
- Cervical osteophytes

Evaluation
- Physical examination
  - Oral cavity, head, neck, and supraclavicular region
  - All cranial nerves with emphasis on nerves V, VII, IX, X, XI, XII
- Review medications for those that can decrease saliva production (eg, anticholinergics)
- Referral to speech-language pathologists
- Diagnostic tests
  - Barium swallow to assess swallowing mechanism; may document aspiration
  - Videofluoroscopy is an alternative to barium studies to assess swallowing mechanism
  - Upper endoscopy
  - Fiberoptic nasopharyngeal laryngoscopy provides detailed evaluation of lesions in oropharynx, hypopharynx, larynx, and proximal esophagus; also visualizes pooled secretions or food
  - Esophageal manometry often used in combination with barium radiography; more useful for assessment of esophageal dysphagia

Treatment
- Identify underlying cause
- Dietary modifications based on recommendation of speech pathologist, occupational therapist, or dietician
- Swallowing rehabilitation, eg, multiple swallows, tilt head back and place bolus on strong side, Mendelsohn's maneuver
- Elevate the head of the bed
- Endoscopic dilation
- Cricopharyngeal myotomy
- Botulinum toxin injection in cricopharyngeal muscle

Food Consistencies
- Pureed: thick, homogenous textures; pudding-like
- Ground/minced: easily chewed without coarse texture; excludes all raw foods except mashed bananas
- Soft or easy to chew: soft foods prepared without a blender; tender meats cut to ≤1-cm pieces; excludes nuts, tough skins, and raw, crispy, or stringy foods
- Modified general: soft textures that do not require grinding or chopping

Fluid Consistencies
- Thin: regular fluids; no change in fluids
- Nectar-like: thin enough to be sipped through a straw or from a cup, but still spillable (eg, eggnog, buttermilk)
- Honey-like: thick enough to be eaten with a spoon, too thick for a straw, not able to independently hold its shape (eg, yogurt, tomato sauce, honey)
- Spoon-thick: pudding-like, must be eaten with a spoon (eg, thick milk pudding, thickened applesauce)

GASTROESOPHAGEAL REFLUX DISEASE (GERD)
Definition
The retrograde movement of the gastric contents in the esophagus due to incompetent lower esophageal sphincter, transient relaxations of the sphincter, or compromise of other antireflux mechanisms.

Evaluation and Assessment
Empiric treatment is appropriate when hx is typical for uncomplicated GERD.
- Endoscopy (if symptoms persist despite initial management, atypical presentation, or longstanding symptoms)
- 24-h pH monitoring

Symptoms Suggesting Complicated GERD and Need for Evaluation
- Dysphagia
- Bleeding
- Weight loss
- Choking (acid causing cough, shortness of breath, or hoarseness)
- Chest pain

Management

Nonpharmacologic:

- Antacids
- Avoid alcohol and fatty foods
- Avoid lying down for 3 h after eating
- Avoid tight-fitting clothes
- Change diet (avoid pepper, spearmint, chocolate, spicy or acidic foods)
- Drink 6–8 oz water with all medications
- Elevate head of the bed (6–8 in)
- Lose weight (if overweight)
- Stop drugs that may promote reflux
- Stop smoking
- Consider surgery

Pharmacologic:

Table 38. Pharmacologic Management of GERD		
Drug	Initial Oral Dosage	Formulations (Excretion)
Proton-Pump Inhibitors		
✔ Esomeprazole (*Nexium*)	20 mg qd × 4 wk	C: ER 20, 40 (L)
✔ Lansoprazole (*Prevacid*)	15 mg qd × 8 wk	C: ER 15, 30; granules for susp: 15, 30/packet (L)
✔ Omeprazole (*Prilosec*)	20 mg qd × 4–8 wk	C: ER 10, 20,* 40; T: enteric-coated 20 (L)
✔ Pantoprazole (*Protonix*)	40 mg qd × 8 wk	T: enteric-coated 20; Inj (L)
✔ Rabeprazole (*AcipHex*)	20 mg qd × 4–8 wk; 20 mg qd maintenance, if needed	T: enteric-coated ER 20 (L)
H₂ Antagonists (for less severe GERD)		
Cimetidine (*Tagamet*)	400 or 800 mg bid	S: 200 mg/20 mL, 300 mg/5 mL with alcohol 2.8%; T: 100, 200,* 300, 400, 800; Inj (K, L)
✔ Famotidine (*Pepcid*)	20 mg bid × 6 wk	S: oral sus 40 mg/5 mL; T: film-coated 10,* 20, 40, oral disintegrating 20, 40; C (gel): 10*; ChT: 10*; Inj (K)
✔ Nizatidine (*Axid*)	150 mg bid	C: 150, 300; T: 75 (K)
✔ Ranitidine (*Zantac*)	150 mg bid	Pk: gran, effervescent (EFFERdose) 150 mg; S: syr 15 mg/mL; T: 75,* 150, 300; T: effervescent (EFFERdose) 150; Inj (K, F)
Mucosal Protective Agent		
Sucralfate (*Carafate*)	1 g qid, 1 h ac and hs	S: oral sus 1 g/10 mL; T: 1 g (F, K)
Prokinetic Agents		
Bethanechol (*Urecholine*)	25 mg qid	T: 5, 10, 25, 50 (unknown)
Metoclopramide† (*Reglan*)	5 mg qid, ac, and hs	S: syr, sugar-free 5 mg/5 mL, conc 10 mg/mL; T: 5, 10; Inj (K, F)

✔ = preferred for treating older adults.
* OTC strength.
† Risk of EPS high in people >65 yr old.
Source: Data from DeVault KR, Castell DO. Updated guidelines for the diagnosis and treatment of gastroesophageal reflux disease. *Am J Gastroenterol.* 1999;94:1430–1442.

PEPTIC ULCER DISEASE
Causes
Helicobacter pylori is the major cause. NSAIDs are the second most common cause.

Diagnosis of *H pylori*
- Endoscopic examination
- Serology
- Urea breath test

Initial Treatment Options
- Empiric anti-ulcer treatment for 6 wk
- Definitive diagnostic evaluation by endoscopy
- Noninvasive testing for *H pylori* and treatment with antibiotics for those that test positive (see **Table 39** for regimens)
- Review patient's chronic medications for drug interactions before selecting regimen; many potential drug interactions and adverse drug events.

Table 39. **FDA-approved Treatments for *H pylori*–induced Ulcerations (all oral routes)**

Lansoprazole 30 mg bid + amoxicillin 1 g bid + clarithromycin 500 mg tid × 10 (or 14) d

or Omeprazole 20 mg bid + clarithromycin 500 mg bid + amoxicillin 1 g bid × 10 d

or Lansoprazole 30 mg bid + clarithromycin 500 mg bid + amoxicillin 1 g bid × 10 d (*Prevpac*)

or Omeprazole 40 mg qd + clarithromycin 500 mg tid × 2 wk, then omeprazole 20 mg qd × 2 wk

or Lansoprazole 30 mg tid + amoxicillin 1 g bid × 2 wk (only for person allergic or intolerant to clarithromycin)

or Ranitidine bismuth citrate (RBC) 400 mg bid + clarithromycin 500 mg tid × 2 wk, then RBC 400 mg bid × 2 wk

or RBC 400 mg bid + clarithromycin 500 mg bid × 2 wk, then RBC 400 mg bid × 2 wk

or Bismuth subsalicylate (*Pepto-Bismol*) 525 mg qid (pc and hs) + metronidazole 250 mg qid + tetracycline 500 mg qid × 2 wk (*Helidac*) + H₂ receptor antagonist or proton-pump inhibitor as directed × 4 wk

Source: http://www.cdc.gov/ulcer/md.htm.
For additional, non-FDA approved regimens, see Howden CW, Hunt RH. Guidelines for the management of *Helicobacter pylori* infection. *Am J Gastroenterol* 1998;93:2330–2338, or http://www.acg.gi.org.

Medications
Bismuth subsalicylate (*Pepto-Bismol*) [T: 324; ChT: 262; S: sus 262 mg/15 mL, 525 mg/15 mL]
Antibiotics: (for complete information, see **Table 52**)
Amoxicillin (*Amoxil*) [C: 250, 500; ChT: 125, 250; S: oral sus 125 mg/5 mL, 250 mg/5 mL]
Clarithromycin (*Biaxin*) [T: film-coated 250, 500; S: oral sus 125 mg/5 mL, 250 mg/5 mL]
Metronidazole (*Flagyl*) [T: 250, 500, 750; C: 375]
Tetracycline (*Achromycin, Sumycin*) [T: 250, 500; S: oral sus 125 mg/5 mL]
Proton-Pump Inhibitors: See **Table 38**.

STRESS-ULCER PREVENTION IN HOSPITALIZED OLDER ADULTS
Risk Factors (in order of prevalence in older adults)
- Hx of GI ulceration or bleed in the past year
- Sepsis

- Multiple organ failure
- Hypotension
- Respiratory failure requiring mechanical ventilation for >48 h
- Kidney failure
- Major trauma, shock, or head injury
- Coagulopathy (platelets <50,000/μL, INR >1.5, or PTT >2 × control)
- Burns over >25% of body surface area
- Hepatic failure
- Intracranial hypertension
- Spinal cord injury
- Tetraplegia

Prophylaxis
- H_2 antagonists (see **Table 38**)
- Proton-pump inhibitors (see **Table 38**)
- Sucralfate (see **Table 38**)
- Antacids
- Enteral feedings

Discontinue H_2 antagonists, proton-pump inhibitors, and other treatments for stress-ulcer prevention before transfer or discharge.

Key Points
- Prophylaxis has not been shown to reduce mortality
- No one regimen has shown superior efficacy
- Choice of regimen depends on access to and function of GI tract and presence of nasogastric suction

IRRITABLE BOWEL SYNDROME (IBS)
Signs and Symptoms
Symptoms should be present ≥12 wk.
Consistent with IBS:
- Abdominal pain
- Bloating
- Constipation
- Diarrhea

Not Consistent with IBS:
- Weight loss
- First onset after age 50
- Nocturnal diarrhea
- Family hx of cancer or inflammatory bowel disease
- Rectal bleeding or obstruction
- Laboratory abnormalities
- Presence of fecal parasites

Diagnosis (of exclusion)
Exclude ischemia, diverticulosis, colon cancer, inflammatory bowel disease by physical examination and testing (colonoscopy, CT scan, or small-bowel series)

Treatment
- Reassurance; not life threatening; focus on relief of physical and emotional symptoms
- Dietary modification
  ○ Avoid foods that trigger symptoms or produce excess gas or bloating
  ○ Consider a trial of a lactose-free diet

- Behavioral interventions: hypnosis, biofeedback, psychotherapy have been shown to be more effective than placebo
- Fiber supplements (see **Table 40**)
  - Synthetic: polycarbophil (*FiberCon* [caplet: 625], others), methylcellulose (*Citrucel, Fiber Ease* [C, sus, pwd])
  - Natural: psyllium (*Metamucil* [C, T, wafer, pwd], others)
- Antispasmodics (short-term use only)
  - Dicyclomine (*Bentyl* [C: 10; T: 20; syr: 10 mg/5 mL; Inj]) 10–20 mg po qid prn (L)
  - Hyoscyamine (*Anazpaz, Levsin, Levsin/SL*, others [T (sl): 0.125, 0.15; T ER, C: 0.375; Inj: 125 sol]) 0.125–0.25 mg po/sl tid–qid prn (L, K)
- Antidiarrheals: may be helpful for diarrhea but not for global IBS symptoms, abdominal pain, or constipation
  - Loperamide (*Imodium A-D* [C, T: 2; sol 1 mg/5 mL]) 4 mg after each loose bowel movement, max 16 mg/24 h
- Antidepressants
  - TCAs and SSRIs may be beneficial for patients with diarrhea or pain. See Depression, p 51, for dosing.
- Serotonin agents
  - Alosetron (*Lotronex* [T: 0.5, 1]): serotonin 3 antagonist; treatment of women with severe diarrhea-predominant IBS who have not responded to conventional therapy; 0.5 mg po bid × 4 wk, increase to 1 mg bid × 4 wk, stop if no response (K, L)
  - Tegaserod (*Zelnorm* [T: 2, 6]): short-term treatment of constipation-predominant IBS in women; 6 mg bid ac × 4–6 wk, may continue an additional 4–6 wk if responding (F, K)

CONSTIPATION
Definition
Infrequent (usually <3 times/wk), incomplete, or painful evacuation of feces

Drugs That Constipate
- Analgesics—opiates
- Antacids with aluminum or calcium
- Anticholinergic drugs
- Antidepressants, lithium
- Antihypertensives
- Antipsychotics
- Barium sulfate
- Bismuth
- Calcium channel blockers
- Diuretics
- Iron

Conditions That Constipate
- Colon tumor or mechanical obstruction
- Dehydration
- Depression
- Diabetes mellitus
- Hypercalcemia
- Hypokalemia
- Hypothyroidism
- Immobility
- Low intake of fiber
- Panhypopituitarism
- Parkinson's disease
- Spinal cord injury
- Stroke
- Uremia

Management of Chronic Constipation
Step 1. Stop all constipating medications, when possible.
Step 2. Increase dietary bran to ≥6–25 g/d, increase fluid intake to ≥1500 mL/d, and increase physical activity; or add bran supplements, provided fluid intake is ≥1500 mL/d. If fiber exacerbates symptoms or is not tolerated, go to Step 3.

Step 3. Add 70% sorbitol solution (15–30 mL qd or bid, max 150 mL/d).
Step 4. Add stimulant laxative (eg, senna, bisacodyl), 2–3 times/wk. (Alternative: Saline laxative, but avoid in renal insufficiency.)
Step 5. Use tap water enema or saline enema 2 times/wk.
Step 6. Use oil-retention enema for refractory constipation.

Table 40. Medications That May Relieve Constipation

Medication	Onset of Action	Starting Dosage	Site and Mechanism of Action
Bulk laxatives			
Methylcellulose (*Citrucel**), psyllium (*Metamucil**)	12–24 h (up to 72 h)	1–2 rounded tsp or packets qd–tid with water or juice	Small and large intestine; holds water in feces; mechanical distention
Polycarbophil (*FiberCon**, others)	12–24 h (up to 72 h)	1250 mg qd–qid	Small and large intestine; holds water in feces; mechanical distention
Osmotic laxatives			
Lactulose (*Cephulac*)	24–48 h	15–30 mL qd–bid	Colon; osmotic effect
Polyethylene glycol (*Miralax*)	48–96 h	17 g pwd qd (~1 tbsp) dissolved in 8 oz water	GI tract; osmotic effect
Sorbitol 70%*	24–48 h	15–30 mL qd–bid	Colon; delivers osmotically active molecules to colon
Saline laxatives			
Magnesium citrate (*Citroma**)	30 min–3 h	120–240 mL × 1	Small and large intestine; attracts, retains water in intestinal lumen
Magnesium hydroxide (*Milk of Magnesia**)	30 min–3 h	30 mL qd–bid	Osmotic effect and increased peristalsis in colon
Sodium phosphate/biphosphate emollient enema (*Fleet**)	2–15 min	14.5-oz enema × 1, repeat prn	Colon, osmotic effect; potential hyperphosphatemia in patients with renal insufficiency
Stimulant laxatives			
Bisacodyl tablet (*Dulcolax**)	6–10 h	5–15 mg × 1	Colon; increases peristalsis
Bisacodyl suppository (*Dulcolax**)	15 min–1 h	10 mg × 1	Colon; increases peristalsis
Senna (*Senokot**)	6–10 h	2 tabs or 1 tsp qhs	Colon; direct action on intestine; stimulates myenteric plexus; alters water and electrolyte secretion
Surfactant laxative			
Docusate (*Colace**)	24–72 h	100 mg qd–bid	Small and large intestine; detergent activity; facilitates admixture of fat and water to soften feces

*Available OTC.

NAUSEA AND VOMITING

Causes
- CNS disorders (eg, motion sickness, intracranial lesions)
- Drugs (eg, chemotherapy, NSAIDs, opioid analgesics, antibiotics, digoxin)
- GI disorders (eg, mechanical obstruction; inflammation of stomach, intestine, or gallbladder; pseudo-obstruction; motility disorders; dyspepsia; diabetic gastroparesis)
- Infections (eg, viral or bacterial gastroenteritis, hepatitis, otitis, meningitis)
- Metabolic conditions (eg, uremia, acidosis, hyperparathyroidism, adrenal insufficiency)
- Psychiatric disorders

Evaluation
- If patient is not seriously ill or dehydrated, can probably wait 24–48 h to see if symptoms resolve spontaneously.
- If patient is seriously ill, dehydrated, or has other signs of acute illness, hospitalize for further evaluation.
- If symptoms persist, evaluate on the basis of the most likely causes.

Pharmacologic Management
Drugs that are useful in the management of nausea and vomiting are listed in **Table 41**.

Table 41. Selected Antiemetics		
Drug	Formulations	Dosages (Metabolism)
Dimenhydrinate* (*Dramamine*)	Inj; S: 12.5 mg/4 mL, 16.62 mg/5 mL; T: 50; ChT: 50	Oral, IM IV; 50–100 mg q 4–6 h, not to exceed 400 mg/d (L)
Meclizine* (*Antivert*)	C: 25, 30; T: 12.5, 25, 50; ChT: 25; T: film-coated 25	Motion sickness: 12.5–25 mg 1 h before travel, repeat dose q 12–24 h if needed; doses up to 50 mg may be needed; vertigo: 25–100 mg/d in divided doses (L)
Metoclopramide (*Reglan*)	Inj; S: oral conc 10 mg/mL, syr, sugar-free, 5 mg/5 mL; T: 5, 10	Chemotherapy-induced emesis, IV: 1–2 mg/kg 30 min before chemotherapy and q 2–4 to q 4–6 h; postoperative nausea and vomiting, IM: 5–10 mg near the end of surgery (K)
Prochlorperazine (*Compazine*)	C: ER 10, 15, 30; Inj; Sp: 2.5, 5, 25; S: syr 5 mg/5 mL; T: 5, 10, 25	Oral or IM: 5–10 mg 3–4 times/d, usual max 40 mg/d; IV: 2.5–10 mg; max 10 mg/dose or 40 mg/d; may repeat dose q 3–4 h as needed; rectal: 25 mg bid (L)

*Available OTC.
Note: All have potential CNS toxicity.

DIARRHEA

Causes
- Drugs (eg, antibiotics [see **Table 52** and next section], laxatives, colchicine)
- Fecal impaction
- GI disorders (eg, irritable bowel syndrome, malabsorption, inflammatory bowel disease)
- Infections (eg, viral, bacterial, parasitic)
- Lactose intolerance

Evaluation
- If patient is not seriously ill or dehydrated and there is no blood in the feces, can probably wait 48 h to see if symptoms resolve spontaneously.
- If patient is seriously ill, dehydrated, or has other signs of acute illness, hospitalize for further evaluation.
- If diarrhea persists, evaluate on the basis of the most likely causes.
- If analgesic drug is suspected, decrease dosage, consider adding antiemetic until tolerance develops, or change to a different analgesic drug.

Pharmacologic Management
Drugs that are useful in the management of diarrhea are listed in **Table 42**.

Table 42. Antidiarrheals		
Drug	**Dosage (Metabolism)**	**Formulations**
✔ Attapulgite* (*Kaopectate*)	1200–1500 mg after each loose bowel movement or q 2 h; 15–30 mL up to 9 × /d, up to 9000 mg/24 h (not absorbed)	S: oral conc 600, 750 mg/15 mL; T: 750; ChT: 300, 600
✔ Bismuth subsalicylate* (*Pepto-Bismol*)	2 tabs or 30 mL q 30 min–1 h prn up to 8 doses/24 h	S: 262 mg/15 mL, 525 mg/15 mL; T: 324; ChT: 262
Diphenoxylate with atropine (*Lomotil*)†	15–20 mg/d of diphenoxylate in 3–4 divided doses; maintenance 5–15 mg/d in 2–3 divided doses (L)	S: oral, diphenoxylate hydrochloride 2.5 mg + atropine sulfate 0.025 mg/5 mL; T: diphenoxylate hydrochloride 2.5 mg + atropine sulfate 0.025 mg
✔ Loperamide* (*Imodium A-D*)	Initial: 4 mg followed by 2 mg after each loose bowel movement, up to 16 mg/d (L)	Caplet: 2; C: 2; T: 2; S: oral, 1 mg/5 mL

✔ = preferred for treating older persons.
* Available OTC.
† Anticholinergic, potentially CNS toxic.

ANTIBIOTIC-ASSOCIATED DIARRHEA
(Antibiotic-associated pseudomembranous colitis [AAPMC])

Definition
A specific form of *Clostridium difficile* pseudomembranous colitis

Risk Factors
Almost any oral or parenteral antibiotic and several antineoplastic agents, including cyclophosphamide, doxorubicin, fluorouracil, methotrexate.

Presentation
- Abdominal pain, cramping
- Dehydration
- Diarrhea (can be bloody)
- Fecal leukocytes
- Fever (100–105°F)
- Hypoalbuminemia
- Hypovolemia
- Leukocytosis

Symptoms appear a few days after starting to 10 wk after discontinuing the offending agent.

Diagnosis
- Isolation of *C difficile* or its toxin from symptomatic patient. Three negative fecal examinations are needed to exclude diagnosis.
- Lower endoscopy; however, lesions may be scattered.

Treatment
- D/C offending agent and/or switch to alternative treatment.
- Metronidazole (*Flagyl*) 250 mg po qid or 500 mg po tid × 10 d or vancomycin 125–500 mg po qid × 10 d.
- Treat diarrhea with cholestyramine resin (eg, *Questran*) 4 g 1–6 ×/d to adsorb toxin.
- Avoid opiates or other agents that slow GI motility.

Recurrence
Relapse seen in 10%–20% of patients 1–4 wk after treatment (spore-producing organism). Re-treat with same regimen or use alternative.

HEARING IMPAIRMENT

DEFINITION
The most common sensory impairment in old age. To quantify hearing ability, the necessary intensity (decibel = dB) and frequency (Hertz) of the perceived pure-tone signal must be described.

EVALUATION
Screening and Evaluation
- Note problems during conversation
- Ask about hearing dysfunction
- Use a standardized questionnaire (see p 220)
- Test with handheld audioscope
- Use whisper test—stand behind patient 2 ft from ear, cover untested ear, fully exhale, whisper an easily answered question
- Refer patients who screen positive for audiologic evaluation

Audiometry
- Documents the dB loss across frequencies
- Determines the pattern of loss (see Classification, below)
- Determines if loss is unilateral or bilateral (**Note:** If speech discrimination is <50%, results with hearing aids may be poor.)

Aggravating Factors
- Sensorineural loss (Weber test lateralizes away from impaired ear, Rinne test normal in both ears)—medication ototoxicity (eg, aminoglycosides, loop diuretics, cisplatin), cerumen impaction (see p 82)
- Conductive loss (Weber test lateralizes toward impaired ear, Rinne test abnormal in impaired ear)—cerumen impaction, external otitis

CLASSIFICATION
Sensorineural Hearing Loss
- Due to cochlear or retrocochlear pathology
- Thresholds for both air and bone conduction increased
- Causes: aging, cranial nerve VIII damage from syphilis, viral meningitis, trauma, vascular events to cranial nerve VIII or cortical tracts, acoustic neuroma, Ménière's disease

Conductive Hearing Loss
- Occurs when sound transmission to inner ear is impaired
- Bone conduction better than air conduction
- Causes: external or middle ear disorders, including otosclerosis; rheumatoid arthritis; Paget's disease

Central Auditory Processing Disorder
- Loss of speech discrimination in excess of that from loss in hearing sensitivity
- Involves the CNS
- Occurs in dementia and infrequently with presbycusis

Presbycusis (Old-age Hearing Loss, a Subtype of Sensorineural Loss)
- Mainly high-frequency loss
- Impaired speech discrimination
- Recruitment (an increase in sensation of loudness)
- Both bone and air conduction affected

MANAGEMENT
Remove Ear Wax
Fill ear canal with 5–10 gtt water and cover with cotton bid × ≥4 d. Liquid must stay in contact with ear for ≥15 min. Hearing may worsen as cerumen expands. Water is as effective as commercial preparations (eg, *Debrox, Cerumenex, Colace*). Use of any of the commercial preparations for >4 d may cause ear irritation.

Table 43. Effects and Rehabilitation of Hearing Loss, by Level of Loss

Level of Loss	Difficulty Understanding	Need for Hearing Aid
0–24 dB	None	None
25–40 dB (mild)	Normal speech	In specific situations
41–55 dB (moderate)	Loud speech	Frequent
56–80 dB (severe)	Anything but amplified speech	For all communication
81 dB or more (profound)	Even amplified speech	Plus speech reading, aural rehabilitation, sign language, or cochlear implants

Source: Data in part from *A Report on Hearing Aids: User Perspectives and Concerns*. Washington, DC: American Association of Retired Persons; 1993:2.

Hearing Devices
Hearing Aids: Appropriate for most hearing-impaired persons; enhance select frequencies; should be individualized for each ear. Amplification in both ears (binaural) provides best speech understanding; unilateral aid may be appropriate if asymmetrical speech discrimination, if hearing-aid care is challenging, or because of cost.
Assistive Listening Devices: Microphone placed close to sound source transmits to headphones or earpiece. Transmission is by wire or wireless (FM or infrared); these systems increase signal-to-noise ratio, which is useful for persons with central auditory processing disorder.
Telephone Device for the Deaf (TDD): Receiver is a keyboard that allows the hearing-impaired person to respond.
Cochlear Implants: Bypass the middle ear, directly innervate auditory nerve. Reserved for severe and profound hearing loss (score ≤40% on the sentence recognition test in the ear to be implanted). Results after age 65 comparable to those in younger people. Failure rate <1%, but patient selection important.

Tips for Communication with Hearing-impaired People
- Stand 2–3 ft away
- Have the person's attention
- Have the person seated in front of a wall, which helps reflect sound
- Use lower-pitched voice
- Speak slowly and distinctly; don't shout
- Rephrase rather than repeat
- Pause at the end of phrases or ideas

TINNITUS
Definition
The perception of sound in the absence of external acoustic stimulation; may be ringing, crackling, or whistling; may be continuous or intermittent

Objective Tinnitus
Noise heard by both patient and examiner (rare); usually due to abnormal blood flow in or around ear (normal anatomic variants or a pathologic condition)

Subjective Tinnitus
- Cannot be heard externally by others (common).
- Normal tinnitus lasts <5 min, <once/week.
- Pathologic tinnitus lasts >5 min, >weekly (usually in people with hearing loss).

Evaluation
- Auscultate the head and neck near ear orbits, mastoids for objective tinnitus.
  - If pulsatile, obtain CT/MRA for vascular cause.
  - If continuous, obtain MRI looking for patulous Eustachian tube; other causes include palatal myoclonus, stapedial muscle spasm.
  - Refer to otolaryngology
- Examine ear canals for cerumen, otitis externa or interna; treat and reassess.
- Assess hearing (as above); unilateral hearing loss and tinnitus suggest acoustic neuroma; obtain MRI.
- Audiometry
  - Low- and high-tone loss supports Ménière's disease.
  - High-tone loss suggests presbycusis.
- Check medication list for drugs associated with tinnitus, eg, NSAIDs, ASA, antibiotics (especially erythromycin), loop diuretics (especially furosemide), chemotherapy, quinine.

Treatment
- Objective tinnitus: refer to otolaryngology.
- Subjective tinnitus without distress:
  - Normal tinnitus: reassure patient.
  - Pathologic tinnitus: educate patient, encourage amplification for those with hearing impairment.
- Subjective tinnitus with distress:
  - Severe complaints about tinnitus are often a sign of depression.
  - Evaluate for depression and treat (see p 51).

ANEMIA

Evaluation

- Some decrease in Hb with age is normal.
- Evaluate persons >65 yr old when Hb <13.
- Evaluate if Hb falls >1 g/dL in 1 yr.
- Physical examination and laboratory tests to look for kidney or liver disease.
- Evaluate GI and GU source if iron deficient.
- Check WBC and peripheral blood smear, and pursue suspected causes as appropriate.
- Combined deficiencies are common in older adults; reasonable to check B_{12}, folate, and iron in all cases.
- Check reticuloctye count and reticulocyte index.
  - Reticulocyte count or index high: adequate response, suspect blood loss or RBC destruction
  - Reticulocyte count or index normal or low: check MCV
    - MCV >100 μm³/cell: see **Figure 4**
    - MCV <100 μm³/cell: see **Figure 5**

Common Anemias of Later Life: Diagnosis and Treatment

Iron deficiency anemia: Usual laboratory values (Fe, TIBC, ferritin) less reliable in presence of inflammatory conditions (see **Figure 5**). Soluble transferrin receptors (sTfR) help differentiate anemia of chronic disease from that of iron deficiency; elevated receptors suggest iron deficiency. The ratio sTfR/log ferritin is the best test for identification of iron deficiency in the presence of chronic disease.

Chronic disease anemia:
- Most common causes in older adults:
  - Acute and chronic infection
  - Chronic inflammation
  - Malignancy
  - Protein calorie malnutrition
  - Unidentified chronic disease
- Laboratory tests: usually low iron, low or normal TIBC, high ferritin, low sTfR
- Type determines treatability:
  - "Rheumatoid arthritis type" responds to erythropoietin at usual dosages (see **Table 44**).
  - "Cancer type" may respond to erythropoietin at high dosages (see **Table 44**).
- Restoring Hb to higher levels improves quality of life, function, and possibly survival.

Combined iron deficiency and anemia of chronic disease:
- Anemia often more severe than in chronic disease alone.
- Ferritin low to normal.
- Iron transferrin and saturation reduced.
- Elevated sTfR log ferritin documents iron deficiency; if sTfR is normal, calculate ratio of sTfR/log ferritin (see **Figure 5**) or give iron trial and check reticulocyte count in 2 wk.

Anemia of renal insufficiency:
- Caused by decreased erythropoietin production; check erythropoietin level.
- Restoring Hb levels increases survival, quality of life, and cognitive function, and decreases hospitalization, LVH, and HF. Treatment is erythropoietin (see **Table 44**).

Figure 4. Evaluation of Hypoproliferative Anemia with High MCV

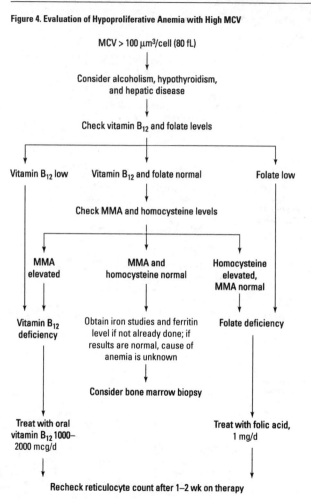

MCV > 100 μm³/cell (80 fL)

↓

Consider alcoholism, hypothyroidism, and hepatic disease

↓

Check vitamin B₁₂ and folate levels

↓

Vitamin B₁₂ low — **Vitamin B₁₂ and folate normal** — **Folate low**

↓ (Vitamin B₁₂ and folate normal)

Check MMA and homocysteine levels

↓

MMA elevated — **MMA and homocysteine normal** — **Homocysteine elevated, MMA normal**

↓ **Vitamin B₁₂ deficiency**

↓ Obtain iron studies and ferritin level if not already done; if results are normal, cause of anemia is unknown

↓ Consider bone marrow biopsy

↓ **Folate deficiency**

↓ **Treat with oral vitamin B₁₂ 1000–2000 mcg/d**

↓ **Treat with folic acid, 1 mg/d**

↓

Recheck reticulocyte count after 1–2 wk on therapy

Source: Balducci L. Epidemiology of anemia in the elderly: Information on diagnostic evaluation. *J Amer Geriatr Soc* 2003; 51(3 Suppl):S2–9. Reprinted with permission.

Figure 5. Evaluation of Hypoproliferative Anemia with Normal or Low MCV

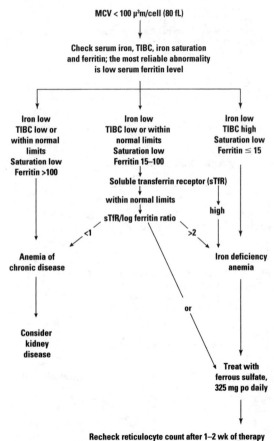

Anemia of B₁₂ and folate deficiency:

- Laboratory tests: anemia or pancytopenia, macrocytosis
- B_{12} deficiency definite at concentrations <100 pg/mL, possible at concentrations of 100–300 pg/mL; check MMA or give trial of B_{12} replacement (see **Figure 5**)
- Treatment: see **Table 44**

Anemia of unknown cause:

- Prevalence: 17% of all anemias after age 65
- May be age-related decline in hematopoietic reserve, low erythropoietin, or poor response to endogenous erythropoietin

PANCYTOPENIA

Unless due to B_{12} deficiency, bone marrow aspirate is indicated; causes include cancer, fibrosis, myelodysplasia, sideroblastic anemia.

Aplastic Anemia

- Increases in prevalence with age
- 50% respond to antithymocyte globulin and cyclosporine

Myelodysplasia

A group of stem cell disorders, refractory anemia with or without ringed sideroblasts.

- Macrocytosis, mild leukopenia, normal or increased platelets
- Cytogenetic abnormalities common, most often 5q deletion
- Treatment supportive
- DiGuglielmo's syndrome related to myelodysplasia; red cell, white cell, and platelet dysplasia often evolves to acute myelogenous leukemia

PRIMARY MYELOPROLIFERATIVE DISORDERS

Polycythemia vera

- Elevated RBC mass
- Normal arterial oxygen saturation
- Splenomegaly, leukocytosis, and thrombocytosis may be seen
- Plasma erythropoietin low
- Treatment: phlebotomy to achieve iron deficiency and hematocrit ≤45 and low-dose ASA

Essential thrombocytosis

- Platelet count >600,000/µL on two occasions ≥1 mo apart
- Normal RBC mass
- Presence of marrow iron
- Absence of myelofibrosis
- Splenomegaly
- No Philadelphia or *bcr-abl* gene rearrangements
- Treatment: For patients at high risk of thrombohemorrhagic events, use ASA and anagrelide (*Agrylin*) or interferon-alpha or hydroxyurea.

Chronic myelogenous leukemia

- Leukocytosis with early myeloid forms evenly distributed in peripheral blood
- Philadelphia chromosome in >95% of cases
- Leukocyte alkaline phosphatase score low
- Treatment: chronic and acute phases—imatinib (*Gleevec*); acute-phase treatment for select patients is stem cell transplantation.

Myelofibrosis
- Pancytopenia
- Splenomegaly and other extramedullary hematopoiesis
- Marrow fibrosis (dry tap)
- Peripheral blood: leukoerythroblastosis, tear-drop cells
- Acute leukemia develops in 5%–20%
- Treatment for patients with symptomatic anemia: androgens, steroids, erythropoietin

Table 44. Treatment of Anemias Associated with Deficiency

Treatment	Formulation and Dosage	Comments
Iron	Ferrous sulfate 325 mg po qd	Higher doses cause more GI adverse events
	Ferrous polysaccharide 150 mg po qd	Fewer GI adverse events
	Iron dextran: Dose (mL) = 0.0442 (desired Hb − observed Hb) × LBW (kg) + (0.26 × LBW). For LBW, see p 1.	For severe deficiency or poor absorption
	Administer test dose at 0.5 mL IM or IV sol (5 gtt/min). Wait 30–45 min. If tolerated, complete dose by slow IM injection (≤50 mg/min). By IV, dilute dose in 500 mL normal saline (45–60 mL/min).	IM administration is painful, done over a few days, problematic for those with low muscle mass
B_{12}	1000 mcg IM every wk × 5, then 1000 mcg IM every mo or 1000 mcg po qd	Monitor K^+ in first wk of treatment
Folate	1 mg po qd	
Erythropoietin	Epoetin alfa (*Epogen, Procrit*) usual dosage 50–150 U/kg SC every wk	Monitor BP, adjust dose based on response; Medicare pays for use in kidney failure and in anemia due to chemotherapy
	Darbepoetin alfa (*Aranesp*) 0.45 mcg/kg every wk	See full prescribing information for titration

INCONTINENCE—URINARY AND FECAL

URINARY INCONTINENCE (UI)
General Information
UI is not a normal part of aging. It is a loss of urine control due to a combination of:
- Genitourinary pathology
- Age-related changes
- Comorbid conditions and medications
- Environmental obstacles

Classification
Potentially Reversible Causes of Incontinence (DRIP Mnemonic)
Delirium

Restricted mobility (illness, injury, gait disorder, restraint)

Infection (acute, symptomatic); **I**nflammation (atrophic vaginitis); **I**mpaction of feces

Polyuria (diabetes mellitus, caffeine intake, volume overload); **P**harmaceuticals (diuretics, autonomic agents, psychotropics)

Common Causes
- **Urge UI:** Detrusor muscle overactivity (uninhibited bladder contractions); small to large volume loss; may be idiopathic or associated with CNS lesions or bladder irritation from infection, stones, tumors. Detrusor hyperactivity with impaired contractility (DHIC) is urge incontinence with a weak detrusor muscle.
- **Stress UI:** Failure of sphincter mechanisms to remain closed during bladder filling (often due to insufficient pelvic support in women and to trauma from prostate surgery in men); loss occurs with increased intra-abdominal pressure.
- **Overflow UI:** Impaired detrusor contractility or bladder outlet obstruction. Impaired contractility—chronic outlet obstruction, diabetes mellitus, vitamin B_{12} deficiency, tabes dorsalis, alcoholism, or spinal disease. Outlet obstruction—in men, BPH, cancer, stricture; in women, prior incontinence surgery or large cystocele.
- **Mixed UI:** Combined urge and stress UI is common in older women. A similar syndrome may develop in men after prostatectomy.
- **Other (rare):** Bladder-sphincter dyssynergia, fistulas, reduced detrusor compliance.

Risk Factors
- Age-related changes (eg, BPH, atrophic urethritis)
- Constipation
- Dementia, depression, stroke, Parkinson's disease
- HF, COPD, or chronic cough
- Impaired ADLs
- Obesity
- Parity

Evaluation
History
- Sudden, compelling urgency suggests urge UI.
- Loss with cough, laugh, or bend suggests stress UI.
- Continuous leakage suggests intrinsic sphincter insufficiency or overflow.
- Onset, frequency, volume, timing, precipitants (eg, caffeine, diuretics, alcohol, cough, medications).

Physical Examination
- Functional status (eg, mobility, dexterity)
- Mental status

- Findings:
  - Bladder distention
  - Cord compression (interosseus muscle wasting, Hoffmann's or Babinski's signs)
  - Rectal mass or impaction
  - Sacral root integrity (anal sphincter tone, anal wink, perineal sensation)
  - Volume overload, edema

Male GU
Prostate consistency; symmetry; in uncircumcised, check phimosis, paraphimosis, balanitis

Female GU
Atrophic vaginitis (see p 188); pelvic support (cystocele, rectocele, prolapse; see p 212)

Testing
- **Bladder Diary:** Record time and volume of incontinent and continent voids, activities and time of sleep; knowing oral intake is sometimes helpful.
- **Standing Full Bladder Stress Test (for patients with symptoms of stress UI):** Relax perineum and cough once—immediate loss suggests stress, several seconds delay suggests detrusor overactivity.
- **Postvoid Residual:** If available, bladder ultrasound after voiding is preferred to catheterization. If >100 mL, repeat; still >100 mL suggests detrusor weakness, neuropathy, medications, fecal impaction, outlet obstruction, or DHIC.
- **Laboratory:** UA and urine C&S; glucose and calcium if polyuric; renal function tests and B_{12} if urinary retention; urine cytology if hematuria or pain.
- **Urodynamic Testing:** Not routinely indicated; indicated before corrective surgery, when diagnosis is unclear, or when empiric therapy is ineffective.

Management
In a stepped approach, treat all transient causes first (DRIP); avoid caffeine, alcohol, and if nocturia is a problem, minimize evening intake of fluids.

Nonpharmacologic Behavioral Therapy (First-line Therapy)
- **Urge and Stress UI:**
  - Bladder retraining, regular voiding (based on bladder diary, or every 2 hr), urgency control—when urgency occurs, sit or stand quietly, focus on letting urge pass, do pelvic muscle contraction, when no longer urgent walk slowly to the bathroom and void. When no incontinence for 2 d, increase voiding interval by 30–60 min until voiding every 3–4 h.
  - Pelvic muscle (Kegel's) exercises—isolate pelvic muscles (avoid thigh, rectal, buttocks contraction); perform 3–10 sets of 10 contractions at max strength daily; progressively longer (up to 10-sec) contractions; follow up and encouragement necessary; consider biofeedback for training if initial instructions are not successful. Learning to use vaginal weights is an alternative method for strengthening pelvic muscles.
- **Cognitively Impaired Persons:** Prompted toileting (ask if patient needs to void, take them to toilet) starting at 2- to 3-h intervals during day; encourage patients to report continence status; praise patient when continent and responds to toileting.
- **Pessaries:** May benefit women with vaginal (see p 212) or uterine prolapse who experience retention or stress UI (see p 89).
- **Electrical Stimulation:** Often effective for urge UI; refer to PT.

- **DHIC:** Treat urge first with behavioral methods; clean intermittent self-catheterization if needed.

Nocturnal Frequency in the Absence of HF

- Two voidings per night is probably normal for older adults.
- Exclude sleep difficulties (see Sleep Disorders, p 199), then consider if the condition is due to excessive output or urinary tract dysfunction.
- Bladder diary with measured voided volumes can be very helpful. If between bedtime and awakening, the patient voids more than one-third of his or her total 24-hr output, this is excessive fluid excretion.
  - All patients should restrict fluid intake 4 h before bedtime.
  - If stasis edema is present, have patient wear pressure-graded stockings.
  - If no stasis edema, a potent, short-acting loop diuretic can be used in the afternoon or early evening to induce a diuresis before bedtime, eg, bumetanide 0.5–1.5 mg titrated to achieve a brisk diuresis.
  - Evaluate for other factors contributing to volume overload or diuresis (eg, HF, poorly controlled diabetes).

Pharmacologic Therapy

There are limited data showing benefit of topical postmenopausal estrogen therapy in urge and possibly stress UI. See **Table 90** for available preparations. See **Table 45** for other therapies.

Table 45. Drugs to Treat Urge or Mixed Urinary Incontinence*

Drug	Dosage	Formulations	Adverse Events (Metabolism)
Oxybutynin (*Ditropan, Ditropan XL, Oxytrol*)	2.5–5.0 mg bid-tid 5–20 mg qd 3.9 mg/d (apply Pch 2 × /wk)	T: 5; S: 5 mg/5 mL SR: 5, 10, 15 transdermal Pch 39 cm²	Dry mouth, blurry vision, dry eyes, delirium/confusion, constipation Pch: Side effects similar to those of placebo; may irritate skin (L)
Tolterodine (*Detrol, Detrol LA*)	2 mg bid 4 mg qd	T: 1, 2 C: ER 2, 4	Dry mouth, blurry vision, dry eyes, constipation, delirium, hallucinations, P450 interactions (L, CYP3A4 and CYP2D6)
Trospium (*Sanctura*)	20 mg qd-bid (on empty stomach) Dose once daily at hs in patients >75 yr old and in those with CrCl <30 mL	T: 20	Dry mouth, constipation, dyspepsia, headache; caution in liver dysfunction (L, K)
Darifenacin (*Enablex*)	7.5–15 mg qd	T: 7.5, 15	Dry mouth, constipation (L, CYP3A4 and CYP2D6)
Solifenacin (*VESIcare*)	5–10 mg qd	T: 5, 10	Max dose 5 mg with ketoconazole or other potent CYP3A4 inhibitors or CrCl <30 mL/min or moderate liver impairment; not recommended with severe liver impairment; blurred vision, constipation, urinary retention, urinary tract infection (L)

For prostate obstruction UI, see benign prostatic hyperplasia, p 171.
* ↑ bladder capacity, ↓ involuntary contractions

Surgical Therapy
- Consider for the 50% of women whose stress UI does not respond adequately to behavioral treatment and exercise.
- Type of surgery depends on type of urethral function impairment, patient-related factors, and coexisting conditions (eg, prolapse).
  - Retropubic colposuspension for prolapse.
  - Periurethral injection for intrinsic sphincter function.
  - Newer minimally invasive techniques (eg, tension-free vaginal tape) should result in substantial improvement or cure in at least 75% of surgically treated patients.

Catheter Care
- Use catheter **only** for chronic urinary retention, to protect wounds such as pressure ulcers, and when requested by patients or families to promote comfort (eg, at end of life).
- Use closed drainage system only; avoid topical or systemic antibiotics or catheters treated with antibiotics. Silver alloy hydrogel catheters reduce UTI by 27% to 73%.
- Bacteriuria is universal; treat only if symptoms (eg, fever, inanition, anorexia, delirium) or if bacteriuria persists after catheter removal.
- Culture best taken from a newly inserted catheter.
- Replace catheter if symptomatic bacteriuria develops, then culture urine from new catheter.
- Nursing-facility patients with catheters should be kept in separate rooms.
- For acute retention, catheterize for 7–10 d, then do voiding trial after catheter removal, never clamping.

Replacing Catheter: Routine replacement not necessary. Changing q 4–6 wk is reasonable to prevent blockage. Patients with recurrent blockage need increased fluid intake and possibly acidification of urine.

FECAL INCONTINENCE (FI)
Definition
Involuntary or inappropriate passing of feces that has an impact on social functioning or hygiene.

Prevalence
Varies by setting. After age 65: 2% of community-dwelling, 14% of hospitalized, 54% of nursing-home residents (38% as a long-term problem).

Risk Factors
Constipation, age >80 yr, female sex (if younger than 80), UI, impaired mobility, dementia, neurologic disease.

Age-related Factors
Decreased strength of external sphincter and weak anal squeeze; possibly increased rectal compliance, decreased resting tone in internal anal sphincter, and impaired anal sensory function.

Causes: FI is commonly multifactorial.
- Overflow: from colonic distention by excessive feces, causing continuous soiling.
- Loose feces: caused by drugs (eg, laxatives, antibiotics), neoplasia, colitis, lactose intolerance.
- Functional incontinence: associated with poor mobility.
- Dementia related: uninhibited rectal contraction, often have UI.
- Anorectal incontinence: weak external sphincter (surgery, multiparity, etc).
- Comorbidity: stroke, diabetes mellitus (autonomic neuropathy), sacral cord dysfunction.

Evaluation
History
- Description of FI (eg, diarrhea, hard feces, etc), including usual bowel habit, change in habit, usual fecal consistency.
- Frequency, urgency, ability to delay, difficulty wiping, post-defecation soiling, ability to distinguish feces and flatus.
- Evacuation difficulties: straining, incomplete emptying, rectal prolapse or pain.
- Functional: communication of needs, need for assistance, toilet access.
- Other: bowel medications, other medications, UI, prior treatment (eg, pads).

Examination
- Examine/palpate abdomen for colonic distention.
- Visually inspect anus.
- Check for prolapse while patient seated on commode.
- Perform rectal examination for tone, volume, and consistency of feces; heme test.
- Observe gait, mobility, dressing, hygiene, mental status.

Laboratory
- TSH, electrolytes, calcium

Bowel investigations
- Abdominal radiograph: may identify colonic distention by excessive feces in the presence of empty rectum
- Colonoscopy: only when pathology suspected (unexplained loose feces, bleeding, etc)
- Anorectal physiology tests: not generally needed for treatment, rarely alter plans even for surgery.

Treatment: Multiple interventions may be required.
Main approach
- Simulate the patient's usual bowel pattern.
- Use rectal evacuants to stimulate evacuation and to establish a bowel pattern.
- Use evacuants in the following order of preference: glycerine suppository, bisacodyl suppository, microenemas (eg, *Enemeez*, docusate 5 mL); phosphate or tap water enemas; digital stimulation for some patients.
- Use antidiarrheals to slow an overactive bowel or to enable planned evacuation with rectal preparations.

Constipation (see p 76): Often plays a role; evaluate (if needed) and treat

Modify fecal consistency to achieve soft, formed feces
- Loose feces: use fiber or loperamide titrated to effect, sometimes as little as qod.

- Hard feces: modify diet; fluids add osmotic agent (MgSO or MgOH are preferred). In poorly mobile people, bran and fiber may exacerbate constipation.

Patient education
- Respond promptly on urge to defecate.
- Use coffee to stimulate the gut.
- Position on toilet to facilitate rectal evacuation: back support, foot stool to achieve squat position.
- Exercise to improve bowel function.
- Those who are able may be taught rectal sphincter exercises (tighten rectal sphincter for 10 sec 50 times/d) using digital rectal examination or biofeedback.

Rectal evacuation and toilet training
- Bowel control is improved with regimens.
- Heed the gastrocolic reflex.
- When no spontaneous bowel action, stimulate with suppositories or enemas (see p 93); those with incompetent sphincters may not retain usual enemas.
- Bed pans should not be used; bedside commodes are not as good as toilets, sani-chairs, or shower chairs.

Nursing-home residents and very disabled older adults: FI is most often due to colonic loading and overflow. Treat as follows:
- Daily enemas until no more results.
- Add a daily osmotic laxative (see **Table 40**) and follow bowel training (above).
- Fecal transit can be stimulated with abdominal massage in direction of colonic transit.

Other therapies
- Manual evacuation may be appropriate in some patients.
- Skin care: Wet wipes better than dry; commercial preparations better than soap and water; toilet tongs and bottom wipers help those with shoulder disease.
- Surgery:
  ○ Full-thickness rectal prolapse usually requires surgery using a transanal approach in frail patients; full continence may not be restored.
  ○ Denervation of the sphincter can be repaired by placation of the puborectalis muscle to the anal canal, which increases the anorectal angle; long-term results are often unsatisfactory.
  ○ Division of the external anal sphincter (as may occur during childbirth) or anal fissure can be surgically repaired; short-term results are good, but long-term results are less satisfactory.
  ○ Selected patients have improved quality of life through creation of a stoma.

PNEUMONIA

Presentation

Can range from subtle signs such as lethargy, anorexia, dizziness, falls, and delirium to septic shock or adult respiratory distress syndrome. Pleuritic chest pain, dyspnea, productive cough, fever, chills, or rigors are not consistently present in older adults.

Evaluation and Assessment

- Physical examination: Respiratory rate >20 breaths/min; low BP; chest sounds may be minimal, absent, or consistent with HF; temperature: 20% are afebrile.
- CXR: Infiltrate may not be present on initial film if the patient is dehydrated.
- Sputum Gram's stain and culture (optional per ATS guidelines)
- CBC with differential: Up to 50% of patients have a normal WBC count, but 95% have a left shift.
- BUN, creatinine, electrolytes, glucose
- Blood culture × 2
- Oxygenation: Arterial blood gas or oximetry
- Test for *Mycobacterium tuberculosis* with acid-fast bacilli stain and culture in selected patients.
- Test for *Legionella* spp in patients who are seriously ill without an alternative diagnosis, are immunocompromised, are nonresponsive to β-lactam antibiotics, have clinical features suggesting this diagnosis, or in outbreak setting. Urinary antigen testing is highly specific for serotype 1 but lacks specificity for other serotypes. Value and use vary by geographic region.
- Thoracentesis (if moderate to large effusion)

Aggravating Factors

- Age-related changes in pulmonary reserve
- Alcoholism
- Altered mental status
- Comorbid conditions that alter gag reflexes or ciliary transport
- COPD or other lung disease
- Heart disease
- Heavy sedation or paralytic agents
- Hyperglycemia (maintain blood glucose between 80 and 110 mg/dL in patients in intensive care)
- Intubation, mechanical ventilation (orotracheal intubation and orogastric tubation preferred)
- Malnutrition
- Medications: Immunosuppressants, sedatives, anticholinergic or other agents that dry secretions, agents that decrease gastric pH
- Nasogastric tubes
- Poor compliance with infection control (eg, hand disinfection)
- Supine positioning (semi-recumbent, 30–45 degrees preferred)

Expected Organisms (in order of frequency of occurrence)

Community-acquired:	*Nursing-home–acquired:*	*Hospital-acquired:*
Streptococcus pneumoniae	*Staphylococcus aureus* (including methicillin-resistant *S aureus*)	Gram-negative bacteria
Respiratory viruses		Anaerobes
Haemophilus influenzae		Gram-positive bacteria
Gram-negative bacteria	Gram-negative bacteria	Fungi
Chlamydia pneumoniae	*S pneumoniae*	
Moraxella catarrhalis	Anaerobes	
Legionella spp	*H influenzae*	
M tuberculosis	Group B streptococcus	
Endemic fungi	*Chlamydia pneumoniae*	

Supportive Management
- Chest percussion
- Inhaled β-adrenergic agonists
- Mechanical ventilation (if indicated)
- Oxygen as indicated
- Rehydration

Empiric Antibiotic Therapy (see Table 52)

Table 46. Treatment of Community-acquired Pneumonia for Immunocompetent Patients by Setting

Clinical Circumstances	Treatment Options
Outpatient, previously healthy	
No recent antibiotic therapy	A macrolide* or doxycycline
Recent antibiotic therapy	A fluoroquinolone ** alone, **or** Azithromycin or clarithromycin plus amoxicillin **or** Azithromycin or clarithromycin plus amoxicillin-clavulanate
Outpatient, with comorbidities	
No recent antibiotic therapy	Azithromycin or clarithromycin or a fluoroquinolone alone
Recent antibiotic therapy	A fluoroquinolone alone, **or** Azithromycin or clarithromycin plus amoxicillin-clavulanate, cefpodoxime, cefprozil, or cefuroxime
Outpatient, suspected aspiration	Amoxicillin-clavulanate or clindamycin
Outpatient, influenza with bacterial superinfection	Amoxicillin, amoxicillin-clavulanate, cefpodoxime, cefprozil, or cefuroxime; **or** A fluoroquinolone
Hospitalized patient	
No recent antibiotic therapy	A fluoroquinolone alone, **or** Azithromycin or clarithromycin plus cefotaxime, ceftriaxone, ampicillin-sulbactam, or ertrapenem
Recent antibiotic therapy	Azithromycin or clarithromycin plus a beta-lactam, **or** A fluoroquinolone alone (regimen will depend on local resistance-sensitivity patterns and previous antibiotic therapy)

(cont.)

Table 46. Treatment of Community-acquired Pneumonia for Immunocompetent Patients by Setting (cont.)

Clinical Circumstances	Treatment Options
Hospitalized patient, intensive care unit	
No concern about *Pseudomonas*	Cefotaxime, ceftriaxone, ampicillin-sulbactam, or ertapenem plus azithromycin or clarithromycin or a fluoroquinolone
No concern about *Pseudomonas* but β-lactam allergy	A fluoroquinolone with or without clindamycin
Concern about *Pseudomonas*	Piperacillin, piperacillin-tazobactam, imipenem, meropenem, or cefepime plus ciprofloxacin; **or** Piperacillin, piperacillin-tazobactam, imipenem, meropenem, or cefepime plus an aminoglycoside plus a fluoroquinolone or a macrolide
Concern about *Pseudomonas* and β-lactam allergy	Aztreonam plus levofloxacin, **or** Aztreonam plus moxifloxacin or gatifloxacin, with or without an aminoglycoside
Nursing-home patient[††]	A fluoroquinolone alone, **or** Amoxicillin-clavulanate plus azithromycin or clarithromycin

* Macrolides: erythromycin, azithromycin, or clarithromycin.
** Fluoroquinolones: moxifloxacin, gatifloxacin, levofloxacin, or gemifloxacin.
† Patients being treated in the nursing home; for treatment of nursing-home patients who are hospitalized, see hospitalized patient or intensive care unit.
‡ Because of the incidence of gram-negative and atypical bacterial pneumonia in nursing-home patients, experts in geriatric infectious disease often recommend expanded gram-negative antibiotic coverage.
Source: Mandell LA, Bartlett JG, Dowell SF, et al. Update of practice guidelines for the management of community-acquired pneumonia in immunocompetent adults. *Clin Infect Dis* 2003;37:1405–1433.

Nursing-home or Hospital-acquired Pneumonia Requiring Parenteral Treatment: Alternative Recommendations

Antipseudomonal cephalosporin (cefepime or ceftazadime) *or*
Antipseudomonal carbepenem (imipenem or meropenem) *or*
β-Lactam/β-lactamase inhibitor (piperacillin-tazobactam)

plus

Antipseudomonal fluoroquinolone (ciprofloxacin or levofloxacin) *or*
Aminoglycoside (amikacin, gentamicin, or tobramycin)

plus

Linezolid or vancomycin (if risk factors for methicillin-resistant *S aureus* are present or if local incidence is high)
For both sets of empiric therapy guidelines, the choice of combination depends on local bacteriologic patterns.

Adapted from: ATS and IDSA Guidelines for the management of adults with hospital-acquired, ventilator-associated, and healthcare-associated pneumonia. *Am J Resp Crit Care Med* 2005;171:388–416.

> Note: The empiric use of vancomycin should be reserved for patients with a serious allergy to β-lactam antibiotics or for patients from environments in which methicillin-resistant *S aureus* is known to be a problem pathogen. For all cases, antimicrobial therapy should be individualized once Gram's stain or culture results are known.

URINARY TRACT INFECTION OR UROSEPSIS

Definition

Bacteriuria is the presence of significant number of bacteria in the urine without reference to symptoms.

- **Symptomatic bacteriuria** usually has signs of dysuria and increased frequency of urination; fever, chills, nausea may be present; pyuria ($>10^5$ cfu/mL) supports the diagnosis of UTI.
- **Asymptomatic bacteriuria** is seen when the same organism(s) ($\geq10^5$ cfu/mL) is found on 2 consecutive cultures in the absence of symptoms of a UTI; no treatment is necessary.

Risk Factors

- Abnormalities in function or anatomy of the urinary tract
- Catheterization or recent instrumentation
- Comorbid conditions (eg, diabetes mellitus, BPH)
- Female gender
- Limited functional status

Assessment and Evaluation

Choice is based on presenting symptoms and severity of illness.

- Urinalysis with culture (do not obtain specimen from catheter bag)
- Blood culture × 2
- BUN, creatinine, electrolytes
- CBC with differential

Expected Organisms

Noncatheterized Patients: Most common: *Escherichia coli*, *Proteus* spp, *Klebsiella* spp, *Providencia* spp, *Citrobacter* spp, *Enterobacter* spp, and *Pseudomonas aeruginosa* if recent antibiotic exposure, known colonization, or known institutional flora

Nursing-Home–Catheterized Patients: *Enterobacter* spp and gram-negative bacteria

Empiric Antibiotic Management

Duration should be at least 7–10 d.

Community-Acquired or Nursing-Home–Acquired Cystitis or Uncomplicated UTI (Oral Route): TMP/SMZ DS, cephalexin, ampicillin, or amoxicillin. Amoxicillin-clavulanate should be reserved for patients with sulfa allergy and for settings with known β-lactam resistance. Fluoroquinolones should be reserved for patients with allergies to sulfa or β-lactams, or for settings with known resistance.

Suspected Urosepsis (IV Route): Third-generation cephalosporin plus aminoglycoside, aztreonam, or fluoroquinolone $\pm$ aminoglycoside.

> Vancomycin should be reserved for patients with a serious allergy to β-lactam antibiotics.

UTI Prophylaxis

Leads to antibiotic resistance; generally not recommended.

HERPES ZOSTER ("SHINGLES")
Definition
Cutaneous vesicular eruptions followed by radicular pain secondary to the recrudescence of varicella zoster virus.

Clinical Manifestations
- Abrupt onset of pain along a specific dermatome (see **Figure 1**)
- Macular, erythematous rash that becomes vesicular and pustular (Tzanck cell test positive) after ~3 d, crusts over and clears in 10–14 d
- Complications: post-herpetic neuralgia, visual loss or blindness if ophthalmic involvement

Pharmacologic Management
When started within 72 h of the rash's appearance, antiviral therapy (see **Table 47**) decreases the severity and duration of the acute illness and possibly shortens the duration and reduces the risk of post-herpetic neuralgias. Corticosteroids may also decrease the risk and severity of post-herpetic neuralgias. (See p 143 for treatment of post-herpetic neuralgia.)

Table 47. Antiviral Treatments for Herpes Zoster			
Agent, Route	**Dosage**	**Formulations**	**Comment**
Acyclovir (*Zovirax*)			
Oral	800 mg 5 ×/d for 7–10 d	T: 400, 800; C: 200; S: 200 mg/5 mL	Reduce dosage when CrCl* <50 mL/min
IV**	7.5–10 mg/kg q 8 h for 7–10 d	500 mg/10 mL	
Famciclovir (*Famvir*)			
Oral	500 mg q 8 h for 7 d	T: 125, 250, 500	Reduce dosage when CrCl* <60 mL/min
Valacyclovir† (*Valtrex*)			
Oral	1000 mg q 8 h for 7 d	C: 500, 1000	Reduce dosage when CrCl* <50 mL/min

* The CrCl listed is the threshold below which the dosage (amount or frequency) should be reduced. See package insert for detailed dosing guidelines.

** Use IV for serious illness, ophthalmic infection, or patients who cannot take oral medication.

† Preferred to po acyclovir; prodrug of acyclovir with serum concentrations equal to those achieved with IV administration.

INFLUENZA
Vaccine Prevention (ACIP Guidelines)
Yearly vaccination is recommended for all adults ≥65 yr old and all residents and staff of nursing homes, or residential or long-term–care facilities. Nursing-home residents admitted during the winter months after the vaccination program has been completed should be vaccinated at admission if they have not already been vaccinated. The influenza vaccine is contraindicated in people who have an anaphylactic hypersensitivity to eggs or any other component of the vaccine. Dose: 0.5 mL IM once in the fall (Oct – Nov) for residents in the northern hemisphere.

Pharmacologic Prophylaxis and Treatment with Antiviral Agents
Indications:
• Prevention (during an influenza outbreak): people who are not vaccinated, are immunodeficient, or may spread the virus
• Prophylaxis: during 2 wk required to develop antibodies for people vaccinated after an outbreak of influenza A
• Reduction of symptoms, duration of illness when started within the first 48 h of symptoms
• During epidemic outbreaks in nursing homes

Duration: Treatment of symptoms: 3–5 d or for 24–48 h after symptoms resolve. Prophylaxis during outbreak: Min 2 wk or until ~1 wk after end of outbreak.

Table 48. Antiviral Treatment of Influenza

Agent	Formulation	Dosage
Amantadine (*Symmetrel*)	C: 100 mg; S: 50 mg/5 mL	100 mg po daily*
✔ Oseltamivir (*Tamiflu*)**	C: 75 mg; S: 12 mg/mL	Treatment: 75 mg po bid × 5 d (75 mg po qd if CrCl 10–30 mL/min); not recommended if CrCl <10 mL/min
		Prophylaxis: 75 mg po qd × ≥7 d up to 6 wk (75 mg po qod if CrCl 10–30 mL/min); not recommended if CrCl <10 mL/min
✔ Rimantadine (*Flumadine*)	T: 100 mg; S: 50 mg/5 mL	100 mg po qd for frail older adults and nursing-home residents
		200 mg po qd for other adults, including those ≥65 yr old
		Decrease dose to 100 mg if adverse events appear
Zanamivir (*Relenza*)**†	Inh: 5 mg/blister	2 × 5-mg inhalations q 12 h × 5 d
		Give doses on 1st d at least 2 h apart

✔ = preferred for treating older adults.
* Dosage adjustments for kidney function, CrCl (mL/min): ≥30 = 100 mg daily; 20–29 = 200 mg 2 ×/wk; 10–19 = 100 mg 3 ×/wk; <10 = 200 mg alternating with 100 mg q 7 d.
** Must be started within 2 d of symptom onset.
† Do not use in patients with COPD or asthma.

TUBERCULOSIS (TB)
TB in older adults may be the reactivation of old disease or a new infection due to exposure to an infected individual. Treatment recommendations differ; if a new infection is suspected or the patient has risk factors for resistant organisms, then bacterial sensitivities must be determined.

Risk or Reactivating Factors
• Chronic institutionalization
• Corticosteroid use
• Diabetes mellitus
• Malignancy
• Malnutrition
• Kidney failure

Risk Factors for Resistant Organisms
- HIV infection
- Homelessness, institutionalization (other than a nursing home)
- IV drug abuse
- Origin from geographic regions with a high prevalence of resistance (New York, Mexico, Southeast Asia)
- Exposure to INH-resistant TB or history of ineffective chemotherapy
- Previous treatment for TB
- AFB-positive sputum smears after 2 mo of treatment
- Positive cultures after 4 mo of treatment

Diagnosis
- PPD with booster 5-TU subdermal; read in 48–72 h; repeat in 1–2 wk if negative (see **Table 49** for interpretation of test results)
- CXR

Treatment
Latent Infection: See **Table 49** and **Table 50**.

Table 49. **Identification of Patients at High Risk of Developing TB Who Would Benefit from Treatment of Latent Infection**

Population	Minimum Induration Considered a Positive Test
Low risk: testing generally not indicated	15 mm
Residents and employees of hospitals, nursing homes, and long-term facilities for older adults, residential facilities for AIDS patients, and homeless shelters	
Recent immigrants (<5 yr) from high-prevalence countries	10 mm
Injection drug users	
People with silicosis; diabetes mellitus; chronic kidney failure; leukemia; lymphoma; carcinoma of the head, neck, or lung; weight loss of ≥10%; gastrectomy or jejunoileal bypass	
Recent contact with TB patients	
Fibrotic changes on CXR consistent with prior TB	
Immunosuppressed (receiving the equivalent of prednisone at ≥15 mg/d for ≥1 mo), organ transplant recipients, patients receiving tumor necrosis factor α inhibitors	5 mm
HIV-positive patients	

Table 50. **Treatment of Latent Tuberculosis**

Drug	Dosage and Duration
INH*	5 mg/kg/d (max 300 mg/d) for 6 or 9 mo; or 15 mg/kg/d (max 900 mg/d) 2 × /wk with directly observed therapy for 6 or 9 mo
RIF	10 mg/kg/d (max 600 mg/d) for 4 mo

Note: INH = isoniazid; RIF = rifampin.
* The preferred treatment for patients not infected with HIV.
Source: Data from: American Thoracic Society. Targeted tuberculin testing and treatment of latent tuberculosis. *Am J Respir Crit Care Med* 2000;161:S221–S247 (also available at http://www.atsjournal.org). *MMWR* 2003; 52:735–739.

Active Infection:

Initial treatment options for adults with active *Mycobacterium tuberculosis* infection in order of evidence-based preference are listed below. Daily observed therapy is preferred for all regimens and must be part of any 5 d/wk regimen. (Note: EMB = ethambutol, INH = isoniazid, PZA = pyrazinamid, RIF = rifampin, RPT = rifapentine)

• INH, RIF, PZA, EMB daily × 8 wk or 5 d/wk × 8 wk, then INH + RIF daily × 18 wk or 5 d/wk × 18 wk or 2 d/wk × 18 wk, or INH + RPT 1 d/wk × 18 wk.

• INH, RIF, PZA, EMB daily × 2 wk, then INH + RIF 2 d/wk × 18 wk or INH + RPT 1 d/wk × 18 wk.

• INH, RIF, PZA, EMB 3 d/wk × 8 wk, then INH + RIF 3 d/wk × 18 wk.

• INH, RIF, EMB daily × 8 wk or 5 d/wk × 8 wk, then INH + RIF daily × 21 wk or 5 d/wk × 31 wk, or 2 d/wk × 31 wk.

Source: http://www.cdc.gov/mmwr/preview/mmwrhtml/rr5211a1.htm#tab2

Table 51. Dosing for Treatment Options for Active Tuberculosis

Agent	Route	Daily	2/Wk	3/Wk
INH	po, IM	5 mg/kg*	15 mg/kg*	15 mg/kg*
RIF	po, IM	600 mg**	600 mg**	600 mg**
RPT	po	10 mg/kg†	—	—
PZA	po	1.5 g (<50 kg)	2.0 g (<50 kg)	2.0 g (<50 kg)
		2 g (51–74 kg)	2.5 g (51–74 kg)	2.5 g (51–74 kg)
		2.5 g (≥75 kg)	3.0 g (≥75 kg)	3.0 g (≥75 kg)
Ethambutol	po	15–25 mg/kg‡	50 mg/kg	30 mg/kg
Streptomycin	IM	10 mg/kg	—	—

* Max: daily = 300 mg; 2/wk = 900 mg; 3/wk = 900 mg
** Max: daily = 600 mg; 2/wk = 600 mg; 3/wk = 600 mg
† Max: daily = 600 mg.
‡ Max: daily = 2.5 g

ANTIBIOTICS

Table 52. Antibiotics

Antimicrobial Class, *Subclass*	Route of Elimination (%)	Dosage	Adjust When CrCl* Is: (mL/min)	Formulations
β-Lactams				
Penicillins				
Amoxicillin (*Amoxil*)	K (80)	po: 250 mg–1 g q 8 h	<50	T: film coated 500, 875 C: 250, 500 ChT: 125, 200, 250, 400 S: 125, 200, 250, 400 mg/5 mL
Ampicillin	K (90)	po: 250–500 mg q 6 h IM/IV: 1–2 g q 4–6 h	<30	C: 250, 500 S: 125, 250 mg/5 mL Inj

(cont.)

Table 52. Antibiotics (cont.)

Antimicrobial Class, *Subclass*	Route of Elimination (%)	Dosage	Adjust When CrCl* Is: (mL/min)	Formulations
Penicillin G	K L (30)	IV: 3–5 × 10⁶ U q 4–6 h IM: 0.6–2.4 × 10⁶ U q 6–12 h	<30	Inj procaine for IM
Penicillin VK	K, L	po: 125–500 mg q 6 h	**	T: 250, 500 S: 125, 250 mg/5 mL
Antipseudomonal Penicillins				
Carbenicillin indanyl sodium (*Geocillin*)	K (80–99)	po: 382–764 mg q 6 h	<50	T: 382
Piperacillin (*Pipracil*)	K, F	IM: 1–2 g q 8–12 h IV: 2–4 g q 6–8 h	<40	Inj
Ticarcillin (*Ticar*)	K	IM, IV: 1–4 g q 4–6 h	<60	Inj
Antistaphylococcal Penicillins				
Dicloxacillin (*Dycill, Pathocil*)	K (56–70)	po: 125–500 mg q 6 h	NA	C: 125, 250, 500 S: 62.5 mg/5 mL
Nafcillin	L	IM: 500 mg q 4–6 h IV: 500 mg–2 g q 4–6 h	NA	Inj
Oxacillin (*Bactocill*)	K	po: 500 mg–1 g q 4–6 h IM, IV: 250 mg–2 g q 6–12 h	<10	C: 250, 500 S: 250 mg/5 mL Inj
Monobactam (antipseudomonal)				
Aztreonam (*Azactam*)	K (70)	IM: 500 mg–1 g q 8–12 h IV: 500 mg–2 g q 6–12 h	<30	Inj
Carbapenem (antipseudomonal)				
Ertrapenem (*Invanz*)	K, F	IM, IV: 1 g q 24 h × 3–14 d IM × 7 d max IV × 14 d max	<30	Inj
Imipenem-Cilastatin (*Primaxin*)	K (70)	IM: 500 mg–1 g q 8–12 h IV: 500 mg–2 g q 6–12 h	<70	Inj
Meropenem (*Merrem IV*)	K (75), L (25)	IV: 1 g q 8 h	≤50	Inj
Penicillinase-resistant Penicillins				
Amoxicillin–Clavulanate (*Augmentin*)	K	po: 250 mg q 8 h, 500 mg q 12 h, 875 mg q 12 h	<30	T: 250, 500, 875 ChT: 125, 200, 250, 400 S: 125, 200, 250, 400 mg/5 mL
Ampicillin–Sulbactam (*Unasyn*)	K (85)	IM, IV: 1–2 g q 6–8 h	<30	Inj

(cont.)

Table 52. Antibiotics (cont.)

Antimicrobial Class, *Subclass*	Route of Elimination (%)	Dosage	Adjust When CrCl* Is: (mL/min)	Formulations
Penicillinase-resistant and Antipseudomonal Penicillins				
Piperacillin–Tazobactam (*Zosyn*)	K	IV: 3.375 g q 6 h	<40	Inj
Ticarcillin–Clavulanate (*Timentin*)	K, L	IV: 3 g q 4–6 h	<60	Inj
First-generation Cephalosporins				
Cefadroxil (*Duricef*)	K (90)	po: 500 mg–1 g q 12 h	<50	C: 500 T: 1 g S: 125, 250, 500 mg/5 mL
Cefazolin (*Ancef, Kefzol*)	K (80–100)	IM, IV: 500 mg–2 g q 8 h	<55	Inj
Cephalexin (*Keflex*)	K (80–100)	po: 250 mg–1 g q 6 h	<40	C: 250, 500 T: 250, 500; 1 g S: 125, 250 mg/5 mL
Cephalothin (*Keflin*)	K (50–75)	IM, IV: 500 mg–2 g q 4–6 h	<50	Inj
Cephapirin (*Cefadyl*)	K (60–85)	IM, IV: 1–3 g q 6 h	<10	Inj
Cephradine (*Anspor*)	K (80–90)	po, IM, IV: 500 mg–2 g q 6 h	<20	C: 250, 500 T: 1 g S: 125, 250 mg/5 mL Inj
Second-generation Cephalosporins				
Cefaclor (*Ceclor*)	K (80)	po: 250–500 mg q 8 h	<50	C: 250, 500 S: 125, 187, 250, 375 mg/5 mL T: ER 375, 500
Cefamandole (*Mandol*)	K	IM, IV: 1–3 g q 6 h	<80	Inj
Cefmetazole (*Zefazone*)	K (85)	IV: 2 g q 6–12 h	<90	Inj
Cefotetan (*Cefotan*)	K (80)	IM, IV: 1–3 g q 12 h or 1–2 g q 24 h (UTI)	<30	Inj
Cefoxitin (*Mefoxin*)	K (85)	IM, IV: 1–2 g q 6–8 h	<50	Inj
Cefprozil (*Cefzil*)	K (60–70)	po: 250–500 mg q 12–24 h	<30	T: 250, 500 S: 125, 250 mg/5 mL
Cefuroxime axetil (*Ceftin*)	K (66–100)	po: 125–500 mg q 12 h IM, IV: 750 mg–1.5 g q 6 h	<20	T: 125, 250, 500 S: 125, 150 mg/5 mL Inj
Loracarbef (*Lorabid*)	K	po: 200–400 mg q 12–24 h	<50	C: 200, 400 S: 100, 200 mg/5 mL

(cont.)

Table 52. Antibiotics (cont.)

Antimicrobial Class, *Subclass*	Route of Elimination (%)	Dosage	Adjust When CrCl* Is: (mL/min)	Formulations
Third-generation Cephalosporins				
Cefdinir (*Omnicef*)	K	po: 300 mg bid or 600 mg qd × 10 d	<30	C: 300 S: 125 mg/5 mL
Cefditoren (*Spectracef*)	K	po: 400 mg bid × 10 d (bronchitis) 400 mg bid × 14 d (pneumonia) 200 mg bid × 10 d (soft tissue or skin)	<50	T: 200
Cefixime (*Suprax*)	K (50)	po: 400 mg q 24 h	<60	T: 200, 400 S: 100 mg/5 mL
Cefoperazone (*Cefobid*)	L, K (25)	IM, IV: 1–2 g q 12 h	Adjust in cirrhosis	Inj
Cefotaxime (*Claforan*)	K, L	IM, IV: 1–2 g q 6–12 h	<20	Inj
Cefpodoxime (*Vantin*)	K (80)	po: 100–400 mg q 12 h	<30	T: 100, 250 S: 50, 100 mg/5 mL
Ceftazidime (*Ceptaz, Fortaz*)	K	IM, IV: 500 mg–2 g q 8–12 h UTI: 250–500 mg q 12 h	<50	Inj
Ceftibuten (*Cedax*)	K (65–70)	po: 400 mg q 24 h	<50	C: 400 S: 100, 200 mg/5 mL
Ceftizoxime (*Cefizox*)	K (100)	IM, IV: 500 mg–2 g q 4–12 h	<80	Inj
Ceftriaxone (*Rocephin*)	K (33–65)	IM, IV: 1–2 g q 12–24 h	NA	Inj
Fourth-generation Cephalosporins				
Cefepime (*Maxipime*)	K (85)	IV: 500 mg–2 g q 12 h	<60	Inj
Aminoglycosides				
Amikacin (*Amikin*)	K (95)	IM, IV: 15–20 mg/kg/d divided q 12–24 h; 15–20 mg/kg q 24–48 h	<60, TDM	Inj
Gentamicin (*Garamycin*)	K (95)	IM, IV: 2–5 mg/kg/d divided q 12–24 h; 5–7 mg/kg q 24–48 h	<60, TDM	Inj ophth sus, oint
Streptomycin	K (90)	IM, IV: 10 mg/kg/d not to exceed 750 mg/d	<50	Inj
Tobramycin (*Nebcin*)	K (95)	IM, IV: 2–5 mg/kg/d divided q 12–24 h; 5–7 mg/kg q 24–48 h	<60, TDM	Inj ophth sus, oint

(cont.)

Table 52. Antibiotics (cont.)

Antimicrobial Class, *Subclass*	Route of Elimination (%)	Dosage	Adjust When CrCl* Is: (mL/min)	Formulations
Macrolides				
Azithromycin (*Zithromax*)	L	po: 500 mg day 1, then 250 mg IV: 500 mg qd	NA	C: 250 S: 100, 200 mg/5 mL, 1 g (single-dose pk) T: 600; Inj
Clarithromycin (*Biaxin, Biaxin XL*)	L K (20–30)	po: 250–500 mg q 12 h ER: 1000 mg q 24 h	<30	S: 125, 250 mg/5 mL T: 250, 500 ER: 500
Dirithromycin (*Dynabac*)	L, F	po: 500 mg qd with food	NA	T: 250
Erythromycin	L	po: Base: 333 mg q 8 h Estolate, stearate or base: 250–500 mg q 6–12 h Ethylsuccinate: 400–800 mg q 6–12 h IV: 15–20 mg/kg/d divided q 6 h	NA	Base: C, T: 250, 333, 500 Estolate: 250 S: 125, 250 mg/5 mL T: 500 Ethylsuccinate: S: 100, 200, 400 mg/5 mL T: 400 ChT: 200 Stearate: T: 250, 500 Inj
Ketolide				
Telithromycin (*Ketek*)	L, K	po: 800 mg q 24 h × 5–10 d	<30	T: 800
Quinolones				
Cinoxacin (*Cinobac*)	K (60)	po: 500 mg bid	<80	C: 250, 500
Ciprofloxacin (*Cipro*)	K (30–50) L F (20–40)	po: 250–750 mg q 12 h ophth: see **Table 96** note IV: 200–400 mg q 12 h	po: <50 IV: <30	T: 100, 250, 500, 750 S: 250 mg/5 mL, 500 mg/5 mL ophth sol: 3.5 mg/5 mL Inj
Enoxacin (*Penetrex*)	K L (15–20)	po: 200 mg q 12 h × 7 d or 400 mg q 12 h × 14 d	≤30	T: 200, 400
Gatifloxacin (*Tequin*)	K (95) F (5)	po, IV: 200–400 mg qd × 7–10 d	<40	T: 200, 400 Inj
Gemifloxacin (*Factive*)	K, L, F	po: 320 mg qd	≤40	T: 320 mg
Levofloxacin (*Levaquin*)	K	po, IV: 250–500 mg q 24 h	<50	T: 250, 500
Lomefloxacin (*Maxaquin*)	K	po: 400 mg q 24 h	<40	T: 400
Moxifloxacin (*Avelox*)	L (~55) F (25) K (20)	po: 400 mg q 24 h	NA	T: 400

(cont.)

Table 52. Antibiotics (cont.)

Antimicrobial Class, *Subclass*	Route of Elimination (%)	Dosage	Adjust When CrCl* Is: (mL/min)	Formulations
Norfloxacin (*Noroxin*)	K (30) F (30)	po: 400 mg q 12 h ophth: see **Table 96** note	<30	T: 400 ophth: 0.3%
Ofloxacin (*Roxin*)	K	po, IV: 200–400 mg q 12–24 h ophth: see **Table 96** note	<50	T: 200, 300, 400 ophth: 0.3% Inj
Sparfloxacin (*Zagam*)	L	po: 400 mg day 1, then 200 mg q 24 h	<50	T: 200
Trovafloxacin (*Trovan*)	L	po, IV: 200 mg q 24 h × 10–14 d	NA	T: 100, 200 Inj
Tetracyclines				
Doxycycline (eg, *Vibramycin*)	K (25) F (30)	po, IV: 100–200 mg/d given q 12–24 h	NA	C: 50, 100 T: 50, 100 S: 25 mg/5 mL, 50 mg/5 mL Inj
Minocycline (*Minocin*)	K	po, IV: 200 mg once, then 100 mg q 12 h	NA	C: 50, 100 S: 50 mg/5 mL; Inj
Tetracycline	K (60)	po, IV: 250–500 mg q 6–12 h	NA	C: 100, 250, 500 T: 250, 500 S: 125 mg/5 mL; Inj ophth: oint, sus topical: oint, sol
Glycycline				
Tigecycline (*Tygacil*)	K, F, L	IV: 100 mg once, then 50 mg q 12 h × 5–14d	NA	Inj
Other Antibiotics				
Chloramphenicol (*Chloromycetin*)	L (90)	po, IV: 50 mg/kg/d given q 6 h; max: 4 g/d	NA	C: 250; topical; ophth; Inj
Clindamycin (*Cleocin*)	L (90)	po: 150–450 mg q 6–8 h; max: 1.8 g/d IM, IV: 1.2–1.8 g/d given q 8–12 h; max: 3.6 g/d	NA	C: 75, 150, 300 S: 75 mg/5 mL crm, vaginal: 2% gel, topical: 1% Inj
Co-trimoxazole (TMP/SMZ, *Bactrim*)	K, L	Doses based on the trimethoprim component: po: 1 double-strength tab q 12 h; IV: sepsis: 20 TMP/kg/d given q 6 h	≤50	T: SMZ 400, TMP 80 double-strength: SMZ 800, TMP 160 S: SMZ 200, TMP 40 mg/5 mL Inj
Daptomycin (*Cubicin*)	K, L	IV: 4 mg/kg q 24 h × 7–14 d	<30	Inj
Linezolid (*Zyvox*)	L (65) K (30)	po: 400–600 mg q 12 h IV: 600 mg q 12 h	NA	T: 400, 600; S: 100 mg/5 mL; Inj

(cont.)

Table 52. Antibiotics (cont.)

Antimicrobial Class, *Subclass*	Route of Elimination (%)	Dosage	Adjust When CrCl* Is: (mL/min)	Formulations
Metronidazole (*Flagyl, MetraGel*)	L (30–60) K (20–40) F (6–15)	po: 250–750 mg q 6–8 h Topical: Apply bid Vaginal: 1 applicator full (375 mg) qhs or bid	≤10	T: 250, 500 ER: 750 C: 375 gel, topical: 0.75% (30 g) gel, vaginal: 0.75% (70 g) Inj
Nitrofurantoin (*Macrodantin*)	L (60) K (40)	po: 50–100 mg q 6 h	Do not use if <40	C: 25, 50, 100 S: 25 mg/5 mL
Quinupristin-dalfopristin (*Synercid*)	L, B, F (75) K (15–19)	Vancomycin-resistant *E faecium*: IV: 7.5 mg/kg q 8 h Complicated skin or skin structure infection: 7.5 mg/kg q 12 h	NA	Inj
Vancomycin (*Vancocin*)	K (80–90)	po: *C difficile:* 125–500 mg q 6–8 h IV: 500 mg–1 g q 8–24 h Peak: 20–40 mcg/mL Trough: 5–10 mcg/mL		C: 125, 250 Inj
Antifungals (see also **Table 32**)				
Amphotericin B (*Fungizone*)	K	IV: test dose: 1 mg infused over 20–30 min; if tolerated, initial therapeutic dose is 0.25 mg/kg; the daily dose can be increased by 0.25-mg/kg increments on each subsequent day until the desired daily dose is reached Maintenance dose: IV: 0.25–1 mg/kg/d or 1.5 mg/kg qod; do not exceed 1.5 mg/kg/d	†	topical: crm, lot, oint 3% Inj
Amphotericin B Lipid Complex (*Abelcet*)	K	2.5–5 mg/kg/d as a single infusion	†	Inj
Amphotericin B Liposomal (*AmBisome*)	K	3–5 mg/kg/d infused over 1–2 h	†	Inj

(cont.)

Table 52. Antibiotics (cont.)

Antimicrobial Class, *Subclass*	Route of Elimination (%)	Dosage	Adjust When CrCl* Is: (mL/min)	Formulations
Amphotericin B Colloidal Dispersion (*Amphotec*)	K	3–4 mg/kg/d infused at 1 mg/kg/h; max dosage 7.5 mg/kg/d	†	Inj
Caspofungin (*Cancidas*)	L	Initial: 70 mg infused over 1 h, then 50 mg/d over 1 h	NA	Inj
Fluconazole (*Diflucan*)	K (80)	po, IV: first dose 50–400 mg, then 50–400 mg qd for 14 d–12 wk, depending on indication Vaginal candidiasis: 150 mg as a single dose	<50	T: 50, 100, 150, 200 S: 10 and 40 mg/mL Inj
Flucytosine (*Ancobon*)	K (75–90)	po: 50–150 mg/kg/d divided q 6 h	<40	C: 250, 500
Griseofulvin (*Fulvicin P/G, Grifulvin V*)	L	po: Microsize: 500–1000 mg/d in single or divided doses Ultramicrosize: 330–375 mg/d in single or divided doses Duration based on indication	NA	Microsize: S: 125 mg/5 mL T: 250, 500 Ultramicrosize: T: 125, 165, 250, 330
Itraconazole (*Sporanox*)	L	po: 200–400 mg/d; doses >200 mg/d should be divided. Life-threatening infections: loading dose: 200 mg tid should be given for the first 3 d of therapy IV: 200 mg bid × 4 d, then 200 mg qd	<30	C: 100 S: 100 mg/10 mL Inj
Ketoconazole (*Nizoral*)	L, F	po: 200–400 mg qd shp: 2/wk × 4 wk with at least 3 d between each shp Topical: apply qd–bid	NA	T: 200 shp: 2% crm: 2%
Miconazole (*Monistat IV*)	L, F	IT: 20 mg q 1–2 d IV: initial: 200 mg, then 1.2–3.6 g/d divided q 8 h for up to 2 wk	NA	Inj

(cont.)

Table 52. Antibiotics (cont.)

Antimicrobial Class, *Subclass*	Route of Elimination (%)	Dosage	Adjust When CrCl* Is: (mL/min)	Formulations
Terbinafine (*Lamisil*)	L, K	po: 250 mg/d × 6–12 wk for superficial mycoses; 250–500 mg/d for up to 16 mo Topical: apply 1–2 times/d for a max of 4 wk	<50	T: 250 mg crm: 1% topical S: 1%
Voriconazole (*VFEND*)	L	IV: loading dose 6 mg/kg q 12 h for 2 doses, then 4 mg/kg q 12 h po: >40 kg: 200 mg q 12 h; ≤40 kg: 100 mg q 12 h If on phenytoin: 5 mg/kg q 12 h, and po: >40 kg: 400 mg q 12 h; ≤40 kg: 200 mg q 12 h	<50 (IV only)	Inj T: 50, 200 mg

Note: NA = not applicable; TDM = adjust dose on basis of therapeutic drug monitoring principles and institutional protocols.

* The CrCl listed is the threshold below which the dosage (amount or frequency) should be adjusted. See package insert for detailed dosing guidelines.

** Dosage should not exceed 250 mg q 6 h in kidney impairment.

† Adjust dosage if decreased kidney function is due to the drug, or give every other day.

ACUTE KIDNEY FAILURE
Definition
An acute deterioration in kidney function defined by decreased urine output or increased values of kidney function tests, or both

Precipitating and Aggravating Factors (Italicized type indicates most common.)
- *Acute tubular necrosis* due to hypoperfusion or nephrotoxins
- Medications (eg, aminoglycosides, radiocontrast materials, NSAIDs, ACE inhibitors)
- Multiple myeloma
- Obstruction (eg, BPH)
- Vascular disease (thromboembolic, atheroembolic)
- *Volume depletion* or redistribution of extracellular fluid (eg, cirrhosis, burns)

Evaluation
- Review medication list
- Catheterize bladder, determine postvoid residual
- Perform UA (see **Table 53** for likely diagnoses)
- Perform renal ultrasonography
- If patient not on diuretics, determine fractional excretion of sodium (FENa):

$$FENa = \left[\frac{urine\ Na/plasma\ Na}{urine\ creatinine/plasma\ creatinine} \right] \times 100$$

(FENa <1% indicates prerenal cause; FENa >3% indicates acute tubular necrosis; FENa 1%–3% is nondiagnostic. Note that some older adults who have prerenal cause may have FENa ≥1% because of age-related changes in sodium excretion.)

If patient receiving diuretics, determine fractional excretion of urea (FEun):

$$FEun = \left[\frac{urine\ urea\ nitrogen/BUN}{urine\ creatinine/plasma\ creatinine} \right] \times 100$$

(FEun ≤35% indicates prerenal azotemia; FEun >50% indicates acute tubular necrosis; FEun 36%–50% is nondiagnostic.)
- Renal biopsy in selected cases.

Table 53. Likely Diagnoses Based on UA Findings	
Findings	**Diagnoses**
Hematuria, RBC casts, heavy proteinuria	Glomerular disease or vasculitis
Granular and epithelial cell casts, free epithelial cells	Acute tubular necrosis
Pyuria, WBC casts, granular or waxy casts, little or no proteinuria	Acute interstitial nephritis, glomerulitis, vasculitis, obstruction, renal infarction
Normal UA	Prerenal disease, obstruction, hypercalcemia, myeloma, acute tubular necrosis

Prevention of Radiocontrast-induced Acute Kidney Failure in High-risk Patients (Cr >1.5, GFR <60 mL/min)
- Nonionic low osmolal contrast agents in low doses
- Avoid closely spaced repeat studies
- Avoid volume depletion and NSAIDs
- Acetylcysteine *(Mucomyst)* (100, 200/mL) 600 mg po bid the day before and the day of procedure
- Sodium bicarbonate (154 mEq/L) 3 mL/kg/h for 1 h before procedure and 1 mL/kg/h for 6 h after procedure

Treatment
- D/C medications that are possible precipitants; avoid contrast dyes.
- If prerenal pattern, treat HF (see p 27) if present. Otherwise, volume repletion. Begin with fluid challenge 500–1000 mL over 30–60 min. If no response, give furosemide 100–400 mg IV.
- If obstructed, leave urinary catheter in place during evaluation and while specific treatment is implemented.
- If acute tubular necrosis, monitor weight daily, record intake and output, and monitor electrolytes frequently. Fluid replacement should be equal to urinary output plus other drainage plus 500 mL/d for insensible losses.
- Dialysis is indicated when severe hyperkalemia, acidosis, or volume overload cannot be managed with other therapies or when uremic symptoms (eg, pericarditis, coagulopathy, or encephalopathy) are present.

CHRONIC KIDNEY FAILURE
Evaluation
- Hx and physical examination: assess for diabetes mellitus, HTN, vascular disease, HF, NSAIDs, contrast dye exposure, angiographic procedures with possible cholesterol embolization, glomerulonephritis, myeloma, BPH or obstructive cancers, current or previous treatment with a nephrotoxic drug, hereditary kidney disease (eg, polycystic)
- Blood tests (CBC, comprehensive metabolic profile, cholesterol, ESR, SPEP, estimate CrCl (see p 1)
- If CrCl 15–59 mL/min, then measure iPTH; if iPTH >100 pg/mL, then measure serum 25-hydroxy vitamin D
- UA and quantitative urine protein (protein:Cr ratio or 24-h urine for protein and Cr); urine immunoelectrophoresis, if indicated
- Renal ultrasound, consider Doppler to exclude renal artery stenosis
- Renal biopsy in selected cases

Treatment
- Attempt to slow progression of kidney failure
  ○ Control BP (target <125/75 if proteinuria or increased Cr); most important
  ○ ACE inhibitor or ARB (see **Table 17**)
  ○ Diabetes control, HbA$_{1c}$ <7
  ○ Moderate dietary protein restriction, 1 g/kg/d (controversial)
  ○ Smoking cessation
  ○ Reduction of proteinuria to <1 g/d, if possible

- Prevent and treat symptoms and complications
  - Treat hyperkalemia if present; restrict orange juice, bananas, potatoes, cantaloupe, honeydew, tomatoes; diuretics and oral bicarbonate can also be helpful.
  - Normalize serum calcium with calcium carbonate (500 mg elemental calcium qd to qid) or calcium citrate if patient is on proton-pump inhibitor or has achlorhydria; if hypocalcemia is refractory, consider calcitriol (*Rocaltrol*) 0.25 mcg/d.
  - Normalize serum phosphate with target goal ≤6 mg/dL; restrict dairy products and cola. When hyperphosphatemia is refractory, begin:
    - If calcium is low, calcium carbonate, calcium citrate, or calcium acetate with meals.
    - If serum calcium is normal or calcium supplementation is ineffective:
      □ Sevelamer (*Renagel*) [T: 400, 800; C: 403].
        - If phosphate 6–7.5 mg/dL, 800 mg po tid with each meal.
        - If phosphate 7.5–9.0 mg/dL, 1200–1600 po tid with each meal.
        - If phosphate >9 mg/dL, 1600 mg po tid with each meal.
      □ Lanthanum carbonate (*Fosrenol*) [ChT:250, 500] at initial dosage of 250–500 mg po tid with each meal, then titrate in increments of 750 mg/d at intervals of 2–3 wk to max of 3750 mg/d.
  - Treat vitamin D insufficiency.
    - If GFR <30 mL/min, iPTH >100 pg/mL, and serum 25-hydroxy vitamin D is <30 ng/mL, then vitamin D (ergocalciferol) 50,000 U po every mo for 6 mo.
    - If iPTH remains >100 pg/mL, then oral vitamin D therapy with calcitriol at 0.25 mcg/d.
  - Correct metabolic acidosis if HCO_3 falls below 18–20 mEq/L with sodium bicarbonate 325–650 mg tid.
  - Treat anemia with iron (if iron-deficient) or erythropoietin-darbopoetin (see **Table 44**).
  - Manage volume overload (see HF, p 27).
  - Prevent and treat cardiovascular disease (see p 24) with target LDL goal <100 mg/dL.
  - Treat secondary hyperparathyroidism; elevated PTH can be treated with calcitriol as mentioned above.
  - Immunize with *Pneumovax* and, before dialysis, hepatitis B vaccines if hepatitis B surface antigen and antibody are negative.
  - Preparation for renal replacement therapy. Educate patients regarding options of hemodialysis, peritoneal dialysis, and kidney transplantation. If estimated GFR <25 mL/min, recommend referral for arteriovenous fistula access. If estimated GFR <20 mL/min, patients can be listed for cadaveric kidney transplant.
- Dialysis is indicated when severe hyperkalemia, acidosis, or volume overload cannot be managed with other therapies or when uremic symptoms (eg, pericarditis, coagulopathy, or encephalopathy) are present.

VOLUME DEPLETION (DEHYDRATION)
Definition
Losses of sodium and water that may be isotonic (eg, loss of blood) or hypotonic (eg, nasogastric suctioning).

Precipitating Factors
- Blood loss
- Diuretics
- GI losses
- Kidney or adrenal disease (eg, renal sodium wasting)
- Sequestration of fluid (eg, ileus, burns, peritonitis)
- Age-related changes (impaired thirst, sodium wasting due to hyporeninemic hypoaldosteronism, and free water wasting due to renal insensitivity to antidiuretic hormone)

Evaluation
Clinical symptoms:
- Anorexia
- Nausea and vomiting
- Orthostatic lightheadedness
- Delirium
- Weakness

Clinical signs:
- Dry tongue and axillae
- Oliguria
- Orthostatic hypotension
- Elevated heart rate
- Weight loss

Laboratory Tests
- Serum electrolytes
- Urine sodium (usually <10 mEq/L) and FENa (usually <1% but may be higher because of age-related sodium wasting)
- Serum BUN and creatinine (BUN:creatinine ratio often >20)

Management
- Daily weight; monitor fluid losses and serum electrolytes, BUN, creatinine
- If mild, oral rehydration of 2–4 L of water/d and 4–8 g Na diet; if poor oral intake, give IV D5W1/2 NS with potassium as needed
- If hemodynamically unstable, give IV 0.9% saline 500 mL bolus and 200 mL/h until systolic BP ≥100 mm Hg and no longer orthostatic. Then switch to D5W1/2 NS. Monitor closely in patients with a hx of HF.

HYPERNATREMIA
Causes
- Pure water loss:
  ○ Insensible losses due to sweating and respiration
  ○ Central (eg, post-traumatic, CNS tumors, meningitis) diabetes insipidus or nephrogenic (eg, hypercalcemia, lithium) diabetes insipidus
- Hypotonic sodium loss:
  ○ Renal causes: osmotic diuresis (eg, due to hyperglycemia), postobstructive diuresis, polyuric phase of acute tubular necrosis
  ○ GI causes: vomiting and diarrhea, nasogastric drainage, osmotic cathartic agents (eg, lactulose)
- Hypertonic sodium gain (eg, treatment with hypertonic saline)
- Impaired thirst (eg, delirious or intubated) or access to water (eg, functionally dependent) may sustain hypernatremia

Evaluation
- Measure intake and output.
- Obtain urine osmolality:
  ○ >800 mOsm/kg suggests extrarenal (if urine Na <25 mEq/L) or remote renal water loss or administration of hypertonic Na+ salt solutions (if urine Na >100 mEq/L).
  ○ <250 mOsm/kg and polyuria suggest diabetes insipidus.

Treatment
• Treat underlying causes.
• Correct slowly over at least 48–72 h using oral (can use pure water), nasogastric (can use pure water), or IV (D5W, 1/2 or 1/4 NS) fluids; correct at rate of no more than 1 mmol/L/h if acute (eg, developing over hours) and at no more than 10 mmol/L/d if of longer duration.
• Correct with NS only in cases of severe volume depletion with hemodynamic compromise; once stable, switch to hypotonic solution.
• When repleting fluids, use the following formula to estimate the effect of 1 L of any infusate on serum Na:

$$\text{Change in serum Na} = \frac{\text{infusate Na} - \text{serum Na}}{\text{total body water} + 1}$$

  ○ Infusate Na (mmol/L): D5W = 0; 1/4 NS = 34; 1/2 NS = 77; NS = 154.
  ○ Calculate total body water as a fraction of body weight (0.5 kg in older men and 0.45 kg in older women).
• Divide treatment goal (usually 10 mmol/L/d) by change in serum Na/L (from formula) to determine amount of solution to be given over 24 h.
• Compensate for any ongoing obligatory fluid losses, which are usually 1–1.5 L/d.
• Divide amount of solution for repletion plus amount for obligatory fluid losses by 24 to determine rate per hour.

HYPONATREMIA
Causes
• With increased plasma osmolality: Hyperglycemia (1.6 mEq/L decrement for each 100 mg/dL increase in plasma glucose)
• With normal plasma osmolality (pseudohyponatremia): Severe hyperlipidemia, hyperproteinemia (eg, multiple myeloma)
• With decreased plasma osmolality:
  ○ With extracellular fluid (ECF) excess: Kidney failure, HF, hepatic cirrhosis, nephrotic syndrome
  ○ With decreased ECF volume: Renal loss from salt-losing nephropathies, diuretics, osmotic diuresis; extrarenal loss due to vomiting, diarrhea, skin losses, and third-spacing (usually urine Na <20 mEq/L, FENa <1%, and uric acid >4 mg/dL)
  ○ With normal ECF volume: Primary polydipsia (urine osmolarity <100 mOsm/kg), hypothyroidism, adrenal insufficiency, SIADH (urine Na >40 mEq/L and uric acid <4 mg/dL)

Management
Treat underlying cause. Specific treatment only if symptomatic (eg, altered mental status, seizures) or severe acute hyponatremia (eg, <120 mEq/L):
• Goal is 0.5 mEq/L/h rise in Na (more rapid correction can result in central pontine myelinolysis); time (in hours) to correct = (140 − Na)/0.5 mEq/L/h.
• Calculate free water excess (liters) = (0.5 × current body weight in kg) × (1 − [Na/140]).
• Target rate of free water removal (L/h) = free water excess/time to correct.
• Replace urine output with 3% saline or isotonic saline.
• Monitor Na closely and taper treatment when >120 mEq/L or symptoms resolve.

SYNDROME OF INAPPROPRIATE SECRETION OF ANTIDIURETIC HORMONE (SIADH)
Definition
Hypotonic hyponatremia (<280 mOsm/kg) with:
- Less than maximally dilute urine (usually >100 mOsm/kg)
- Elevated urine sodium (usually >40 mEq/L)
- Normal volume status
- Normal kidney, adrenal, and thyroid function

Precipitating Factors, Causes
- Drugs (eg, SSRIs, venlafaxine, chlorpropamide, carbamazepine, oxcarbazepine, NSAIDs, barbiturates)
- Neuropsychiatric factors (eg, neoplasm, subarachnoid hemorrhage, psychosis, meningitis)
- Postoperative state, especially if pain or nausea
- Pulmonary disease (eg, pneumonia, tuberculosis, acute asthma)
- Tumors (eg, lung, pancreas, thymus)

Evaluation
- BUN, creatinine, serum cortisol, TSH
- CXR
- Review of medications
- Neurologic tests as indicated
- Urine sodium and osmolality

Management
Acute Treatment: See hyponatremia management (p 115).
Chronic Treatment:
- D/C offending drug or treat precipitating illness.
- Restrict water intake to 1000–1500 mL/d.
- Liberalize salt intake.
- Demeclocycline (*Declomycin*) 150–300 mg bid [T: 150, 300] (may be nephrotoxic in patients with liver disease).

HYPERKALEMIA
Causes
- Kidney failure
- Addison's disease
- Hyporeninemic hypoaldosteronism
- Renal tubular acidosis
- Acidosis
- Diabetic hyperglycemia
- Hemolysis, tumor lysis, rhabdomyolysis
- Medications (potassium-sparing diuretics, ACE inhibitors, trimethoprim-sulfamethoxazole, β-blockers, NSAIDs, cyclosporine, tacrolimus, pentamidine, heparin, digoxin toxicity)
- Pseudohyperkalemia from extreme thrombocytosis or leukocytosis
- Transfusions of stored blood
- Constipation

Evaluation
• ECG; peaked T waves typically occur when K^+ exceeds 6.5 mEq/L. Acute changes of K^+ are more likely than chronic elevations to cause ECG changes.

Treatment
Minor elevations
• K^+ <6 mEq/L without ECG changes:
  ○ Low-potassium diet
  ○ Oral diuretics (eg, oral torsemide or bumetanide, combined oral loop and thiazide-like diuretics; metolazone is the most K^+ wasting); avoid hypovolemia
  ○ Oral $NaHCO_3$ (650–1300 mg bid)
  ○ Reduce or D/C medications that increase K^+
• K^+ 6–6.5 mEq/L without ECG changes: above treatments plus sodium polystyrene sulfonate (*SPS, Kayexelate*) 15–30 g po qd to qid, or prn as enema 30–50 g in 100 mL of dextrose; full effect takes 4–24 h
• K^+ 6.5 mEq/L with peaked T waves but no other ECG changes; hospitalization is decided case-by-case based on acuteness of onset, cause, and other patient factors.
Absolute indications for hospitalization
• K^+ >8.0 mEq/L
• ECG changes other than peaked T waves (eg, prolonged PR, loss of P waves, widened QRS)
• Acute deterioration of kidney function
Inpatient management of hyperkalemia
• Antagonism of cardiac effects of hyperkalemia (most rapid-acting acute therapy; use only for severe hyperkalemia with significant ECG changes when too dangerous to wait for redistribution therapies to work)
  ○ 10% calcium gluconate IV infused over 2–3 min (20–30 min if on digoxin) with ECG monitoring; effect lasts 30–60 min, may repeat if needed
• Reduction of serum K^+ by redistribution into cells (acute therapy; can be used in combination with calcium gluconate, and different redistribution therapies can be combined depending on severity of hyperkalemia)
  ○ Insulin (regular) 10 U in 500 mL of 10% dextrose over 30–60 min or bolus insulin (regular) 10 U IV followed by 50 mL of 50% dextrose
  ○ Albuterol 0.5 mg in 100 mL of 5% dextrose given over 10–15 min or nebulized 10–20 mg in 4 mL of NS over 10 min (should not be used as single agent)
  ○ Sodium bicarbonate use is controversial
• Removal of potassium from body (definitive therapy; work more slowly)
  ○ Diuretics (eg, oral torsemide or bumetanide, IV furosemide, combined oral loop and thiazide-like diuretics; metolazone is the most K^+ wasting). Avoid hypovolemia.
  ○ Fludrocortisone (*Florinef*) 0.1–0.3 mg/d
  ○ Sodium polystyrene sulfonate (*SPS, Kayexalate*) 15–30 g po qd to qid or pr as enema 30–50 g in 100 mL of dextrose; full effect takes 4–24 h
  ○ Dialysis

MALNUTRITION

DEFINITION
There is no uniformly accepted definition of malnutrition in older adults. Some commonly used definitions include the following:

Community-dwelling Older Adults
- Involuntary weight loss (eg, ≥10 lb over 6 mo, ≥4% over 1 yr)
- Abnormal body mass index (eg, BMI >27; BMI <22)
- Hypoalbuminemia (eg, ≤3.8 g/dL)
- Hypocholesterolemia (eg, <160 mg/dL)
- Specific vitamin or micronutrient deficiencies (eg, vitamin B_{12})

Hospitalized Patients
- Dietary intake (eg, <50% of estimated needed caloric intake)
- Hypoalbuminemia (eg, <3.5 g/dL)
- Hypocholesterolemia (eg, <160 mg/dL)

Nursing-home Patients (Triggered by the Minimum Data Set)
- Weight loss of ≥5% in past 30 d; ≥10% in 180 d
- Dietary intake <75% of most meals

EVALUATION
Multidimensional Assessment
In the absence of valid nutrition screening instruments, clinicians should focus on whether the following issues may be affecting nutritional status:
- Economic barriers to securing food
- Availability of sufficiently high-quality food
- Dental problems that preclude ingesting food
- Medical illnesses that
  ○ interfere with digestion or absorption of food
  ○ increase nutritional requirements
  ○ require dietary restrictions (eg, low-sodium diet or npo)
- Functional disability that interferes with shopping, preparing meals, or feeding
- Food preferences or cultural beliefs that interfere with adequate food intake
- Poor appetite
- Depressive symptoms

Anthropometrics
Weight on each visit and yearly height (see p 1)

Biochemical Markers
Serum Proteins: All may drop precipitously because of trauma, sepsis, or major infection.
- Albumin (half-life 18–20 d) has prognostic value in all settings.
- Transferrin (half-life 7 d)
- Prealbumin (half-life 48 h) may be valuable in monitoring nutritional recovery.

Serum Cholesterol (Low or Falling Levels): Has prognostic value in all settings but may not be nutritionally mediated.

MANAGEMENT
Calculating Basic Energy (Caloric) and Fluid Requirements
- WHO energy estimates for adults 60 yr old and older:
  - Women (10.5) (weight in kg) + 596
  - Men (13.5) (weight in kg) + 487
- Harris-Benedict energy requirement equations:
  - Women 655 + (9.6) (weight in kg) + (1.7) (height in cm) − (4.7) (age in yr)
  - Men 66 + (13.7) (weight in kg) + (5.0) (height in cm) − (6.8) (age in yr)

Depending on activity and physiologic stress levels, these basic requirements may need to be increased (eg, 25% for sedentary or mild, 50% for moderate, and 100% for intense or severe activity or stress).
- Fluid requirements for older adults without heart or kidney disease are approximately 30 mL/kg/d.

Appetite Stimulants
- No drugs are FDA approved to promote weight gain in older adults.
- Dronabinol and megestrol acetate (not covered by Medicare Part D) have been effective in promoting weight gain in younger adults with specific conditions (eg, AIDS, cancer).
- A minority of patients receiving mirtazapine report appetite stimulation and weight gain.
- All drugs used for appetite have substantial potential adverse events.

Nutritional Supplements
Protein and energy supplements in older adults at risk of malnutrition appear to have beneficial effects on weight gain and mortality, and shorten length of stay in hospitalized patients.

Many formulas are available (see **Table 54** and **Table 55**). Read the content labels and choose on the basis of calories/mL, protein, fiber, lactose, and fluid load.
- Oral: Many (eg, *Carnation Instant Breakfast, Health Shake*) are milk-based and provide approximately 1.0–1.5 calories/mL.
- Enteral: Commercial preparations have between 0.5 and 2.0 calories/mL; most contain no milk (lactose) products. For patients who need fluid restriction, the higher concentrated formulas may be valuable, but they may cause diarrhea. Because of reduced kidney function with aging, some recommend that protein should contribute no more than 20% of the formula's total calories. If formula is sole source of nutrition, consider one that contains fiber (25 g/d is optimal).

Table 54. **Examples of Lactose-free Oral Products**

Product	Kcal/mL	mOsm	Protein (g/L)	Water (mL/L)	Na (mEq/L)	K (mEq/L)	Fiber (g/L)
Low residue							
*Boost Basic**	1.06	650	37.0	850	37.0	41.0	0
Boost Plus	1.50	670	61.0	780	37.0	38.0	<1

(cont.)

Table 54. Examples of Lactose-free Oral Products (cont.)

Product	Kcal/mL	mOsm	Protein (g/L)	Water (mL/L)	Na (mEq/L)	K (mEq/L)	Fiber (g/L)
Ensure**	1.06	590	35.2	800	34.9	37.7	0
Ensure Plus	1.50	525	54.9	720	41.9	44.8	0
Nu Basics	1.00	480	35.0	842	38.0	32.0	0
Nu Basics Plus	1.50	620	42.4	776	50.8	48.0	0
Low volume (packaged as 45-mL supplements; nutrients are provided per serving)							
Resource Benecalorie	330	NA	7.0	0	15.0	0	0
Epulor	320	418	4.0	0	10.0	0	0
High fiber (can also be given enterally)							
Boost with Fiber	1.00	480	43.0	850	31.0	41.0	12.0
Ensure Fiber with FOS	1.06	500	36.0	780	37.0	40.0	12.0
Clear liquid							
CitriSource	0.76	700	37.0	876	10.0	1.6	0
Resource	1.06	430	33.0	842	24.0	1.3	0
Diabetes formulations							
ChoiceDM beverage	0.93	400	39.0	850	37.0	46.5	11
Glucerna shake	0.93	530	40.0	800	37.0	43.0	12
Enlive	1.25	671	40.0	764	11.6	4.1	0

NA = not available
* Also has "pudding" product that has 240 Kcal/5 oz and 0 fiber
** Also has "pudding" product that has 170 Kcal/4 oz and 1 g fiber/serving

Table 55. Examples of Lactose-free Enteral Products

Product	Kcal/mL	mOsm	Protein (g/L)	Water (mL/L)	Na (mEq/L)	K (mEq/L)	Fiber (g/L)
Diabetes formulations							
ChoiceDM TF	1.06	300	45.0	850	37.0	47.0	14.4
Glucerna	1.00	355	41.8	853	40.5	40.2	14.4
Low residue							
Isocal	1.06	270	34.0	850	23.0	34.0	0
Osmolite	1.06	300	37.2	841	28.0	26.0	0
Nutren 1.0	1.00	315	40.0	852	38.1	32.0	0
Low volume							
Deliver	2.00	640	75.0	710	35.0	43.0	0
Nutren 2.0	2.00	745	80.0	700	56.5	49.2	0
TwoCal HN	2.00	730	83.5	701	63.5	62.7	0
High fiber							
Jevity	1.06	310	44.4	830	40.0	40.0	14.4
Ultracal	1.06	310	44.0	850	40.0	41.0	14.4
Nutren 1.0 with fiber	1.00	320	40.0	840	38.1	32.0	14.0

Important Drug-enteral Interactions

- Soybean formulas increase fecal elimination of thyroxine; time administration of thyroxine and enteral nutrition as far apart as possible.
- Enteral feedings reduce absorption of phenytoin; administer phenytoin at least 2 h after a feeding and delay feeding at least 2 h after phenytoin is administered; monitor levels and adjust dosages, as necessary.
- Check with pharmacy about suitability and best way to administer sustained-release, enteric-coated, and micro-encapsulated products (eg, omeprazole, lansoprazole, diltiazem, fluoxetine, verapamil).

Tips for Successful Tube Feeding

- Gastrostomy tube feeding may be either intermittent or continuous.
- Jejunostomy tube feedings must be continuous.
- Continuous tube feeding is associated with less frequent diarrhea but with higher rates of tube clogging.
- To prevent clogging and to provide additional free water, flushing with at least 30–60 mL of water 4–6 times a day is recommended. Sometimes sugar-free carbonated beverages, cranberry juice, or meat tenderizer can restore patency to clogged tubes.
- Diarrhea, which develops in 5%–30% of people receiving enteral feeding, may be related to the osmolality of the formula, the rate of delivery, high sorbitol content in liquid medications (eg, APAP, lithium, oxybutynin, furosemide), or other patient-related factors such as antibiotic use or impaired absorption.
- To help prevent aspiration, maintain ≥30-degree elevation of the head of the bed during continuous feeding and for at least 2 h after bolus feedings.
- Do not administer bulk-forming laxatives (eg, methylcellulose or psyllium) through feeding tubes.
- Check gastric residual volume before each bolus feeding and hold feeding for at least 1 h if residual is more than half of previous feeding volume. Metoclopramide (*Reglan*) 5–10 mg [5 mg/5 mL] qid may be useful for high gastric residual volume problems once mechanical obstruction has been excluded.

Parenteral Nutrition

Indicated in those with digestive dysfunction precluding enteral feeding. Delivers protein as amino acids, carbohydrate as dextrose, and fat as lipid emulsions.
Peripheral Parenteral Nutrition: For short-term use; requires rotation of peripheral IV site q 72 h; solution osmolarity of <900 mOsm/L is recommended to reduce risk of phlebitis (see **Table 56**).
Total Parenteral Nutrition: Must be administered through a central catheter, which may be inserted peripherally.

Table 56. Caloric Value and Osmolarity of Parenteral Solutions

Solution	Caloric Value (Kcal/L)	Osmolarity (mOsm/L)
Dextrose (%)		
5	170	250
10	340	500
20	680	1000

(cont.)

Table 56. Caloric Value and Osmolarity of Parenteral Solutions (cont.)		
Solution	Caloric Value (Kcal/L)	Osmolarity (mOsm/L)
Lipid emulsions (%)		
10	1100	230
20	2200	330–340

Source: Bçikston SJ. In: Ewald GA, McKenzie CR. *Manual of Medical Therapeutics.* 28th ed. Boston: Little, Brown;1995:36.
Copyright © 1995 by Little, Brown & Company. Reprinted with permission.

SHOULDER PAIN: DIFFERENTIAL DIAGNOSIS AND TREATMENT

Rotator Cuff Tendinitis, Subacromial Bursitis, or Rotator Tendon Impingement on Clavicle

Dull ache radiating to upper arm. Painful arc (on abduction 60–120 degrees and external rotation) is characteristic. Also can be distinguished by applying resistance against active range of motion while immobilizing the neck with hand.

Treatment: Identify and eliminate provocative, repetitive injury (eg, avoid overhead reaching). A brief period of rest and immobilization with a sling may be helpful. Pain control with APAP or NSAIDs (**Table 57**), home exercises or PT (especially assisted range of motion and wall walking), and corticosteroid injections (see p 129) may be useful.

Rotator Cuff Tears

Mild to complete; characterized by diminished shoulder movement. If severe, patients do not have full range of active or passive motion. The "drop arm" sign (the inability to maintain the arm in an abducted 90-degree position) indicates supraspinatus and infraspinatus tear. Weakness of external rotation (elbows flexed, thumbs up with examiner's hands outside patient's elbows; patient is asked to resist inward pressure) is common. MRI establishes diagnosis.

Treatment: If due to injury, a brief period of rest and immobilization with a sling may be helpful. Pain control with APAP or NSAIDs (**Table 57**), home exercises or PT (especially assisted range of motion and wall walking) may be useful. If no improvement after 6–8 wk of conservative measures, consider surgical repair.

Bicipital Tendinitis

Pain felt on anterior lateral aspect of shoulder, tenderness in the groove between greater and lesser tuberosities of the humerus. Pain is elicited on resisted flexion of shoulder, flexion of the elbow, or supination (external rotation) of the hand and wrist with the elbow flexed at the side.

Treatment: Identify and eliminate provocative, repetitive activities (eg, avoid overhead reaching). A period of rest (at least 7 d with no lifting) and corticosteroid injections (see p 129) are major components of therapy. After rest period, PT should focus on stretching biceps tendon (eg, putting arm on doorframe and hyperextending shoulder, with some external rotation).

Frozen Shoulder (Adhesive Capsulitis)

Loss of passive external (lateral) rotation, abduction, and internal rotation of the shoulder to <90 degrees. Usually follows three phases: painful (freezing) phase lasting wks to a few mo; adhesive (stiffening) phase lasting 4–12 mo; resolution phase lasting 6–24 mo.

Treatment: Avoid rest and begin PT and home exercises for stretching the arm in flexion, horizontal adduction, and internal and external rotation. Corticosteroid injections (see p 129) may reduce pain and permit more aggressive PT. Consider surgical manipulation under anesthesia or arthroscopic dilation of capsule.

BACK PAIN: DIFFERENTIAL DIAGNOSIS AND TREATMENT
Acute Lumbar Strain (Low Back Pain Syndrome)
Acute pain frequently precipitated by heavy lifting or exercise. Pain may be central or more prominent on one side and may radiate to sacroiliac region and buttocks. Pain is aggravated by motion, standing, and prolonged sitting, and relieved by rest. Sciatic pain may be present even when neurologic examination is normal.
Treatment: Most can continue normal activities. If a patient obtains symptomatic relief from bed rest, generally 1–2 d lying in a semi-Fowler position or on side with the hips and knees flexed with pillow between legs will suffice. Treat muscle spasm with the application of ice, preferably in a massage over the muscles in spasm. APAP or NSAIDs (**Table 57**) can be used to control pain. As pain diminishes, encourage patient to begin isometric abdominal and lower-extremity exercises. Symptoms often recur. Education on back posture, lifting precautions, and abdominal muscle strengthening may help prevent recurrences.

Acute Disk Herniation
Over 90% of cases have herniation at L4–L5 or L5–S1 levels, resulting in unilateral impairment of ankle reflex, toe and ankle dorsiflexion, and pain (commonly sciatic) on straight leg raising (can be tested from sitting position by leg extension). Pain is acute in onset and varies considerably with changes in position.
Treatment: Initially same as acute lumbar strain (above). If unresponsive, administer epidural injection of a combination of a long-acting corticosteroid with an epidural anesthetic. Consider surgery if recurrence or neurologic signs persist beyond 6–8 wk after conservative treatment. The value of epidural injections and surgery for pain without neurologic signs is controversial. (See **Table 2** and **Table 3**.)

Osteoarthritis and Chronic Disk Degeneration
Characterized by aching pain aggravated by motion and relieved by rest. Occasionally, hypertrophic spurring in a facet joint may cause unilateral radiculopathy with sciatica.
Treatment: Identify and eliminate provocative activities. Education on back posture, lifting precautions, and abdominal muscle strengthening. APAP or NSAIDs (**Table 57**). Corticosteroid injections may be useful. Consider opioids and other pain treatment modalities for chronic refractory pain (see p 151).

Unstable Lumbar Spine
Severe, sudden, short-lasting, frequently recurrent pain often brought on by sudden, unguarded movements. Pain is reproduced when moving from the flexed to the erect position. Pain is usually relieved by lying supine or on side. Impingement on nerve roots by spurs from facet joints or herniated disks can cause similar complaints, although symptoms in these conditions usually worsen over time. Symptoms can mimic disk herniation or degeneration, or osteoarthritis. Lumbar flexion radiographs can be diagnostic.
Treatment: Abdominal and paraspinal exercises, lumbosacral corset. Surgery only in severe cases.

Lumbar Spinal Stenosis
Symptoms increase on spinal extension (eg, with prolonged standing, walking downhill, lying prone) and decrease with spinal flexion (eg, sitting, bending forward while

walking, lying in the flexed position). Only symptom may be fatigue or pain in legs when walking (pseudo-claudication). May have immobility of lumbar spine, pain with straight leg raises, weakness of muscles innervated by L4 through S1 (see **Table 3**). Over 4 yr, 15% improve, 15% deteriorate, and 70% remain stable.

Treatment: APAP or NSAIDs (**Table 57**) and exercises to reduce lumbar lordosis are sometimes beneficial. Corticosteroid injections may be useful. Surgical intervention is more effective than conservative treatment in relieving moderate or severe symptoms; however, recurrence of pain several years after surgery is common.

Vertebral Compression Fracture

Immediate onset of severe pain; worse with sitting or standing; sometimes relieved by lying down.

Treatment: See Osteoporosis, p 145. Bed rest, analgesia, and mobilization as tolerated. Calcitonin may provide symptomatic improvement. May require hospitalization to control symptoms. Percutaneous vertebroplasty or kyphoplasty may be effective for pain relief in refractory cases.

Nonrheumatic Pain (eg, Tumors, Aneurysms)

Gradual onset, steadily expanding, often unrelated to position and not relieved by lying down. Night pain when lying down is characteristic. Upper motor neuron signs may be present. Involvement is usually in thoracic and upper lumbar spine.

HIP PAIN: DIFFERENTIAL DIAGNOSIS AND TREATMENT

Trochanteric Bursitis

Pain in lateral aspect of the hip that usually worsens when patient sits on a hard chair, lies on the affected side, or rises from a chair or bed; pain may improve with walking. Local tenderness over greater trochanter is often present, and pain is often reproduced on resisted abduction of the leg or internal rotation of the hip. However, trochanteric bursitis does not result in limited range of motion, pain on range of motion, pain in the groin, or radicular signs.

Treatment: Identify and eliminate provocative activities. Check for leg length discrepancy, prescribe orthotics if appropriate. Injection of a combination of a long-acting corticosteroid with an anesthetic is most effective treatment.

Osteoarthritis

"Boring" quality pain in the hip, often in the groin, and sometimes referred to the back or knee with stiffness after rest. Passive motion is restricted in all directions if disease is fairly advanced. In early disease, pain in the groin on internal rotation of the hip is characteristic.

Treatment: See also Osteoarthritis, p 129. Elective total hip replacement is indicated for patients who have radiographic evidence of joint damage and moderate to severe persistent pain or disability, or both, that is not substantially relieved by an extended course of nonsurgical management.

Guideline for the Management of Pain in Osteoarthritis, Rheumatoid Arthritis, and Juvenile Chronic Arthritis, 2nd ed., American Pain Society, 2002.

Hip Fracture

Sudden onset, usually after a fall, with inability to walk or bear weight, frequently radiating to groin or knee.

Treatment: Treatment is surgical with open reduction and internal fixation, hemiarthroplasty, or total hip replacement, depending on site of fracture and amount of displacement. For patients who were nonambulatory before the fracture, conservative management is an option.

Nonrheumatic Pain

Referred pain from viscera, radicular pain from the lower spine, avascular necrosis, Paget's disease, metastasis. Treatment based on identified etiology.

PLANTAR FASCIITIS
Definition

Strain or inflammation in plantar fascia causing foot pain that is worse when beginning to walk; 80% resolve spontaneously within 1 yr.

Causes/Risk Factors

- Jumping
- Running
- Rheumatic diseases
- Obesity
- Flat feet
- Plantar spurs

Evaluation

Examiner should dorsiflex toes and then palpate plantar fascia to elicit pain points; posterior heel pain is uncommon and suggests other diagnosis.

Treatment
Nonpharmacologic

- Rest and icing
- Exercises (calf plantar fascia stretch, foot/ankle circles, toe curls)
- Prefabricated silicone heel inserts
- Shoes (running, arch support, crepe sole)
- Short-leg walking cast
- Surgery (rarely needed)

Pharmacologic

- NSAIDs (short duration, 2–3 wk)
- Corticosteroid (eg, methylprednisolone 20–40 mg) and analgesic (eg, 1% lidocaine) injection of fascia; use only if conservative measures fail

CARPAL TUNNEL SYNDROME
Definition

Painful tingling or hypoesthesia, or both, in one or both hands in distribution innervated by median nerve

Causes

- Repetitive activities
- Diabetes mellitus
- Thyroid disease
- Amyloidosis
- Rheumatoid arthritis
- Space-occupying lesions (eg, lymphoma)
- Trauma (eg, Colles' fracture)

Evaluation and Assessment
Physical Examination:
• Decreased sensation in palm, thumb, index finger, middle finger, and thumb side of ring finger
• Weak handgrip
• Tapping over the median nerve at the wrist causes pain to shoot from wrist to hand (Tinel's sign)
• Acute flexion of wrist for 60 sec (Phalen's test) should also cause pain
Laboratory Studies:
• Fasting glucose
• TSH
• Nerve conduction velocity testing confirms diagnosis

Treatment
Nonpharmacologic:
• Redesign work or leisure activities to avoid repetitive movements
• Splinting in neutral position, especially at night
• Surgery (more effective than splinting)
Pharmacologic:
• Injectable corticosteroids, eg, methylprednisolone 15 mg (more effective than oral)
• Oral corticosteroids, eg, prednisone 20 mg/d for 1 wk followed by 10 mg/d for a second wk

RHEUMATOID ARTHRITIS
Diagnosis
Diagnosis established if ≥4 of the following 7 criteria are met (ACR):
1. Morning stiffness in and around the joints, lasting ≥1 hr before max improvement and present for ≥6 wk.
2. Arthritis of 3 or more joint areas simultaneously with soft-tissue swelling or fluid (not bony overgrowth alone), observed by a physician and present for ≥6 wk; the 14 possible joint areas are right or left proximal interphalangeal (PIP) joints, metacarpophalangeal (MCP) joints, wrist, elbow, knee, ankle, and metatarsophalangeal (MTP) joints.
3. Arthritis of hand joints (as defined above) in a wrist, MCP, or PIP joint and present for ≥6 wk.
4. Symmetric arthritis defined as simultaneous involvement of the same joint areas (see #2 above) on both sides of the body (bilateral involvement of PIPs, MCPs, or MTPs is acceptable without absolute symmetry) and present for ≥6 wk.
5. Rheumatoid nodules (which are subcutaneous) over bony prominences or extensor surfaces, or in juxta-articular regions, observed by a physician.
6. Serum rheumatoid factor present (anti-cyclic citrullinated peptide [anti-CCP] may be positive before rheumatoid factor but is not currently a criterion for the diagnosis of RA).
7. Radiographic changes typical of RA on posteroanterior hand and wrist radiographs, which must include erosions or unequivocal bony decalcification localized to or most marked adjacent to the involved joints (osteoarthritis changes alone do not qualify).

Management
Nonpharmacologic
• Patient education
• Exercise
• Physical and occupational therapy
• Splints and orthotics
• Surgery for severe functional abnormalities due to synovitis or joint destruction
Pharmacologic
All patients with established disease should be offered disease-modifying anti-rheumatoid drugs (DMARDs) as soon as possible; goal is to induce remission and then lower dosages to maintain remission.
• Analgesics (see **Table 57** and Pain, p 148)
• NSAIDs (see **Table 57**)
• Glucocorticoids (eg, prednisone ≤15 mg/d or equivalent) with osteoporosis prevention measures (see Osteoporosis, p 145)
• DMARDs (may use ≥1 class; no clear guidelines on which combinations are best and which patients need combination therapy)
  ○ Hydroxychloroquine [T: 200], begin 200–400 mg/d; dose at <6.5 mg/kg/d to reduce risk of retinal toxicity; annual eye examination to screen for retinal toxicity; contraindicated in G6PD deficiency.
  ○ Sulfasalazine (*Azulfidine, Azulfidine* EN-tabs) [T: 500], to avoid GI upset, begin at 500 mg/d, increasing dose by 500 mg every 3–4 d until taking 2–3 g/d split between 2 doses; check CBC and LFTs q 8 wk.
  ○ Methotrexate (*Rheumatrex* [T: 2.5], *Trexall* [T: 5, 7.5, 10, 15]), 10–25 mg/wk, adjust dosage for renal impairment; may cause oral ulcers, hepatotoxicity, pulmonary toxicity, cytopenias, thrombocytopenia (rare), and anemia (rare); avoid in patients with liver disease; check CBC, LFTs q 8 wk; folic acid 1 mg/d should be given with methotrexate to reduce adverse events.
  ○ Leflunomide (*Arava*) [T: 10, 20], begin 100 mg/d × 3 d, then 20 mg/d; may cause hepatotoxicity, cytopenias, thrombocytopenia (rare), and anemia (rare); avoid in patients with liver disease; check CBC, LFTs q 8 wk.
  ○ Anticytokine therapies: increased risk of serious infections and reactivation of latent infections; check PPD and make sure patient is up to date on all vaccinations before starting; hold therapy for any infection.
    ▪ Anti-TNF-alpha agents:
      □ Etanercept (*Enbrel*) 50 mg SC once/wk or 25 mg SC twice/wk
      □ Infliximab (*Remicade*) 3 mg/kg IV in conjunction with methotrexate; repeat in 2–6 wk, then q 8 wk
      □ Adalimumab (*Humira*) 40 mg SC every other week, or 40 mg SC every wk if not taking methotrexate
    ▪ Interleukin-1 receptor antagonist: Anakinra (*Kineret*) 100 mg SC daily

OSTEOARTHRITIS
Nonpharmacologic Approaches
- Superficial heat: Hot packs, heating pads, paraffin, or hot water bottles (moist heat is better).
- Deep heat: Microwave, shortwave diathermy, or ultrasound.
- Biofeedback and transcutaneous electrical nerve stimulation.
- Exercise (especially water-based), PT, OT: Strengthening, stretching, range of motion, functional activities.
- Weight loss: Especially for low back, hip, and knee arthritis.
- Splinting: Avoid splinting for long periods of time (eg, >6 wk) because periarticular muscle weakness and wasting may occur. Bracing (eg, neoprene sleeves over the knee) to correct malalignment is often helpful.
- Assistive devices: Cane should be used in the hand contralateral to the affected knee or hip.
- Surgical intervention (eg, debridement, meniscal repair, prosthetic joint replacement).
- Acupuncture as an adjunct to NSAIDs or analgesics for knee osteoarthritis or chronic low back pain.

Pharmacologic Intervention (see Figure 6)
Topical Analgesics: Liniment, capsaicin cream, lidocaine 5% Pch *(Lidoderm).*
Intra-articular Bursal and Trigger-point Injections:
- Corticosteroids: May be particularly effective if monoarticular symptoms (eg, methylprednisolone acetate, triamcinolone acetonide, and triamcinolone hexacetonide [longest acting]); 20–40 mg for large joints (eg, knee, ankle, shoulder), 10–20 mg for wrists and elbows, and 5–15 mg for small joints of hands and feet; often mixed with lidocaine 1% or its equivalent (in equal volume with corticosteroids) for immediate relief.
- Hyaluronan: Sodium hyaluronate *(Hyalgan)* injections weekly for 5 wk or hylan G-F 20 *(Synvisc)* 3 injections 1 wk apart for knee osteoarthritis.

Nutriceuticals: Glucosamine (500 mg tid) or chondroitin (400 mg tid), or both, have been effective for some patients. Combination tabs and timed-release formulations (1500 mg and 1200 mg, respectively) are available. Clinical trials in the United States are ongoing.

NSAIDs: Often provide pain relief but have higher rates of adverse events (see **Table 57**). Misoprostol *(Cytotec)* 100–200 mg qid with food [T: 100, 200], or a proton-pump inhibitor (see **Table 38**) may be valuable prophylaxis against NSAID-induced ulcers in high-risk patients. Selective COX-2 inhibitors have lower likelihood of causing gastroduodenal ulcers than nonselective NSAIDs. All may increase INR in patients receiving warfarin.

Oral Opioids: Use requires careful risk-benefit analysis (see **Table 69**).

Figure 6. Pharmacologic Management of Osteoarthritis*

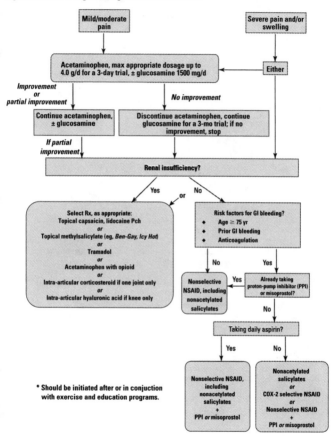

* Should be initiated after or in conjunction with exercise and education programs.

Source: Adapted from original material courtesy of Catherine MacLean, MD, PhD. Reprinted with permission.

Table 57. **APAP and NSAIDs**

Class, Drug	Usual Dosage for Arthritis	Formulations	Comments (Metabolism, Excretion)
✔APAP (*Tylenol*)	650 mg q 4–6 h	T: 80, 325, 500, 650; C: 160, 325, 500; S: elixir 120/5 mL, 160/5 mL, 167/5 mL, 325/5 mL; S: 160/5 mL, 500/15 mL; Sp: 120, 325, 600	Drug of choice for chronic musculoskeletal conditions; no anti-inflammatory properties; hepatotoxic above 4 g/d; at high doses (≥2 g/d) may increase INR in patients receiving warfarin; reduce dose 50%–75% if liver or kidney disease or if harmful or hazardous alcohol intake (L, K)
Extended release (*Tylenol ER*)	1300 mg tid	ER: 650	
ASA	650 mg q 4–6 h	T: 81, 325, 500, 650, 975; Sp: 120, 200, 300, 600	(K)
Extended release (*Ext Release Bayer 8 Hour,* * *ZORprin*)	1300 mg tid or 1600–3200 mg bid	CR: 650, 800	
Enteric-coated*	1000 mg qid	T: 81, 162, 325, 500, 650, 975	
Nonacetylated Salicylates			Do not inhibit platelet aggregation; fewer GI and renal adverse events; no reaction in ASA-sensitive patients; monitor salicylate concentrations
✔Choline magnesium salicylate (*Tricosal, Trilisate, CMT*)	3 g/d in 1, 2, or 3 doses	T: 500, 750, 1000; S: 500 mg/5mL	(K)
✔Choline salicylate (*Arthropan*)	4.8–7.2 g/d divided	S: 870 mg/5 mL	(L, K)
✔Magnesium salicylate* (eg, *Backache, Doan's, Mobigesic, Momentum*)	2 tabs q 6–8 h, max 4800 mg qd	T: 467, 580, 600	Avoid in kidney failure
✔Salsalate (eg, *Disalcid, Mono-Gesic, Salflex*)	1500 mg to 4 g/d in 2 or 3 doses	T: 500, 750; C: 500	(K)
✔Sodium salicylate*	325–650 mg q 4 h	T: 325, 650	
Nonselective NSAIDs			
Diclofenac (*Cataflam, Voltaren*)	50–150 mg/d in 2 or 3 doses	T: 50, enteric coated 25, 50, 75, ER 100	(L)
(*Voltaren-XR*)	100 mg/d	T:100	(L)

(cont.)

Table 57. APAP and NSAIDs (cont.)

Class, Drug	Usual Dosage for Arthritis	Formulations	Comments (Metabolism, Excretion)
✔Enteric coated 50 mg with 200 mcg misoprostol (*Arthrotec 50*);	1 tab bid–tid		(L)
75 mg with 200 mcg misoprostol (*Arthrotec 75*)	1 tab bid		(L)
Diflunisal (*Dolobid*)	500–1000 mg/d in 2 doses	T: 250, 500	(K)
✔Etodolac (*Lodine*)	200–400 mg tid–qid	T: 400, 500; ER 400, 500, 600	Fewer GI adverse events (L)
(*Lodine XL*)	400–1000 mg/d	C: 200, 300	
Fenoprofen (*Nalfon*)	200–600 mg tid–qid	C: 200, 300; T: 600	Higher risk of GI adverse events (L)
Flurbiprofen (*Ansaid*)	200–300 mg/d in 2, 3, or 4 doses	T: 50, 100	(L)
✔Ibuprofen (eg, *Advil, Motrin, Nuprin*)**	1200–3200 mg/d in 3 or 4 doses	T: 100, 200, 300, 400, 600, 800; ChT: 50, 100; S: 100 mg/5 mL	Fewer GI adverse events (L)
✔Ketoprofen (*Actron, Orudis*)	50–75 mg tid	T: 12.5; C: 25, 50, 75	(L)
Sustained release (*Actron 200,** Oruvail*)	200 mg/d	C: 100, 150, 200	(L)
Ketorolac (*Toradol*)	10 mg q 4–6 h, 15 mg IM or IV q 6 h	T: 10 Inj	Duration of use should be limited to 5 d (K)
Meclofenamate sodium	200–400 mg/d in 3 or 4 doses	C: 50, 100	High incidence of diarrhea (L)
Mefenamic acid (*Ponstel*)	50–100 mg tid–qid 250 mg qid	T: 50, 100 C: 250	(L)
Meloxicam (*Mobic*)	7.5–15 mg/d	T: 7.5, 15	Has some COX-2 selectivity (L)
✔Nabumetone (*Relafen*)	500–1000 mg bid	T: 500, 750	Fewer GI adverse events (L)
✔Naproxen (*Aleve,** Naprosyn*)	220–500 mg bid	T: 220**, 250, 375, 500; S: 125 mg/5 mL	(L)
Delayed release (*EC-Naprosyn*)	375–500 mg bid	T: 375, 500	(L)
Extended release (*Naprelan*)	750–1000 mg daily	T: 375, 500, 750	(L)
Naproxen sodium (*Anaprox*)	275 mg or 550 mg bid	T: 275, 550	(L)
✔Oxaprozin (*Daypro*)	1200 mg/d	C: 600	(L)
Piroxicam (*Feldene*)	10 mg/d	T: 10, 20	Can cause delirium (L)

(cont.)

Table 57. APAP and NSAIDs (cont.)

Class, Drug	Usual Dosage for Arthritis	Formulations	Comments (Metabolism, Excretion)
Sulindac (*Clinoril*)	150–200 mg bid	T: 150, 200	May have higher rate of renal impairment (L)
Tolmetin (*Tolectin*)	600–1800 mg/d in 3 or 4 doses	T: 200, 600; C: 400	(L)
Selective COX-2 Inhibitor			
✔Celecoxib (*Celebrex*)	100–200 mg bid	C: 100, 200	Less GI ulceration; do not inhibit platelets; may increase INR if taking warfarin; avoid if moderate or severe hepatic insufficiency; may induce renal impairment; contra-indicated if allergic to sulfonamides (L)

✔ = preferred for treating older adults.

  * Also available without prescription in a lower tab strength.

 ** Available without a prescription.

GOUT
Definition
Urate crystal disease that may be expressed as acute gouty arthritis, usually in a single joint of foot, ankle, knee, or olecranon bursa; or chronic arthritis.

Precipitating Factors
• Alcohol, heavy ingestion
• Allopurinol, stopping or starting
• Binge eating
• Dehydration
• Diuretics
• Fasting
• Infection
• Serum uric acid concentration, any change up or down
• Surgery

Evaluation of Acute Gouty Arthritis
Joint aspiration to remove crystals and microscopic examination to establish diagnosis; serum urate (can be normal during flare).

Management
Treatment of Acute Gouty Flare: Experts differ regarding order of choices:
• Intra-articular injections (see p 129)
• NSAIDs (see **Table 57**)
• Colchicine (more toxic in older adults; more effective if given within 24 hr of symptom onset)
  ○ Oral 0.5–0.6 mg (1 tab) q 1–2 h until symptoms abate, GI toxicity develops, or max dose of 6 mg/24-h period has been given.
  ○ IV 1–2 mg in 10–20 mL NS given over 3–5 min
    ▪ may repeat the following day
    ▪ contraindicated in patients who have had recent oral colchicine

- avoid in patients with kidney or liver disease
- potential for severe bone marrow toxicity
- Prednisone 20–40 mg po qd until response, then rapid taper
- ACTH 75 IU SC or cosyntropin (*Cortrosyn*) 75 mcg SC; may repeat daily for 3 d

Treatment of Hyperuricemia After Acute Flare: Colchicine 0.5–0.6 mg/d for 2–4 wk before beginning any treatment in **Table 58** and continued until serum urate has returned to normal.

Table 58. Medications Useful in Managing Chronic Gout

Drug	Usual Dosage	Formulations	Comments (Metabolism, Excretion)
✔Allopurinol (*Zyloprim, Lopurin*)	100–200 mg qd	T: 100, 300	Do not initiate during flare; reduce dose in renal or hepatic impairment; increase dose by 100 mg every 2–4 wk to normalize serum urate level; monitor CBC; rash is common (K)
Colchicine*	0.5–0.6 mg	T: 0.5, 0.6; Inj	Follow CBC (L)
Losartan *(Cozaar)*	12.5–100 mg qd–bid	T: 25, 50, 100	Modest uricosuric effect that plateaus at 50 mg/d; may be useful in patients with HTN or HF
Probenecid* (*Benemid*)	500–1500 mg in 2–3 divided doses	T: 500	Adjust dose to normalize serum urate level or increase urine urate excretion; inhibits platelet function; may not be effective if renal impairment (K, L)
Sulfinpyrazone (*Anturane*)	50 mg po bid to 100 mg qid	T: 100; C: 200	Inhibits platelet function; may not be effective if renal impairment (K)

✔ = preferred for treating older adults.
* Probenecid (**500** mg) and colchicine (**0.5** mg) combinations (*ColBenemid, Col-Probenecid, Proben-C*) are available.

PSEUDOGOUT

Definition
Crystal-induced arthritis (especially affecting wrists and knees) associated with calcium pyrophosphate.

Risk Factors
- Advanced osteoarthritis
- Diabetes mellitus
- Gout
- Hemochromatosis
- Hypercalcemia
- Hyperparathyroidism
- Hypomagnesemia
- Hypophosphatemia
- Hypothyroidism
- Neuropathic joints
- Older age

Precipitating Factors
- Acute illness
- Dehydration
- Minor trauma
- Surgery

Evaluation of Acute Arthritis
Joint aspiration and microscopic examination to establish diagnosis; radiograph indicating chondrocalcinosis (best seen in wrists, knees, shoulder, symphysis pubis).

Management of Acute Flare
See Gout, management (p 133). Colchicine is less effective in pseudogout.

POLYMYALGIA RHEUMATICA, GIANT CELL (TEMPORAL) ARTERITIS
Definitions and Evaluation
Polymyalgia Rheumatica: Proximal limb and girdle stiffness without tenderness but with constitutional symptoms (eg, fatigue, malaise, weight loss) and sedimentation rate elevated to >50 mm/hr (7%–22% will have normal sedimentation rate), and C-reactive protein; consider ultrasound to demonstrate effusions within shoulder bursae if diagnosis is uncertain.
Giant Cell (Temporal) Arteritis: Medium to large vessel vasculitis that presents with symptoms of polymyalgia rheumatica, headache, scalp tenderness, jaw or tongue claudication, visual disturbances, TIA or stroke, and elevated sedimentation rate and C-reactive protein. The presence of synovitis suggests an alternative diagnosis. Giant cell arteritis is confirmed by temporal artery biopsy.

Management
- Polymyalgia rheumatica management is low-dose (eg, 5–20 mg/d) prednisone or its equivalent. Consider adding methotrexate po 10 mg/wk and folate 5–7.5 mg/d, which may have a steroid-sparing effect. After 2–4 wk, begin gradual taper to lowest dose that will control symptoms and C-reactive protein or sedimentation rate. Some patients with milder symptoms may respond to NSAIDs alone. Monitor symptoms and C-reactive protein or sedimentation rate. Maintain therapy for ≥1 yr to prevent relapse. Consider osteoporosis prevention medication (see p 145).
- Giant cell arteritis treatment should not be delayed while waiting for pathologic diagnosis from temporal artery biopsy. Begin prednisone (1.0–1.5 mg/kg/d) or its equivalent while biopsy and pathology are pending. Consider adding methotrexate po 10 mg/wk and folate 5–7.5 mg/d, which may have a steroid-sparing effect. If no visual loss, then begin prednisone (20–40 mg/d) or equivalent for 2 wk and if symptoms are controlled, gradually reduce dosage. Use low-dosage aspirin (81–100 mg/d) to reduce risk of visual loss, TIA, or stroke. Combine with PPI or misoprostol. Maintain therapy for ≥1 yr to prevent relapse. Consider osteoporosis prevention medication (see p 145). Monitor for development of thoracic aortic aneurysm with CXR yearly for up to 10 yr.

NEUROLOGIC DISORDERS

TREMORS

Table 59. Classification of Tremors

Tremor Type	Hz	Associated Conditions	Features	Treatment
Cerebellar	3–5	Cerebellar disease	Present only during movement; ↑ with intention; ↑ amplitude as target is approached	Symptomatic management
Essential	4–12	Familial in 50% of cases	Varying amplitude; common in upper extremities, head, neck; ↑ with antigravity movements, intention, stress, medications	Long-acting propranolol or atenolol (see **Table 20**); or primidone (*Mysoline*) 100 mg qhs start, titrate to 0.5–1.0 g/d in 3–4 divided doses [T: 50, 250; S: 250 mg/5 mL]; or gabapentin (see **Table 63**)
Parkinson's	3–7	Parkinson's disease, parkinsonism	"Pill rolling;" present at rest; ↑ with emotional stress or when examiner calls attention to it; commonly asymmetric	See Parkinson's disease (p 139)
Physiologic	8–12	Normal	Low amplitude; ↑ with stress, anxiety, emotional upset, lack of sleep, fatigue, toxins, medications	Treatment of exacerbating factor

DIZZINESS

Table 60. Classification of Dizziness

Primary Symptom	Features	Duration	Diagnosis	Management
Dizziness	Lightheadedness 1–30 min after standing	Seconds to minutes (E)	Orthostatic hypotension	See **Table 37**
	Impairment in >1 of the following: vision, vestibular function, spinal proprioception, cerebellum, lower-extremity peripheral nerves	Occurs with ambulation (C)	Multiple sensory impairments	Correct or maximize sensory deficits; PT for balance and strength training
	Unsteady gait with short steps; ↑ reflexes and/or tone	Occurs with ambulation (C)	Ischemic cerebral disease	Aspirin; modification of vascular risk factors; PT
	Provoked by head or neck movement; reduced neck range of motion	Seconds to minutes (E)	Cervical spondylosis	Behavior modification; reduce cervical spasm and inflammation

(cont.)

		Table 60. Classification of Dizziness (cont.)		
Primary Symptom	Features	Duration	Diagnosis	Management
Drop attacks	Provoked by head or neck movement, reduced vertebral artery flow seen on Doppler or angiography	Seconds to minutes (E)	Postural impingement of vertebral artery	Behavior modification
Vertigo	Brought on by position change, positive Dix-Hallpike test	Seconds to minutes (E)	Benign paroxysmal positional vertigo	Epley's maneuver to reposition crystalline debris; exercises provoking symptoms may be of help
	Acute onset, nonpositional	Days	Labyrinthitis (vestibular neuronitis)	Methylprednisolone, 100 mg po qd × 3 d with subsequent gradual taper over 3 wk to improve vestibular function recovery; meclizine (**Table 41**) for acute symptom relief
	Low-frequency sensorineural hearing loss and tinnitus	Minutes to hours (E)	Ménière's disease	Meclizine for acute symptom relief; diuretics and/or salt restriction for prophylaxis
	Vascular disease risk factors, cranial nerve abnormalities	10 min to several hours (E)	TIAs	Aspirin; modification of vascular risk factors

Note: C = chronic; E = episodic.

MANAGEMENT OF ACUTE STROKE
Attempt to Diagnose Cause
Examination:
- Cardiac (murmurs, arrhythmias, enlargement)
- Neurologic (serial examinations)
- Optic fundi
- Vascular (carotids and other peripheral pulses)

Tests:
- ABG
- Brain imaging
- BUN
- CBC
- LFTs
- Creatinine
- ECG
- Glucose
- Electrolytes
- ESR
- PT, PTT, INR

Transesophageal echocardiography is preferred over transthoracic echocardiography for detection of cardiogenic emboli. Carotid duplex and transcranial Doppler studies can detect carotid and vertebrobasilar embolic sources, respectively. Magnetic resonance angiography is indicated if one is considering emergent thrombolytic therapy to reverse stroke progression within 6 h of onset of symptoms (thrombolytic therapy is of unproven benefit in older adults).

Provide Supportive Care
• Do not lower BP if SBP <220 or if DBP <120; higher BP should be lowered *gently*.
• Correct metabolic and hydration imbalances.
• Detect and treat coronary ischemia, HF, arrhythmias.
• Monitor and treat for hypoxia and hyperthermia.
• Monitor for depression.
• Refer to rehabilitation when medically stable.

Stop or Reverse Progression
Acute Noncardioembolic Stroke, Progressing Stroke, Crescendo TIAs, or TIA: Use ASA, 160–325 mg/d, begun within 48 h of onset. The benefit of emergent thrombolytic therapy is unproven in older adults and should be considered on a case-by-case basis. Anticoagulants are not recommended.
Cardioembolic Stroke: Wait at least 48 h after symptom onset to begin anticoagulation (see also p 18).
Hemorrhagic Stroke: Supportive care.

STROKE PREVENTION
Risk Factor Modification
• Stop smoking.
• Reduce SBP (goal <140 mm Hg).
• Lower serum LDL (goal <130 mg/dL; <100 mg/dL for those with prior stroke, TIA, CAD, diabetes mellitus).
• Start anticoagulation (see p 18) or antiplatelet therapy for atrial fibrillation.

Antiplatelet Therapy for Patients With Prior TIA or Stroke
• First-line therapy is ASA 81–325 mg qd.
• Clopidogrel (*Plavix*) 75 mg qd [T: 75] if intolerant to ASA or ASA ineffective.
• Ticlopidine (*Ticlid*) 250 mg bid [T: 250]; monitor CBC and differential.
• Addition of a combination form of ASA and long-acting dipyridamole (*Aggrenox*) 1 tab bid [T: 25/200] may provide additional benefit.
• In the absence of atrial fibrillation, warfarin therapy is no more effective and is associated with more bleeding than ASA in preventing strokes.

Table 61. Treatment Options for Carotid Stenosis

Presentation	% Stenosis	Preferred Treatment	Comments
Prior TIA or stroke	≥70	CE	CE superior to medical therapy only if patient is reasonable surgical risk and facility has track record of low complication rate for CE (<5%)
Prior TIA or stroke	50–69	CE or MM	Serial carotid Doppler testing may identify rapidly developing plaques
Prior TIA or stroke	<50	MM	CE of no proven benefit in this situation
Asymptomatic	≥80	CE or MM	CE should be considered only for the most healthy
Asymptomatic	<80	MM	CE of no proven benefit in this situation

Note: CE = carotid endarterectomy (or carotid angioplasty with stent placement in selected patients); MM = medical management.

PARKINSON'S DISEASE
Parkinson's Disease Diagnosis Requires:
• Bradykinesia, eg,
  ○ Slowness of initiation of voluntary movements (eg, glue-footedness when starting to walk)
  ○ Reduced speed and amplitude of repetitive movements (eg, tapping index finger and thumb together)
  ○ Difficulty switching from one motor program to another (eg, multiple steps to turn during gait testing)
• **and** one or more of the following:
  ○ Muscular rigidity (eg, cogwheeling)
  ○ 4–6 Hz resting tremor
  ○ Impaired righting reflex (eg, retropulsed during sternal nudge)

Nonpharmacologic Management
• Patient education is essential, and support groups are often helpful; see p 240 for telephone numbers, Web sites.
• Monitor for orthostatic hypotension (see **Table 37** for management).
• Exercise program
• Surgical therapies can be considered for disabling symptoms refractory to medical therapy. Tremor can be improved by thalamotomy or thalamic stimulation (fewer adverse events). Dyskinesias can be treated by pallidotomy or pallidal and subthalamic stimulation.

Pharmacologic Treatment (see Table 62)
• Begin treatment when symptoms interfere with function.
• Start at low dose and titrate upward gradually.
• Monitor orthostatic BP during titration of medications.

Table 62. Drugs for Parkinson's Disease

Class, Drug	Initial Dosage	Formulations	Comments (Metabolism, Excretion)
Dopamine			
✔ Carbidopa-levodopa* (*Sinemet*)	1/2 tab of 25/100 qd or bid	T: 10/100, 25/100, 25/250	Mainstay of Parkinson's disease therapy; increase dose by 1/2-1 tab q 1-2 wk to achieve minimal target dose of 1 tab tid; then titrate upward gradually as needed; watch for GI adverse events, orthostatic hypotension, confusion (L)
✔ Sustained-release carbidopa-levodopa* (*Sinemet CR*)	1 tab qd	T: 25/100, 50/200	Useful at daily dopamine requirement ≥300 mg; slower absorption than carbidopa-levodopa; can improve motor fluctuations (L)
Carbidopa-levodopa & entacapone (*Stalevo*)	1 tab qd	T: 12.5/50/200; 25/100/200; 37.5/150/200	Should be used only after individual dosages of carbidopa, levodopa, and entacapone have been established (L, K)

(cont.)

Table 62. Drugs for Parkinson's Disease (cont.)

Class, Drug	Initial Dosage	Formulations	Comments (Metabolism, Excretion)
Dopamine Agonists			More CNS adverse events than dopamine
Bromocriptine (*Parlodel*)	1.25 mg qd or bid	T: 2.5; C: 5	Increase by 1.25-mg increments every 2–5 d, titrating to effective dose (10–30 mg/d); very expensive (L)
Pergolide (*Permax*)	0.05 mg qd	T: 0.05, 0.25, 1	Increase by 0.05 mg q 2–3 d, titrating to effective dose (1–3 mg/d); expensive; may cause restrictive valvular heart disease (K)
✔ Pramipexole* (*Mirapex*)	0.125 qd	T: 0.125, 0.25, 0.5, 1, 1.5	Increase gradually to effective dose (0.5–1.5 mg tid) (K)
✔ Ropinirole* (*Requip*)	0.25 mg qd	T: 0.25, 0.5, 1, 2, 3, 4, 5	Increase gradually to effective dose (up to 1–8 mg tid) (L)
Catechol O-Methyl-transferase (COMT) Inhibitors			Adjunctive therapy with L-dopa
✔ Tolcapone (*Tasmar*)	100 mg tid	T: 100, 200	Monitor LFTs q 6 mo (L, K)
✔ Entacapone (*Comtan*)	200 mg with each L-dopa dose	T: 200	Watch for nausea, orthostatic hypotension (K)
Anticholinergics			
Benztropine (*Cogentin*)	0.5 mg po qd	T: 0.5, 1, 2	Can cause confusion and delirium; helpful for drooling (L, K)
Trihexyphenidyl (*Artane, Trihexy*)	1 mg qd	T: 2, 5; S: 2 mg/5 mL	Same as above (L, K)*
Dopamine Reuptake Inhibitor			
Amantadine (*Symmetrel*)	100 mg qd–bid	T: 100; C: 100; S: 50 mg/5 mL	Useful in early and late Parkinson's disease; watch closely for CNS adverse events; do not D/C abruptly (K)
MAO B Inhibitor			
Selegiline (*Carbex, Eldepryl*)	5 mg bid qam and noon	T: 5	Symptomatic benefit; not proved to be neuroprotective; expensive (L, K)

✔ = preferred for treating older adults.

* = first-line therapy.

SEIZURES

Classification
- Generalized: All areas of brain affected with alteration in consciousness.
- Partial: Focal brain area affected, not necessarily with alteration in consciousness; can progress to generalized type.

Evaluation, Assessment
Initial:
- History: Neurologic disorders, trauma, drug and alcohol use
- Physical examination: General, with careful neurologic

- Routine tests: BUN, calcium, CBC, creatinine, ECG, EEG, electrolytes, glucose, head CT, LFTs, magnesium
- Tests as indicated: Head MRI, lumbar puncture, oxygen saturation, urine toxic or drug screen

Common Causes:

- Advanced dementia
- CNS infection
- Drug or alcohol withdrawal

- Idiopathic causes
- Metabolic disorders
- Prior stroke (most common)

- Toxins
- Trauma
- Tumor

Management

- Treat underlying causes.
- Institute antiepileptic therapy (see **Table 63**). Virtually all antiepileptic drugs can cause sedation and ataxia.

Table 63. Antiepileptic Therapy in Older Adults

Drug	Dosage (mg)	Target Blood Concentration (mcg/mL)	Formulations	Comments (Metabolism, Excretion)
Carbamazepine (*Tegretol*) (*Tegretol XR*)	200–600 bid	4–12	T: 200 ChT: 100 S: 100/5 mL T: 100, 200, 400 C: CR 200, 300	Many drug interactions; mood stabilizer; may cause SIADH, thrombocytopenia, leukopenia (L, K)
Gabapentin (*Neurontin*)	300–600 tid	NA	C: 100, 300, 400 T: 600, 800 S: 250/5 mL	Used as adjunct to other agents; adjust dosage on basis of CrCl (K)
Lamotrigine (*Lamictal*)	100–300 bid	2–4	T: 25, 100, 150, 200 ChT: 2, 5, 25	Prolongs PR interval; risk of severe rash; when used with valproic acid, begin at 25 mg qod, titrate to 25–100 mg bid (L, K)
Levetiracetam (*Keppra*)	500–1500 q 12 h	NA	T: 250, 500, 750	Reduce dosage in renal impairment: CrCl 30–50: 250–750 q 12 h CrCl 10–30: 250–500 q 12 h CrCl <10: 500–1000 q 24 h
Oxcarbazepine (*Trileptal*)	300–1200 bid	NA	T: 150, 300, 600 ChT: 2, 5, 25 S: 300/5 mL	Can cause hyponatremia, leukopenia (L)
Phenobarbital (*Luminal*)	30–60 bid–tid	20–40	T: 15, 16, 30, 32, 60, 100 S: 20/5 mL	Many drug interactions; not recommended for use in older adults (L)
Phenytoin (*Dilantin*)	200–300 qd	5–20*	C: 30, 100 ChT: 50 S: 125/5 mL	Many drug interactions; exhibits nonlinear pharmacokinetics (L)
Tiagabine (*Gabitril Filmtabs*)	2–12 bid–tid	NA	T: 2, 4, 12, 16, 20	Adverse-event profile in older adults less well described (L)

(cont.)

Table 63. Antiepileptic Therapy in Older Adults (cont.)

Drug	Dosage (mg)	Target Blood Concentration (mcg/mL)	Formulations	Comments (Metabolism, Excretion)
Topiramate (*Topamax*)	25–100 qd–bid	NA	T: 25, 100, 200 C, sprinkle: 15, 25	May affect cognitive functioning at high doses (L, K)
Valproic acid (*Depacon, Depakene, Depakote*)	250–750 bid–tid	50–100	T: ER 125, 250, 500 C: 125, 250 S: 250/5 mL	Can cause weight gain, tremor, hair loss; several drug interactions; mood stabilizer; monitor LFTs and platelets; SR preparation (*Depakote ER*) also available [T: 500] (L)
Zonisamide (*Zonegran*)	100–400 qd	NA	C: 100	Anorexia; contraindicated in patients with sulfonamide allergy

Note: NA = not available.

* Phenytoin is extensively bound to plasma albumin. In cases of hypoalbuminemia or marked renal insufficiency, calculate adjusted phenytoin concentration (C):

$$C_{adjusted} = \frac{C_{observed}\,(mcg/mL)}{0.2 \times albumin\,(g/dL) + 0.1}$$

If creatinine clearance <10 mL/min, use:

$$C_{adjusted} = \frac{C_{observed}\,(mcg/mL)}{0.1 \times albumin\,(g/dL) + 0.1}$$

Obtaining a free phenytoin level is an alternative method of monitoring phenytoin in cases of hypoalbuminemia or marked renal insufficiency.

APHASIA

Table 64. Aphasias in Which Repetition Is Impaired

Type	Fluency	Auditory Comprehension	Associated Neurologic Deficits	Comments
Broca's	−	+	Right hemiparesis	Patient aware of deficit; high rate of associated depression; message board helpful for communication
Wernicke's	+	−	Often none	Patient frequently unaware of deficit; speech content usually unintelligible; therapy often focuses on visually based communication
Conduction	+	+	Occasional right facial weakness	Patient usually aware of deficit; speech content usually intelligible
Global	−	−	Right hemiplegia with right field cut	Most commonly due to left middle cerebral artery thrombosis, which has a poor prognosis for meaningful speech recovery

Note: + = present; − = absent

PERIPHERAL NEUROPATHY
Diagnosis
See **Figure 7**.

Treatment
Prevention of Complications:
• Protect distal extremities from trauma—appropriate shoe size, daily foot inspections, good skin care, avoidance of barefoot walking.
• Maintain tight glycemic control in diabetic neuropathy.
Treatment of Painful Neuropathy: Start at low dosage, increase as needed and tolerated:
• Nortriptyline (*Aventyl, Pamelor*) 10–100 mg qhs [T: 10, 25, 50, 75]; desipramine (*Norpramin*) 10–75 mg qam [T: 10, 25, 50, 75]
• Gabapentin (*Neurontin*) can begin 100–200 mg qhs but may need up to 100–600 mg tid [C: 100, 300, 400; T: 600, 800; S: 250/5 mL]
• Pregabalin *(Lyrica)* 75–300 mg po bid [C: 25, 50, 75, 100, 150, 200, 225, 300]
• Other oral agents that may be effective include:
  ○ Carbamazepine (*Tegretol*) 200–400 mg tid [T: 200; ChT: 100; S: 100 mg/5 mL]; (*Tegretol XR*) 200 mg bid [T: 100, 200, 400; C: CR 200, 300]
  ○ Duloxetine (*Cymbalta*) 60 mg qd [C: 20, 30, 60]
  ○ SSRIs (**Table 28**) have not been shown to be as effective as tricyclics
  ○ Lamotrigine (*Lamictal,* see **Table 63**) 400–600 mg/d
  ○ Opioids (**Table 69**); watch for adverse events of itching, mood changes, weakness, confusion
  ○ Tramadol (*Ultram,* see **Table 69**) 200–400 mg/d
• Topical agents that may be effective include:
  ○ Capsaicin cream (eg, *Zostrix*) 0.075% applied tid–qid [0.025%, 0.075%]
  ○ Transcutaneous electrical nerve stimulation
  ○ Lidocaine 5% Pch (*Lidoderm*) 1–3 patches covering the affected area up to 24 h/d [700-mg Pch]

Figure 7. Diagnosis of Peripheral Neuropathy

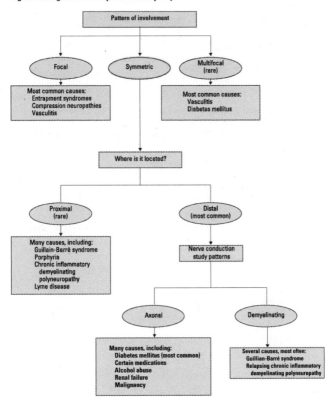

Source: Data from Poncelet AN. An algorithm for the evaluation of peripheral neuropathy. *Am Fam Phys.* 1998;57(4):755–764.

OSTEOPOROSIS

COMMONLY USED DEFINITIONS
- Established osteoporosis: occurrence of a minimal trauma fracture of any bone (WHO).
- Osteoporosis: a skeletal disorder characterized by compromised bone strength (bone density and bone quality) predisposing to an increased risk of fracture (NIH Consensus Development Panel. Osteoporosis prevention, diagnosis, and therapy. *JAMA* 2001; 285 (6):785–795.)
- Osteoporosis: BMD 2.5 SD or more below that of younger normal individuals (T score) (WHO). Some experts prefer to use Z score, which compares an individual with a population adjusted for age, sex, and race. For each SD decrement in BMD, hip fracture risk increases about 2-fold; for each SD increment in BMD, hip fracture risk is about halved.

RISK FACTORS FOR OSTEOPOROTIC FRACTURE
- Previous fracture as adult
- Dementia
- Depression
- Low calcium intake
- Impaired vision
- Low physical activity
- Fracture in 1st-degree relative
- Frailty
- Alcoholism
- Female sex
- Weight <127 lb if female
- Cigarette smoking
- Early menopause (<45 yr)
- Recurrent falls

TOXINS AND MEDICATIONS THAT CAN CAUSE OR AGGRAVATE OSTEOPOROSIS
- Alcohol (>2 drinks/d)
- Anticonvulsants
- Corticosteroids
- Heparin
- Lithium
- Nicotine (ie, smoking)
- Phenytoin
- Thyroxine (if overreplaced or in suppressive dosage)

EVALUATION
BMD at least once after age 65 (see **Table 75**). Uncertain how often to repeat. Some suggest in 3 yr for patients with osteopenia and in 5 yr for those with normal bone density. The value of monitoring BMD in persons already receiving treatment is unproved. Some experts recommend excluding secondary causes (serum 25-hydroxy vitamin D, serum PTH, TSH, calcium, phosphorus, albumin, alkaline phosphatase, bioavailable testosterone in men, kidney and liver function tests, CBC, UA, electrolytes, protein electrophoresis). Less consensus on 24-h urinary calcium excretion, cortisol, antibodies associated with gluten-enteropathy.

MANAGEMENT
Universal Recommendations
- Calcium 1200 mg/d. For most patients, calcium carbonate is sufficient and least expensive. For patients on proton-pump inhibitors (see **Table 38**) or who have achlorhydria, calcium citrate should be used.
- Vitamin D 800 IU
- Avoid tobacco
- Weight-bearing exercise
- Falls prevention
- No more than moderate alcohol use

Pharmacologic Prevention
- Most organizations have recommended initiating pharmacologic management in women with BMD T scores below −2 in the absence of risk factors and in women with T scores below −1.5 if other risk factors are present.

- Regimens:
  ○ Bisphosphonates
    ▪ Alendronate (*Fosamax*) 5 mg/d or 35 mg/wk [T: 5, 10, 35, 40, 70; 70 sol] (must be taken fasting with water; patient must remain upright and npo for ≥30 min after taking; do not use if CrCl <35 mL/min; relatively contraindicated in GERD) **or**
    ▪ Ibandronate *(Boniva)* 150 mg/mo [T: 150] (must be taken fasting with water; patient must remain upright and npo for ≥60 min after taking; do not use if CrCl <30 mL/min) **or**
    ▪ Risedronate (*Actonel*) 35 mg/wk or 5 mg/d [T: 5, 30, 35] (must be taken fasting or ≥2 h after evening meal; patient must remain upright and npo for 30 min after taking; do not use if CrCl <30 mL/min) **or**
  ○ Raloxifene (*Evista*) 60 mg/d [T: 60] **or**
  ○ Estrogen in selected patients (see **Table 99** for dosing).

Nonpharmacologic Treatment
Vertebroplasty (injection of bone cement into a collapsed vertebra) or kyphoplasty (inflation of a balloon before cement injection) has short-term improvements in pain and function in case studies and nonrandomized controlled studies; long-term benefits for pain, function, and vertebral height are uncertain.

Pharmacologic Treatment Regimens for Those with Prior Osteoporotic Fractures
- Bisphosphonates
  ○ Alendronate (*Fosamax*) 10 mg/d or 70 mg/wk [T: 5, 10, 35, 40, 70; 70 sol] (must be taken fasting with water; patient must remain upright and npo for ≥30 min after taking; do not use if CrCl <35 mL/min; relatively contraindicated in GERD) **or**
  ○ Ibandronate *(Boniva)* 150 mg/mo [T: 150] (must be taken fasting with water; patient must remain upright and npo for ≥60 min after taking; do not use if CrCl <30 mL/min) **or**
  ○ Risedronate (*Actonel*) 35 mg/wk or 5 mg/d [T: 5, 30, 35] (must be taken fasting or ≥2 h after evening meal; patient must remain upright and npo for 30 min after taking; do not use if CrCl <30 mL/min) **or**
- Raloxifene (*Evista*) 60 mg/d [T: 60] **or**
- Calcitonin (*Calcimar, Cibacalcin, Miacalcin, Osteocalcin, Salmonine*) 100 IU/d SC [Inj: human (*Cibacalcin*) 0.5 mg/vial; salmon 200 units/mL] or 200 IU (*Miacalcin*) [200 units/activation] intranasally, alternate nostrils every other day. May also be helpful for analgesic effect in patients with acute vertebral fracture (see also p 125) **or**
- Estrogen in selected patients (see **Table 99** for dosing).
- Teriparatide (*Forteo*) 20 mcg/d for up to 24 mo [Inj 3 mL, 28-dose disposable pen device] for high-risk patients; contraindicated in patients with Paget's disease or prior skeletal radiation therapy (L, K).

Table 65. Bone Outcomes of Drugs for Osteoporosis Based on Randomized Clinical Trials*

Drug	Spine BMD and Fracture	Hip BMD	Hip Fracture	All Nonspinal Fractures
Estrogen**	improved	improved	reduced	no effect
Raloxifene	improved	improved	no data	no effect

(cont.)

Table 65. Bone Outcomes of Drugs for Osteoporosis Based on Randomized Clinical Trials* (cont.)

Drug	Spine BMD and Fracture	Hip BMD	Hip Fracture	All Nonspinal Fractures
Alendronate	improved	improved	reduced	reduced
Ibandronate	improved	improved	no data	no effect
Risedronate	improved	improved	reduced	reduced
Calcitonin (nasal)	improved	no effect	no effect	no effect
Teriparatide	improved	improved	no data	reduced

* The populations studied, sample sizes of individual studies, and duration of follow-up vary considerably; hence, this summary must be interpreted cautiously. Moreover, several randomized clinical trials are currently in progress and new findings may appear.
** The least expensive of the drugs listed.

Table 66. Effects on Other Outcomes, Level of Evidence,* and Risks of Drugs for Osteoporosis

Drug	CHD Risk Factors	CHD Prevention	CHD Treatment	Breast Cancer	Deep-vein Thrombosis	Other
Estrogen**	improved–R	↑ risk–R	no effect–R	↑ risk–R	↑ risk–R	↑ Vaginal bleeding, stroke, PE; ↓ colorectal cancer–R
Raloxifene	improved–R	↓ risk–R†	↓ risk–R	↓ risk–R	↑ risk–R	↑ Hot flushes–R
Alendronate	no data	no data	no data	no data	no data	Esophagitis; bone, joint, or muscle pain; osteonecrosis of jaw; occipital inflammation
Ibandronate	no data	no data	no data	no data	no data	Esophagitis; bone, joint, or muscle pain; osteonecrosis of jaw; occipital inflammation
Risedronate	no data	no data	no data	no data	no data	Esophagitis; bone, joint, or muscle pain; osteonecrosis of jaw; occipital inflammation
Calcitonin (nasal)	no data	no data	no data	no data	no data	Rhinitis in 10%–12%

* The populations studied, sample sizes of individual studies, and duration of follow-up vary considerably; hence, this summary must be interpreted cautiously. Moreover, several randomized clinical trials are currently in progress and new findings may appear.
** In the Women's Health Initiative estrogen-alone trial, only stroke and pulmonary embolism risk were increased.
† Reduced risk demonstrated for high-risk women only.
Note: CHD = coronary heart disease; R = randomized clinical trial.

PAIN

DEFINITION
An unpleasant sensory and emotional experience associated with actual or potential tissue damage (International Association for Study of Pain taxonomy)

Acute Pain
Distinct onset, usually evident pathology, short duration; common causes: trauma, postsurgical pain

Persistent Pain
Pain due to ongoing nociceptive, neuropathic, or mixed pathophysiologic processes, often associated with functional and psychologic impairment; can fluctuate in character and intensity over time (see **Table 67**).

Type of Pain and Examples	Source of Pain	Typical Description	Effective Drug Classes and Treatment
Nociceptive: somatic			
Arthritis, acute postoperative, fracture, bone metastases	Tissue injury, eg, bones, soft tissue, joints, muscles	Well localized, constant; aching, stabbing, gnawing, throbbing	Nonopioids, NSAIDs, opioids Physical and cognitive-behavioral therapies
Nociceptive: visceral			
Renal colic, bowel obstruction	Viscera	Diffuse, poorly localized, referred to other sites, intermittent, paroxysmal; dull, colicky, squeezing, deep, cramping; often accompanied by nausea, vomiting, diaphoresis	Nonopioids, NSAIDs, opioids Physical and cognitive-behavioral therapies
Neuropathic			
Cervical or lumbar radiculopathy, post-herpetic neuralgia, trigeminal neuralgia, diabetic neuropathy, post-stroke syndrome, herniated intervertebral disc	Peripheral or central nervous system	Prolonged, usually constant, but can be paroxysmal; sharp, burning, pricking, tingling, squeezing; associated with other sensory disturbances, eg, paresthesias and dysesthesias; allodynia, hyperalgesia, impaired motor function, atrophy, or abnormal deep tendon reflexes	Tricyclic antidepressants, anticonvulsants, opioids, topical anesthetics Physical and cognitive-behavioral therapies
Undetermined			
Myofascial pain syndrome, somatoform pain disorders	Poorly understood	No identifiable pathologic processes or symptoms out of proportion to identifiable organic pathology; widespread musculoskeletal pain, stiffness, and weakness	Antidepressants, antianxiety agents Physical, cognitive-behavioral, and psychological therapies

Table 67. Types of Pain, Examples, and Treatment

EVALUATION

Key Points, Approach

- Perform comprehensive evaluation of cause of pain, pain characteristics, and impact of physical and psychosocial function.
- Consider patient's report as the most reliable evidence of pain intensity.
- Assess for pain on each presentation (older adults may be reluctant to report pain).
- Use synonyms for pain (eg, burning, aching, soreness, discomfort).
- Use a standard pain scale (see p 225); adapt for sensory impairments (eg, large print, written versus spoken).
- Assess cognitively impaired patients by:
  - Using simple tools or questions with yes/no answers.
  - Using a structured approach to assessment and management (see **Figure 8**).
  - Asking caregiver about recent changes in function, gait, behavior patterns, mood.
- Reassess regularly for improvement, deterioration, and complications/adverse events and document.

History and Physical Examination

- Focus on a complete examination of pain source.
- Distinguish new illness from chronic condition.
- Analgesic history: effectiveness and adverse events, current and previous prescription drugs, OTC drugs, "natural" remedies.
- Assess effectiveness of prior nondrug treatments.
- Laboratory and diagnostic tests to establish etiologic diagnosis.

Characteristics of Pain Complaint

Provocative (aggravating) and **P**alliative (relieving) factors
Quality (eg, burning, stabbing, dull, throbbing)
Region (eg, pain map)
Severity (eg, scale of 0 for no pain to 10 for worst pain possible; see p 225)
Timing (eg, when pain occurs, frequency and duration)

Psychosocial Assessment

Depression (see p 217, 219 for screens), anxiety, mental status (see p 215 for screen). Impact on family or significant other. Enabling behaviors by others (eg, oversolicitousness, codependency, reinforcing debility).

Assess for Risk of Addiction with Opioid Use

- Addiction is rare in those without prior hx of substance abuse.
- Risk factors include men who exceed 4 drinks/d or 16 drinks/wk; women who exceed 3 drinks/d or 12 drinks/wk; admission to marijuana or hashish use in the past year; hx of alcohol abuse, drug abuse, or significant psychiatric illness.
- Observe for behavior that may suggest non-adherence to prescribed medication schedule (eg, early refill requests, frequent lost prescriptions).
- Record any suspicious drug-seeking or other aberrant behaviors observed or reported by others, along with action(s) taken.
- Document evaluation process, rationale for long-term opioid therapy, and periodic review of patient status.

Figure 8. Pain Assessment in Older Adults with Severe Cognitive Impairment

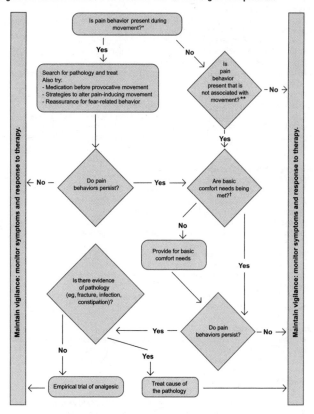

* Examples: grimacing, guarding, combativeness, groaning with movement; resisting care
** Examples: agitation, fidgeting, sleep disturbance, diminished appetite, irritability, reclusiveness, disruptive behavior, rigidity, rapid blinking
† Examples: toileting, thirst, hunger, visual or hearing impairment

Sources: Data from American Geriatrics Society. The management of persistent pain in older persons. *J Amer Geriatr Soc* 2002; 50 (6, Suppl: S205–S240); and Weiner D, Herr K, Rudy T, eds. Persistent Pain in Older Adults: An Interdisciplinary Guide for Treatment, 2002, Copyright Springer Publishing Company, Inc., New York 10036.

Functional Assessment
ADLs, impact on activities (see pp 215–216, for screens) and quality of life.

Brief Pain Inventory
Use for comprehensive assessment of pain and its impact (see p 227).

MANAGEMENT
Goal: To find optimal balance in pain relief, functional improvement, and adverse events.

Acute Pain and Short-term Management
• Use fixed schedule of APAP, NSAIDs (consider nonselective versus COX-2 inhibitors depending on risk factors and comorbidities, see **Figure 6**), or opioids.
• Include nonpharmacologic strategies (eg, relaxation, heat or cold).
• Patient-controlled analgesia (PCA): Requires patient comprehension of PCA instructions
  ○ Indications
    ▪ Acute pain (eg, postoperative pain, trauma)
    ▪ Persistent pain in patients who are npo
  ○ Dosing strategies (see **Table 68**)
    ▪ Titrate up PCA dose 25%–50% if pain still not well controlled after 12 h
    ▪ Unless patient is awakened by pain during sleep, continuous opioid infusion not recommended because of increased risk of drug accumulation and toxicity.
    ▪ If basal rate used, hourly monitoring of sedation and respiratory status is warranted.
    ▪ D/C PCA when patient able to take oral analgesics or unable to self medicate due to altered mental status or physical limitations.

Table 68. **Typical Initial Dosing of PCA for Older Adults with Severe Pain**

Drug (usual concentration)	Usual Dose Range*	Usual Lockout (min)
Morphine (1 mg/mL)	0.5–2.5 mg	5–10
Hydromorphone (0.2 mg/mL)	0.05–0.3 mg	5–10

* For opioid-naive patients, consider lower end of dose range.

Persistent Pain
• Use multidisciplinary assessment and treatment (eg, pharmacists, physical therapists, psychologists) when possible.
• Educate patient for self-management and coping.
• Combine drug and nondrug strategies.
• Anticipate and attend to depression and anxiety.

Nonpharmacologic Treatment
• Educate patient and caregiver.
  ○ Explain difference between addiction, physical dependence, and tolerance.
  ○ http://www.ampainsoc.org/advocacy/opioids2.htm
• Emphasize self-administered therapies (eg, heat, cold, massage, liniments and topical agents, distraction, relaxation, music).
• Prescribe exercise, especially for persistent pain (see p 170).
• Add therapy taught and/or conducted by professionals (eg, coping skills, biofeedback, imagery, hypnosis) as needed.

- When appropriate, obtain:
  - Rehabilitation medicine consult (OT, PT) for mechanical devices to minimize pain and facilitate activity (eg, splints), transcutaneous electrical nerve stimulation, range-of-motion and ADL programs.
  - Psychiatric pain management consult for somatization or severe mood or personality disorder.
  - Anesthesia pain management consult for possible interventional therapy (eg, neuroaxial analgesia, injection therapy, neuromodulation) when more conservative approaches are ineffective.
  - Pain or chemical dependency specialist referral for management of at-risk patients and ongoing chemical dependency, "chemical coping," aberrant drug-related behaviors, and drug withdrawal.

Pharmacologic Treatment
Selection of Agent(s):
- Base initial choice of analgesic on the severity and type of pain; consider cost, availability, patient preference, comorbidity, and impairments (see **Figure 6**):
  - Consider nonopioids for mild pain (rating 1–3) (see **Table 57**).
  - Consider low-dose combination agents (see **Table 69**) for mild to moderate pain (rating 4–6).
  - Consider potent and titratable opioid agonists (see **Table 69**) for more severe pain (rating 7–10).
  - Consider adjuvant drugs (see **Table 72**) alone or in conjunction with opioids or nonopioids for neuropathic pain and other selected chronic conditions.
  - Select agents with lowest adverse-event profiles.
- Select least invasive route (usually oral) and fast-onset, short-acting analgesics for episodic or breakthrough pain.
- Use long-acting or sustained-release analgesics for continuous pain after stabilizing dose with short-acting opioid.
- Avoid long-term use of nonselective NSAIDs for chronic conditions.
- Consider COX-2 inhibitor for patients who would benefit from anti-inflammatory drug therapy on a continuous, long-term basis based on risk/benefit assessment (see Musculoskeletal Disorders, p 123).
- Consider fixed-dose combinations (eg, APAP and hydrocodone or tramadol) for mild to moderate pain; do not exceed max dose for nonopioid.
- Avoid using multiple opioids or nonopioids.
- Drugs with long half-life or depot effects (eg, methadone, levorphanol, transdermal fentanyl) should be used and titrated cautiously, with close supervision of effects; duration of effect may exceed usual dose intervals because of reduced metabolism and clearance.
- Methadone is an option if other long-acting agents are not affordable but should be used with extreme caution.

Adjustment of Dosage:
- Begin with lowest dose possible, usually 25%–50% adult dose, increasing slowly.
- Titrate dose on basis of persistent need for and use of medications for breakthrough pain. If using ≥3 doses of breakthrough pain medication per day, consider increased dose of sustained-release medication.
- Dose to therapeutic ceiling of nonopioid or NSAID as limited by drug adverse events or risk factors.

- Increase opioid dose until pain relief achieved or adverse events unmanageable before changing drugs (there is no max dose or analgesic ceiling with opioids).
- Use morphine equivalents as a common denominator for all dose conversions to avoid errors, and titrate to effectiveness.
- When changing opioids, decrease equivalent analgesic dose by 25%–50% because of incomplete cross-tolerance.
- Administer around-the-clock for continuous pain.
- Reassess, re-examine, and readjust therapy frequently until pain is relieved.
- Opioid analgesics should not be discontinued abruptly. Gradual tapering is necessary to avoid withdrawal symptoms. Decreasing the daily dose by 10%–20% each day for 10 d can wean most patients without adverse responses. Tapering may require conversion to short-acting opioids. For patients at cardiovascular risk, a slower taper, with close monitoring for sympathetic hyperactivity is recommended, and low-dose clonidine may be useful in preventing some of the physiological (and symptomatic) stress related to opioid withdrawal.

Management of Adverse Events:

- Anticipate, prevent, and vigorously treat adverse events; expect older adults to be more sensitive to adverse events.
- Warn patient about risk of sedation with opioids and that gradual resolution occurs within a week.
- Warn about risk of APAP toxicity and importance of including all OTC products with APAP in daily total (not to exceed 4 g/d in healthy older adults, 2 g/d in frail older adults or those with reduced CrCl).
- Begin prophylactic, osmotic, or stimulant laxative when initiating opioid therapy (see **Table 40**); if patient taking in sufficient fluids, cautiously increase fiber or psyllium; titrate laxative dose up with opiate dose. (See also p 76.)
- Monitor for sedation, delirium, urinary retention, constipation, respiratory depression, and nausea; tolerance develops to mild sedation, nausea, and impaired cognitive function. Reduce dose and/or consider adding drug to counter adverse drug events if troublesome until tolerance develops.
- On long-term NSAID use, monitor periodically for GI blood loss, renal insufficiency, and other drug-drug and drug-disease interactions.
- Avoid the following drugs: carisoprodol, chlorzoxazone, cyclobenzaprine, indomethacin, meperidine, metaxalone, methocarbamol, nalbuphine, pentazocine, propoxyphene (see also p 236 for CMS criteria regarding inappropriate drug use).

			Table 69. **Opioid Analgesic Drugs**		
Class, Drug	MS Equiv* (Route)	Starting Oral Dosage in Opioid-naive Patients	Formulations	Indication for Pain**
Codeine	200 mg (po)	15 mg q 4–6 h	T: 15, 30, 60; S: 15/5 mL; Inj	A
Codeine & APAP†	200 mg (po)	1–2 15/325 tabs q 4–6 h; if 1 tab used, add 325 mg APAP	T: 15/325, 30/325, 60/325, 30/500, 30/650, 7.5/300, 15/300, 30/300, 60/300; S: 12/120/5 mL	A

(cont.)

Table 69. Opioid Analgesic Drugs (cont.)

Class, Drug	MS Equiv* (Route)	Starting Oral Dosage in Opioid-naive Patients	Formulations	Indication for Pain**
Hydrocodone & APAP† (eg, Lorcet, Lortab, Vicodin)	30 mg (po)	5–10 mg q 4–6 h	T: 10/325, 5/400, 7.5/400, 10/400, 2.5/500, 5/500, 7.5/500, 10/500, 7.5/650, 7.5/750, 10/650, 10/660; C: 5/500; S: 2.5/167/5 mL (contains 7% alcohol)	A
Hydrocodone & ASA (eg, Lortab ASA)	30 mg (po)	5 mg q 4–6 h	T: 5/500	A
Oxycodone (Oxy IR, Roxicodone)	20–30 mg (po)	2.5–5 mg q 3–4 h	T: 5, 15, 30; C: 5; S: 5 mg/mL, 20 mg/mL	A
Oxycodone & APAP† (Percocet, Tylox)	20 mg (po)	2.5–5 mg oxycodone q 6 h	T: 2.5/325, 5/325, 5/500, 7.5/325, 7.5/500, 10/325, 10/650; C: 5/500; S: 5/325/5 mL	A
Oxycodone & ASA (Percodan)	20 mg (po)	2.25–4.5 mg oxycodone q 6 h	T: 2.25/325, 4.5/325	A
Morphine (MSIR, Astramorph PF, Duramorph, Infumorph, Roxanol, OMS Concentrate, MS/L, RMS, MS/S)	30 mg (po), 10 mg (IV, IM, SC)	5 mg (po), 1– 2 mg (IV) q 4–6 h	C: 15, 30; soluble T: 15, 30; S: 10 mg/5 mL, 20 mg/5 mL, 100 mg/5 mL, 4 mg/mL, 20 mg/mL; Sp: 5, 10, 20, 30; Inj	B
Hydromorphone (Dilaudid, Hydrostat)	7.5 mg (po), 1.5 mg (IV, IM/SC), 6 mg (rectal)	0.5–1 mg q 3–4 h	T: 2, 4, 8; S: 5 mg/5 mL; Sp: 3; Inj	B
Oxymorphone (Numorphan)	1 mg (IV, IM, SC), 10 mg (rectal)	0.5 mg IM, IV, SC q 4–6 h	Sp: 5; Inj	B
Tramadol (Ultram)	150–300 mg (po)	25–50 mg q 4–6 h; not >300 mg for age 75+	T: 50	B
Tramadol & APAP† (Ultracet)	37.5/325 mg (po)	2 tabs po q 4–6 h; max 8 tabs/d‡	T: 37.5/325	B

* MS Equiv = morphine sulphate (MS) equivalent dose: morphine equivalency = dose of opioid equivalent to 10 mg of parenteral morphine or 30 mg of oral morphine with chronic dosing. The parenteral:oral ratio is greater (1:6) during acute dosing, ie, 10 mg IM MS = 60 mg po MS.
** A = mild to moderate pain; B = moderate to severe pain.
† Caution: total APAP dose should not exceed 4 g/d.
‡ Treatment not to exceed 5 d; if CrCl <30 mL/min, max is 2 tab q 12 h, not to exceed 5 d.

Table 70. Opioids for Opioid-tolerant Patients

Class, Drug	MS Equiv* (Route)	Starting Oral Dose	Formulations	Indication for Pain**
Short-acting				
Hydrocodone & ibuprofen (eg, Vicoprofen)	30 mg	7.5/200	T: 7.5/200	A
Fentanyl (Actiq)	NA	Suck on 200 mcg loz over 15 min, effect begins within 10 min	Loz on a stick: 200, 400, 600, 800, 1200, 1600 mcg	B

(cont.)

Table 70. Opioids for Opioid-tolerant Patients (cont.)

Class, Drug	MS Equiv* (Route)	Starting Oral Dose	Formulations	Indication for Pain**
Long-acting				
ER Morphine (*MS Contin, Kadian, Oramorph SR, Avinza*)	30 mg (po) MS Contin, Kadian, Oramorph SR; 60 mg (po) Avinza	20–30 mg q 24 h, 15 mg q 12 h (*MS Contin* CR and XR tabs), 20 mg q 24 h (*Kadian* SR caps), 15 mg q 24 h (*Oramorph SR*), 30 mg q 24 h (*Avinza* caps)	T: CR 15, 30, 60, 100, 200, XR 15, 30, 60; C: SR 5, 20, 30, 60, 100; C: 30, 60, 90, 120; T: SR 15, 30, 60, 100 (tab must be swallowed whole)	B
ER Oxycodone (*OxyContin*)	20–30 mg (po)	20 mg q 24 h, 10 mg q 12 h	T: CR 10, 20, 40, 80, 160	B
Transdermal fentanyl† (*Duragesic*)	NA (see package insert)	25 mcg/h or higher (if able to tolerate 50 mg oral morphine equiv/24 h)	12 mcg/h, 25 mcg/h, 50 mcg/h, 75 mcg/h, 100 mcg/h	B

* MS Equiv = morphine sulphate (MS) equivalent dose: morphine equivalency = dose of opioid equivalent to 10 mg of parenteral morphine or 30 mg of oral morphine with chronic dosing. The parenteral:oral ratio is greater (1:6) during acute dosing, ie, 10 mg IM MS = 60 mg po MS. NA = not applicable.

** A = mild to moderate pain; B = moderate to severe pain.

† Caution: Active ingredient accumulates in subcutaneous fat; thus, duration of action may be >17 hr. Do not use in opioid-naive patients. Not recommended for treatment of acute pain.

Methadone Prescribing and Monitoring

- Use with extreme caution and only with expertise and monitoring ability because of highly variable half-life and risk of dose accumulation.
- Relative potency of methadone is highly variable in patients already tolerant to other opioids.
- Reduce equivalent analgesic dose by 75%–90% and provide immediate-release, short-acting opioid supplementation for rescue analgesia if conversion leads to underdosing.
- Dosing intervals start at q 6 h and may be increased over time to q 8–12 h.
- Do not increase dose more frequently than every 4 d.
- Assure patient has reliable caregiver (educated with patient) to monitor for mental status changes, especially progressive sedation. If observed, instruct to hold dose and contact health care provider.
- Follow-up by telephone in 3–5 d after initial treatment and titration or dose conversion; office visit in 1–2 wk.
- Do baseline ECG (if not within last year) to monitor for QT$_C$ prolongation.

Table 71. Daily Oral Morphine Dose Equivalents and Conversion to Oral Methadone

Daily Oral Morphine Dose Equivalents	Conversion Ratio of Oral Morphine to Oral Methadone
<100 mg	3:1 (ie, 3 mg morphine:1 mg methadone)
101–300 mg	5:1

(cont.)

Table 71. Daily Oral Morphine Dose Equivalents and Conversion to Oral Methadone (cont.)

Daily Oral Morphine Dose Equivalents	Conversion Ratio of Oral Morphine to Oral Methadone
301–600 mg	10:1
601–800 mg	12:1
801–1000 mg	15:1
>1001 mg	20:1

Adapted from Gazelle G, Fine PG. Methadone for pain: #75. *J Palliative Med* 2004;7(2):303–304.

Table 72. Adjuvant Drugs for Pain Relief in Older Adults

Class, Drug	Formulations	Starting Dosage	Comments
Anticonvulsants (see **Table 63** and p 143)			If one does not work, try another
Antidepressants (see **Table 28**)			Use low-dose desipramine or nortriptyline; data on SSRIs lacking
Duloxetine (*Cymbalta*)	C: 20, 30, 60	30 mg q 24 h	For management of pain associated with diabetic peripheral neuropathy; most common adverse effects: nausea, dry mouth, constipation, diarrhea, urinary hesitancy; significant drug-drug interactions: check labeling for prescribing information for all patients
Corticosteroids (see **Table 34**)			Low-dose medical management may be helpful in inflammatory conditions
Counterirritants			
✔Camphor-menthol-phenol (*Sarna*)*	lot: camphor 5%, menthol 5%, phenol 5%	prn	May be effective for arthritic pain, but effect limited when pain affects multiple joints; can cause skin injury, especially if used with heat or occlusive dressing
✔Camphor and phenol (*Campho-Phenique*)*	S: camphor 5%, phenol 4.7%	prn	
✔Methylsalicylate and menthol (*Ben-Gay* oint,* *Icy Hot* crm*)	methylsalicylate 18.3%, menthol 16%	3–4 × /d	Apply to affected area

(cont.)

Table 72. Adjuvant Drugs for Pain Relief in Older Adults (cont.)

Class, Drug	Formulations	Starting Dosage	Comments
(*Ben-Gay* extra strength crm*)	methylsalicylate 30%, menthol 10%	3–4 × /d	Apply to affected area
✔Trolamine salicylate (*Aspercreme* rub*)	trolamine salicylate 10%	≤4 × /d	Apply to affected area
Other			
Baclofen (*Lioresal*)	T: 10, 20; Inj	2.5–5 mg 2–3 × /d	Probably increased sensitivity and decreased clearance; monitor for weakness, urinary dysfunction; avoid abrupt discontinuation because of CNS irritability
✔Capsaicin (eg, *Capsin, Capzasin, No Pain-HP, R-Gel, Zostrix*)	crm, lot, gel, roll-on: 0.025%, 0.075%	3–4 × /d	Renders skin and joints insensitive by depleting and preventing reaccumulation of substance P in peripheral sensory neurons; may cause burning sensation up to 2 wk; instruct patient to wash hands after application to prevent eye contact; do not apply to open or broken skin
✔Lidocaine (*Lidoderm*)	transdermal Pch 5%	12 h on, 12 h off; up to 24 h on	Apply over affected area; used for neuropathic pain, may be helpful for low back pain, osteoarthritis

✔ = preferred for treating older adults.
* Available OTC.
Note: Various adjuvant classes are useful for the treatment of neuropathic pain. TCAs are often helpful for migraine or tension headaches and arthritic conditions. Baclofen is particularly useful for muscle-related problems, such as spasms.

PALLIATIVE AND END-OF-LIFE CARE

DEFINITION
"Palliative care is an approach to care which improves quality of life of patients and their families facing life-threatening illnesses, through the prevention and relief of suffering by means of early identification and impeccable assessment and treatment of pain and other problems, physical, psychosocial, and spiritual." (WHO, 2002)

PRINCIPLES
- Support, educate, and treat both patient and family.
- Address physical, psychologic, social, and spiritual needs.
- Use multidisciplinary team (physicians, nurses, social workers, chaplain, pharmacist, physical and occupational therapists, dietitian, family and caregivers, volunteers).
- Focus on symptom management, comfort, meeting goals, completion of "life business," healing relationships, and bereavement.
- Make care available 24 h/d, 7 d/wk.
- Educate, plan, and document advance directives; health care proxy; family awareness of decisions.
- Coordinate care among various providers. Help integrate potentially curative, disease-modifying, and palliative therapies.
- Offer bereavement support.
- Provide therapeutic environment (palliation can be given in any location).
- Advocate comprehensive palliative care for all dying patients.

QUALITY OF LIFE
Ways to help patient and family enhance quality of life at the end of life:
- Communicate, listen
- Teach stress management, coping
- Use all available resources
- Support decision making
- Encourage conflict resolution
- Help complete unfinished business
- Urge focus on nonillness-related affairs
- Urge a focus on one day at a time
- Help anticipate grief, losses
- Help focus on attainable goals
- Encourage spiritual practices
- Promote physical, psychologic comfort

END-OF-LIFE DECISIONS
Follow principles involved in informed decision making (see **Figure 2**).

Hospice Referral
- Patients, families, or other health care providers can refer, but a physician's certification of limited life expectancy (prognosis of ≤6 mo for most hospice programs; a requirement for the Medicare Hospice Benefit and Medicaid programs) is required for admission to a hospice program (see **Table 73**).
- Referral is appropriate when curative treatment is no longer indicated (ie, ineffective, adverse events too burdensome) and life is limited to months.
- Hospice must be accepted by the patient or family, or both, and can be rescinded at any time.
- Hospice provides palliative medications, durable medical supplies and equipment, team member visits as needed and desired by patient and family (physician, nurses, home health aide, social worker, chaplain), and volunteer services.

- Optimal hospice care requires adequate time in the program; referral when death is imminent does not take full advantage of hospice care.
- Hospice care is usually delivered in patient's home, but it can be delivered in a nursing home or residential care facility (long-term care, assisted living) or in an inpatient setting (hospice-specific or contracted facility) if acuity or social circumstances warrant.

Table 73. Typical Trajectory and Hospice Eligibility for Selected Diseases

Disease	Typical Determinants for Hospice Eligibility*
Cancer	Clinical findings of malignancy with widespread, aggressive, or progressive disease evidenced by increasing symptoms, worsening laboratory values, and/or evidence of metastatic disease Impaired performance status with a Palliative Performance Scale (PPS; see p 229) value of ≤70% Refuses further curative therapy or continues to decline in spite of definitive therapy
Dementia	FAST Scale Stage 7 (loss of speech, locomotion, and consciousness; see p 230) **and** Comorbid or secondary conditions that contribute to structural or functional impairments suggesting a prognosis of ≤6 mo
Failure to thrive	BMI (kg/m^2) <22 Karnofsky (see p 229) or PPS value <40%
End-stage heart disease	Optimally treated with diuretics and vasodilators, which may include ACE inhibitors or combination of hydralazine and nitrates **or** has angina pectoris at rest, resistant to standard nitrate treatment and is either not candidate for or declines invasive procedures **and** Significant symptoms of recurrent HF at rest and classified as NYHA Class IV (ie, unable to carry on any physical activity without symptoms, symptoms present at rest, symptoms increase if any physical activity is undertaken) Additional support needed for treatment-resistant symptomatic supraventricular or ventricular arrhythmia, history of cardiac arrest or resuscitation or unexplained syncope, brain embolism of cardiac origin, concomitant HIV disease, documented ejection fraction of ≤20%
End-stage pulmonary disease	Disabling dyspnea at rest, poorly or unresponsive to bronchodilators, resulting in decreased functional capacity, eg, bed to chair existence, fatigue, and cough (documentation of FEV$_1$, after bronchodilator, <30% of predicted is objective evidence for disabling dyspnea, but is not necessary to obtain) **and** Progression of end-stage pulmonary disease, as evidenced by *prior* increased visits to emergency department or *prior* hospitalization for pulmonary infections and/or respiratory failure (documentation of serial decrease of FEV$_1$ >40 mL/yr is objective evidence for disease progression, but is not necessary to obtain) **and** Hypoxemia at rest on room air, as evidenced by pO$_2$ ≤55 mm Hg or O$_2$ sat ≤88% or hypercapnia, as evidenced by pCO$_2$ ≥50 mm Hg Additional support needed for cor pulmonale and right heart failure secondary to pulmonary disease, unintentional progressive weight loss of >10% of body weight over preceding 6 mo, resting tachycardia >100 beats/min
Acute renal failure	Not seeking dialysis or renal transplant CrCl <10 mL/min (<15 mL/min for diabetes) Serum creatinine >8.0 mg/dL (>6.0 mg/dL for diabetes) Additional support needed for comorbid conditions such as malignancy, chronic lung disease (eg, mechanical ventilation), advanced cardiac disease, advanced liver disease

(cont.)

Table 73. Typical Trajectory and Hospice Eligibility for Selected Diseases (cont.)

Disease	Typical Determinants for Hospice Eligibility*
Chronic renal failure	Not seeking dailysis or renal transplant CrCl <10 mL/min (<15 mL/min for diabetes) Serum creatinine >8.0 mg/dL (>6.0 mg/dL for diabetes) Additional support needed for following signs and symptoms of renal failure: uremia, oliguria (<400 mL/day), intractable hyperkalemia (>7.0) not responsive to treatment, uremic pericarditis, hepatorenal syndrome

* May vary depending on fiscal intermediary; additional supportive indications available for most diagnoses. Adapted from Palmetto GBA (http://www.palmettogba.com)

Advance Directives
Designed to respect patient's autonomy and determine his/her wishes about future life-sustaining medical treatment if unable to indicate wishes.

Oral Statements
• Conversations with relatives, friends, clinicians are most common form; should be thoroughly documented in medical record for later reference.
• Properly verified oral statements carry same ethical and legal weight as those recorded in writing.

Instructional Advance Directives (DNR Orders, Living Wills)
• Written instructions regarding the initiation, continuation, withholding, or withdrawal of particular forms of life-sustaining medical treatment.
• May be revoked or altered at any time by the patient.
• Clinicians who comply with such directives are provided legal immunity for such actions.

Durable Power of Attorney for Health Care or Health Care Proxy
A written document that enables a capable person to appoint someone else to make future medical treatment choices for him or her in the event of decisional incapacity (see Figure 2).

Key Interventions, Treatment Decisions to Include in Advance Directives
• Resuscitation procedures
• Mechanical respiration
• Chemotherapy, radiation therapy
• Dialysis
• Simple diagnostic tests
• Pain control
• Blood products, transfusions
• Intentional deep sedation

Withholding or Withdrawing Therapy
• There is no ethical or legal difference between withholding an intervention (not starting it) and withdrawing life-sustaining medical treatment (stopping it after it has been started).
• Beginning a treatment does not preclude stopping it later; a time-limited trial may be appropriate.
• Palliative care should not be limited, even if life-sustaining treatments are withdrawn or withheld.
• Decisions on artificial feeding should be based on the same criteria applied to use of ventilators and other medical treatment.

Euthanasia
- Active euthanasia: direct intervention, such as lethal injection, intended to hasten a patient's death; a criminal act of homicide.
- Passive euthanasia: withdrawal or withholding of unwanted or unduly burdensome life-sustaining treatment; appropriate in certain circumstances.
- Assisted suicide: the patient's intentional, willful ending of his or her own life with the assistance of another; a criminal offense in most states.

MANAGEMENT OF COMMON END-OF-LIFE SYMPTOMS
Pain
- The most distressing symptom for patients and caregivers.
- If intent is to relieve suffering, the risk that sufficient medication appropriately titrated will produce an unintended effect (hastening death) is morally acceptable (double effect).
- Primary goal: to alleviate suffering at end of life. See Pain (p 148) for assessment and interventions.
- Alternate routes may be needed, eg, transdermal, transmucosal, rectal, vaginal, topical, epidural, and intrathecal.
- Recommend expert pain management consult if pain not adequately relieved with standard analgesic guidelines and interventions.
- Additional treatment may include:
  ○ radionuclides and bisphosphonates (for metastatic bone pain).
  ○ treatments (eg, radiotherapy, chemotherapy) directed at source of pain.
- Pain crisis: Sedation at end of life for intractable pain and suffering is an important option to discuss with patients. Ketamine (*Ketalar*) 0.1 mg/kg IV bolus. Repeat as needed q 5 min. Follow with infusion of 0.015 mg/kg/min IV (if IV access not available, SC at 0.3–0.5 mg/kg). Decrease opioid dose by 50%. A benzodiazepine may be useful. Observe for problems with increased secretions and treat (see p 163).

Weakness, Fatigue
Nonpharmacologic:
- Modify environment to decrease energy expenditure (eg, placement of phone, bedside commode, drinks).
- Adjust room temperature to patient's comfort.
- Teach reordering tasks to conserve energy (eg, eating first, resting, then bathing).
- Modify daily procedures (eg, sitting while showering rather than standing).
Pharmacologic:
- Treat remediable causes such as pain, medication toxicity, insomnia, anemia, and depression.
- Consider psychostimulants (eg, dextroamphetamine [*Dexedrine*] 2.5 mg po qam or bid, methylphenidate [*Ritalin*] 5–10 mg po qam or bid, or modafinil [*Provigil*] 200 mg qam); monitor for signs of psychosis, agitation, or sleep disturbance.

Dysphagia (see also p 71)
Nonpharmacologic:
- Feed small, frequent amounts of pureed or soft foods.
- Avoid spicy, salty, acidic, sticky, and extremely hot or cold foods.

- Keep head of bed elevated for 30 min after eating.
- Instruct patient to wear dentures and to chew thoroughly.
- Use suction machine when necessary.

Pharmacologic:
- For painful mucositis: 1:2:8 mixture of diphenhydramine elixir: lidocaine [2%–4%]: magnesium-aluminum hydroxide (eg, *Maalox*) as a swish-and-swallow suspension before meals.
- For candidiasis: clotrimazole 10-mg troches, 5 doses/d, **or** fluconazole 150 mg po followed by 100 mg po qd × 5 d.
- For severe halitosis: antimicrobial mouthwash; fastidious oral and dental care; treat putative respiratory tract infection with broad-spectrum antibiotics.

Dyspnea
Nonpharmacologic:
- Teach positions to facilitate breathing, elevate head of bed.
- Teach relaxation techniques.
- Eliminate smoke and allergens.
- Assure brisk air circulation (facial breeze) with a room fan; oxygen is indicated only for symptomatic hypoxemia (ie, SaO_2 <90% by pulse oximetry).

Pharmacologic:
- Opioids: oral morphine concentration (20 mg/mL: 1/4 to 1/2 mL sl, po; repeat in 10–15 min prn); nebulized morphine 2.5 mg in 2–4 mL NS **or** fentanyl 25–50 mcg in 2–4 mL NS; **or** IV morphine 1 mg or equivalent opioid q 5–10 min.
- Bronchodilators (see **Table 86**).
- Diuretics, if evidence of volume overload (see **Table 20**).
- Anxiolytics (eg, lorazepam po, sl, SC 0.5–2 mg q 2–4 h or prn); titrate slowly to effect.

Constipation (see p 76)
Most common cause: adverse effects of opioids, medications with anticholinergic adverse effects (see **Table 40**). Use stimulant or osmotic laxative.

Bowel Obstruction
Indications for Radiographic Evaluation:
- To differentiate between constipation and mechanical obstruction
- To confirm the obstruction, determine site and nature if surgery is being considered

Nonpharmacologic Management:
- Nasogastric intubation: only if surgery is being considered, for high-level obstructions, and poor response to pharmacotherapy
- Percutaneous venting gastrostomy: for high-level obstructions and profuse vomiting not responsive to antiemetics
- Palliative surgery
- Hydration: IV or hypodermoclysis

Pharmacologic Management (aimed at specific symptoms):
- Nausea and vomiting: haloperidol (*Haldol*) po, IM 0.5–5 mg (≤10 mg) q 4–8 h prn; ondansetron (*Zofran*) IV (over 2–5 min) 4 mg q 12 h, po 8 mg q 12 h [Inj; T: 4, 8, 24; S: 4 mg/5 mL], but costly; see also **Table 41**.

- Spasm, pain, and vomiting: scopolamine IM, IV, SC 0.3–0.65 mg q 4–6 h prn; oral 0.4–0.8 mg q 4–8 h prn; transdermal 2.5 cm^2 Pch applied behind the ear q 3 d [Inj; T: 0.4; Pch 1.5 mg] or hyoscyamine (*Levsin/SL*) sl [T: 0.125; S: 0.125 mg/mL] 0.125–0.25 tid–qid.
- Diarrhea and excessive secretions: loperamide (*Imodium A-D*) see **Table 42**; octreotide (*Sandostatin*) SC 0.15–0.3 mg q 12 h [Inj], very expensive.
- Pain: see **Table 69**.
- Inflammation due to malignant obstruction: dexamethasone (*Decadron*) po: 4 mg qid × 5–7 d.

Excessive Secretions
Nonpharmacologic: Positioning and suctioning, as needed
Pharmacologic: Glycopyrrolate 0.1–0.4 mg IV,SC q 4 h prn **or** scopolamine 0.3–0.6 mg SC prn **or** transdermal scopolamine Pch q 72 h **or** atropine 0.3–0.5 mg SC, sl, nebulized q 4 h prn

Cough
See p 184.

Nausea, Vomiting
See p 78.

Malnutrition, Dehydration
See also Malnutrition (p 118) and volume depletion (p 113).
Nonpharmacologic:
- Educate patient and family on effects of disease progression resulting in lack of appetite and weight loss.
- Promote interest, enjoyment in meals (eg, alcoholic beverage if desired, involve patient in meal planning, small frequent feedings, cold or semi-frozen nutritional drinks).
- Good oral care is important.
Pharmacologic:
- Corticosteroids: Dexamethasone 1–2 mg po tid; methylprednisolone 1–2 mg po bid; prednisone 5 mg po tid.
- Hormone therapy: Megestrol acetate 200–800 mg qd.

Altered Mental Status, Delirium
See Delirium (p 43).

Anxiety, Depression
- Provide opportunity to discuss feelings, fears, existential concerns
- Referral to appropriate team members (spiritual, nursing)
- Medicate (see Anxiety, p 21, and Depression, p 51).

Source: Fine P. *Hospice Companion—Processes to Optimize Care During the Last Phase of Life.* 2d ed. Scottsdale, AZ: VistaCare, Inc.; 2000.

PREOPERATIVE CARE
Cardiac Risk Assessment

Figure 9. Reducing Cardiac Risk in Noncardiac Surgery

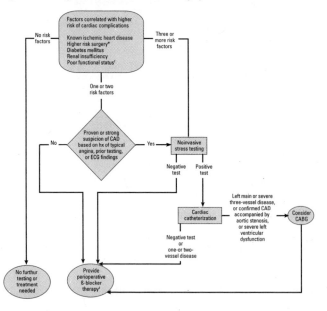

* Intraperitoneal, intrathoracic, or suprainguinal vascular procedures
† Inability to walk 4 blocks or climb 2 flights of stairs
‡ In addition to β-blocker therapy, strongly consider perioperative statin therapy.

Source: Adapted from Fleisher LA, Eagle KA. Lowering cardiac risk in noncardiac surgery. *N Engl J Med* 2001;
345:1677–1682. Copyright © 2001, Massachusetts Medical Society. All rights reserved. Adapted with permission 2003.

Pulmonary Risk Assessment
Assessing the patient for risk of pulmonary complications (respiratory failure,
pneumonia, atelectasis) includes the following risk factors:
Smoking: To lower risk, patients should quit at least 8 wk before surgery.
COPD: Bronchodilators, physical therapy, antibiotics, and corticosteroids given
preoperatively can reduce risk.

ASA Class: III—severe systemic disease; IV—life-threatening systemic disease; V—moribund.
Surgical Site: Upper abdominal, thoracic, >3-h surgeries pose the greatest increased risk.

Note: Routine spirometry has not been shown to be useful in risk assessment.

Other Assessments
Anticoagulation Status: See pp 18–20.
Cognitive Status: Unrecognized dementia is a risk factor for postoperative delirium. Measure preoperative cognitive status with Mini-Cog (see p 215) or MMSE.
Nutritional Status: Poor nutritional status can impair wound healing. Measure height, weight, serum albumin.
Routine Laboratory Tests: Recommended: Hb, hematocrit, electrolytes, creatinine, BUN, ECG, CXR, albumin. Optional: CBC, platelets, ABG, PT, PTT.
Cataract Surgery: Routine laboratory testing or cardiopulmonary risk assessment is unneccessary for cataract surgery performed under local anesthesia.
Advance Directives: Establish or update.

PERIOPERATIVE MANAGEMENT
β-Blocker Use
For patients at risk of cardiac complications (see **Figure 9**), begin β-blocker agent (eg, atenolol or bisoprolol) po 1–2 wk before surgery to achieve heart rate <70 beats/min. Continue therapy until 2 wk after surgery, with a goal of <80 beats/min in the postoperative period. Withhold β-blockers if heart rate is <55 beats/min; SBP <100; or the patient has asthma, decompensated HF, or third-degree heart block.

Statin Use
Statins have been associated with lower perioperative mortality in patients with known or suspected CAD undergoing noncardiac surgery. Unless there is a contraindication, pre-and perioperative administration of statins (see **Table 19**), regardless of LDL cholesterol levels, is recommended.

Endocarditis Prophylaxis
Depends on cardiac condition and type of procedure (see pp 168–169).

DVT Prophylaxis (see Table 12)

Common Problems to Monitor
- Confusion (see p 43)
- Intra- and postoperative coronary events: postoperative ECG to check
- Malnutrition (see p 118)
- Pain (see p 148)
- Polypharmacy: review medications daily
- Pulmonary complications: minimized by incentive spirometry, coughing, early ambulation
- Rehabilitation: encourage early mobility
- Skin breakdown (see p 189)

DISCHARGE PLANNING
- Ideally, all team members should participate in discharge planning, beginning early in the hospitalization.
- Physician should provide discharge summary and orders, including medications.
- Site of care after discharge should be warranted by patient's needs (see **Table 74**).
- See also Housing Alternatives, p 5.

Table 74. Sites of Post-hospital Care		
Site	**Requirements**	**Funding**
Inpatient rehabilitation facility or transitional care unit of a nursing home	Patient can tolerate 3 h of rehabilitation therapy/d requiring multiple disciplines (eg, PT, OT, speech therapy)	Medicare Part A pays 100% of charges for days 1–20, patient pays $114/d (in 2005) for days 21–100 with Part A covering the rest, patient pays 100% after day 100
Skilled nursing facility	Patient requires skilled nursing care and cannot tolerate 3 h of therapy/d	Same as above for rehabilitation services associated with hospitalization; long-term stays principally financed out-of-pocket or by Medicaid
Home	Physician must certify that patient is able to only occasionally leave the home at great effort	Medicare Part A pays for most nonphysician professional services (eg, nursing, OT, PT); very limited coverage for attendant care (eg, cooking, cleaning)
Home, assisted living	Patient able to manage ADLs independently or with informal help	Medicare Part B pays for 80% of most outpatient medical services
Hospice (home or facility-based); see also housing alternatives, p 5	Physician must certify that patient's life expectancy <6 mo (see **Table 73**)	Medicare Part A pays for most professional services and medications related to terminal illness; physician services covered under Part B

PREVENTION

PREVENTIVE TESTS AND PROCEDURES

Table 75. Recommended Primary and Secondary Disease Prevention for People Aged 65 and Older

Preventive Strategy	Frequency
USPSTF* Recommendations for Primary Prevention	
Bone mineral density (women)	at least once after age 65
BP screening	yearly
Diabetes mellitus screening	at least once in people with HTN or hyperlipidemia
Influenza immunization	yearly
Lipid disorder screening	every 5 yr, more often in CAD, diabetes mellitus, PAD, prior stroke
Obesity (height and weight)	yearly
Pneumonia immunization	once at age 65**
Smoking cessation	at every office visit
Tetanus immunization	every 10 yr
USPSTF* Recommendations for Secondary Prevention	
Abdominal aortic aneurysm ultrasonography	once between age 65–75 in men who have ever smoked
Alcohol abuse screening	unspecified but should be done periodically
Depression screening	yearly
FOBT/sigmoidoscopy/colonoscopy	yearly/every 5 yr/every 10 yr
Hearing impairment screening	yearly
Mammography, clinical breast examination***	every 1–2 yr
Pap smear[†]	at least every 3 yr
Visual impairment screening	yearly
Other[‡] Recommendations for Primary Prevention	
ASA to prevent MI	daily
Calcium (1200 mg) and vitamin D (400–800 IU) to prevent osteoporosis	daily
Measurement of serum C-reactive protein	at least once in people with one CAD risk factor
Omega-3 fatty acids to prevent MI, stroke	at least 2x/wk (see MI care, p 27)
Multivitamin	1–2/d
Other[‡] Recommendations for Secondary Prevention	
Skin examination	yearly
Breast self-examination	monthly
Cognitive impairment screening	yearly
Electron-beam computed tomography	at least once in people with multiple CAD risk factors
Glaucoma screening	yearly
Inquiry about falls	yearly
PSA and digital rectal examination	yearly
TSH in women	yearly

* US Preventive Services Task Force. See http://www.ahrq.gov/clinic/uspstfix.htm.

** Consider repeating pneumococcal vaccine every 6–7 yr.

*** Mammograms to age 70 are almost universally recommended; many organizations, including the USPSTF, recommend that mammography should be continued in women over 70 who have a reasonable life expectancy.

[†] Pap smear testing can be stopped in most women after age 65. See p 209. Women without a cervix should not have pap smears.

[‡] Not endorsed by USPSTF for all older adults, but recommended in selected patients or by other professional organizations.

The USPSTF recommends **against** screening for:
- Asymptomatic bacteriuria with urinalysis
- Bladder cancer with hematuria, bladder tumor antigen, NMP22 urinary enzyme immunoassay, or urine cytology measurement
- CAD with ECG, exercise treadmill test, or electron-beam computerized tomography in people with few or no CAD risk factors
- Ovarian cancer with transvaginal ultrasonography or CA-125 measurement
- Pancreatic cancer with ultrasonography or serologic markers

ENDOCARDITIS PROPHYLAXIS (AHA GUIDELINES)
Antibiotic Regimens Recommended (see **Table 76**)

Cardiac Conditions Requiring Prophylaxis
High-risk Category: Prosthetic heart valves, previous endocarditis, surgical systemic pulmonary shunts
Moderate-risk Category: Acquired valvular dysfunction (eg, rheumatic heart disease), hypertrophic cardiomyopathy, mitral valve prolapse with valvular regurgitation and/or thickened leaflets, most congenital heart malformations

Procedures Warranting Prophylaxis
Dental: Extractions, periodontal procedures, implants and reimplants, root canals, subgingival placement of antibiotic fibers or strips, initial placement of orthodontic bands but not brackets, intraligamentary local anesthetic injections, teeth cleaning during which bleeding is expected
Respiratory Tract: Tonsillectomy and/or adenoidectomy, rigid bronchoscopy, surgery involving respiratory mucosa
GI Tract: Esophageal varices sclerotherapy, esophageal stricture dilation, endoscopic retrograde cholangiography with biliary obstruction, biliary tract surgery, surgery involving intestinal mucosa
GU Tract: Prostatic surgery, cystoscopy, urethral dilation

Cardiac Conditions Not Requiring Prophylaxis
Previous CABG surgery; mitral valve prolapse without valvular regurgitation; physiologic, functional, or innocent heart murmurs; previous rheumatic fever without valvular dysfunction; cardiac pacemakers; implanted defibrillators; isolated secundum atrial septal defect; surgical repair of atrial or ventricular septal defect

Procedures Not Warranting Prophylaxis
Dental: Restorative dentistry, local anesthetic injections, intracanal endodontic treatment, rubber dam placement, suture removal, placement of removable prosthodontic or orthodontic appliances, oral impressions, fluoride treatments, oral radiographs, orthodontic appliance adjustment
Respiratory Tract: Endotracheal intubation, flexible bronchoscopy (prophylaxis optional for high-risk patients), ear tube insertion
GI Tract: Transesophageal echocardiography, endoscopy (prophylaxis optional for high-risk patients)

GU Tract: Vaginal hysterectomy (prophylaxis optional for high-risk patients), urethral catheterization of uninfected tissue
Other: Cardiac catheterization, balloon angioplasty

Table 76. Endocarditis Prophylaxis Regimens

Situation	Regimen
Dental, oral, respiratory tract, or esophageal procedures	
Standard general prophylaxis	Amoxicillin 2.0 g po 1 h before procedure
Unable to take oral medications	Ampicillin 2.0 g IM or IV ≤30 min before procedure
Allergic to penicillin	Clindamycin 600 mg, cephalexin 2.0 g, cefadroxil 2.0 g, azithromycin 500 mg, or clarithromycin 500 mg po 1 h before procedure
Allergic to penicillin and unable to take oral medications	Clindamycin 600 mg or cefazolin 1.0 g IM or IV ≤30 min before procedure
GU or GI procedures	
High-risk patients	Ampicillin 2.0 g IM or IV + gentamicin 1.5 mg/kg IV or IM (not to exceed 120 mg) ≤30 min before procedure; 6 h later, ampicillin 1.0 g IM or IV or amoxicillin 1.0 g po
High-risk patients allergic to ampicillin or amoxicillin	Vancomycin 1.0 g IV over 1–2 h + gentamicin 1.5 mg/kg IV or IM (not to exceed 120 mg); complete injection or infusion ≤30 min before procedure
Moderate-risk patients	Amoxicillin 2.0 g po 1 h before procedure or ampicillin 2.0 g IM or IV ≤30 min before procedure
Moderate-risk patients allergic to ampicillin or amoxicillin	Vancomycin 1.0 g IV over 1–2 h, complete infusion ≤30 min before procedure

Note: See **Table 52** for details about antibiotics.
Source: Dajani AS, Taubert KA, Wilson W, et al. Prevention of bacterial endocarditis: Recommendations by the American Heart Association. *JAMA.* 1997;277:1794–1801. Copyright 1997, American Medical Association. All rights reserved. Reprinted with permission.

PROPHYLAXIS FOR DENTAL PATIENTS WITH TOTAL JOINT REPLACEMENTS (TJR)
Conditions Requiring: Inflammatory arthropathies (eg, rheumatoid arthritis, systemic lupus erythematosus); disease-, drug-, or radiation-induced immunosuppression; type 1 diabetes mellitus; first 2 yr after TJR; previous prosthetic joint infection; malnourishment; hemophilia
Conditions Not Requiring: Patients >2 yr after TJR who do not have one of the above conditions; patients with pins, plates, or screws
Dental Procedures Warranting: see those listed on p 168 for endocarditis
Suggested Prophylactic Regimens: (all given 1 h before procedure)
• Not allergic to penicillin: Amoxicillin, cephalexin, or cephradine 2.0 g po
• Not allergic to penicillin and unable to take oral medications: Ampicillin 2.0 g or cefazolin 1.0 g IM or IV

• Allergic to penicillin: Clindamycin 600 mg po
• Allergic to penicillin and unable to take oral medications: Clindamycin 600 mg IV

EXERCISE PRESCRIPTION
Before Giving an Exercise Prescription
Screen patient for:
• Musculoskeletal problems: Decreased flexibility, muscular rigidity, weakness, pain, ill-fitting shoes
• Cardiac disease: Consider stress test if patient is beginning a vigorous exercise program and is sedentary with ≥ 2 cardiac risk factors (male gender, HTN, smoking, diabetes mellitus, dyslipidemia, obesity, family hx, sedentary lifestyle).

Individualize the Prescription
Specify short- and long-term goals; include the following components:
Flexibility: Static stretching; daily, >15 sec per muscle group
Endurance: Walking, cycling, swimming at 50%–75% of max HR (220 – age for men; 220 – [0.6 × age] for women); 3–4 ×/wk; goal of 20–30 min duration
Strength: Muscle resistance (weight training); 3 sets (8–15 repetitions) per muscle group 2–3 ×/wk
Balance: Tai Chi, dance, yoga, postural awareness; 1–3 ×/wk
Patient Information: See http://www.niapublications.org/exercisebook/index.asp. See also Assessment and Management of Falls, p 66.

BENIGN PROSTATIC HYPERPLASIA
Evaluation
Detailed medical hx focusing on physical examination of the urinary tract, including a digital rectal examination and a focused neurologic examination; UA; measurement of serum creatinine. Measurement of PSA is optional.

Management
Mild Symptoms: (eg, AUA score ≤7; see p 230) watchful waiting
Moderate to Severe Symptoms: (eg, AUA score ≥8) medical or surgical treatment
Medical Treatment: Combining drugs from different classes may be more effective than single-agent therapy.

- **α_1-Blockers**
  Nonselective and selective agents are equally effective. (Note: sildenafil [*Viagra*], vardenafil [*LEVITRA*], or tadalafil [*Cialis*] can cause hypotension in men receiving α_1-blockers.)
  - **Nonselective** (less expensive):
    - Terazosin (*Hytrin*) increase dosage as tolerated—days 1–3, 1 mg/d hs; days 4–7, 2 mg; days 8–14, 5 mg; day 15 and beyond, 10 mg [T: 1, 2, 5, 10]
    - Doxazosin (*Cardura*) start 0.5 mg with max of 16 mg/d [T: 1, 2, 4, 8]
    - Prazosin (*Minipress*) start 1 mg/d (first dose hs) or bid with max 20 mg/d [T: 1, 2, 5]
  - **Selective** (fewer side effects):
    - Tamsulosin (*Flomax*) 0.4 mg 30 min after the same meal each day and increase to 0.8 mg if no response in 2–4 wk [T: 0.4]
    - Alfuzosin ER (*Uroxatral*) 10 mg after the same meal every day [T: 10]
- **5-α Reductase inhibitors:**
  - Finasteride (*Proscar*) 5 mg/d [T: 5]*
  - Dutasteride (*Avodart*) 0.5 mg/d [C: 0.5]

Surgical Management: Indicated if recurrent UTI, recurrent or persistent gross hematuria, bladder stones, or renal insufficiency are clearly secondary to BPH or as indicated by severe symptoms (AUA score >16), patient preference, or ineffectiveness of medical treatment.** For men with moderate symptoms (AUA scores 8–15), surgical therapy is more effective than watchful waiting, but the latter is a reasonable alternative. Surgical options are:

- Transurethral resection of the prostate (TURP).
- Transurethral incision of the prostate (TUIP), which is limited to prostates with an estimated resected tissue weight (if done by TURP) of ≤30 g.
- Open prostatectomy for large glands (>50 g).
- Urethral stents may be an option for poor surgical candidates.
- For laser prostatectomy, microwave therapy, and electrovaporization, data to support effectiveness and safety are limited.

---

* May reduce risk of developing prostate cancer by 20%–25% but increases risk of developing high-grade prostate cancer.

** Source: McConnell JD, Barry MJ, Bruskewitz RC, et al. *Benign Prostatic Hyperplasia: Diagnosis and Treatment.* Clinical Practice Guideline No. 8. Rockville, MD: Agency for Health Care Policy and Research, Public Health Service, US Dept. of Health and Human Services, February 1994. AHCPR Publication No. 94-0582.

PROSTATE CANCER

Evaluation

Predicting extent of disease:
- PSA (see **Table 75**)
- Biopsy
- Digital rectal examination
- CT abdomen and pelvis (selectively)
- Bone scan (selectively)

Histology

- Gleason score 2–6 has low 15–20 yr morbidity and mortality; watchful waiting usually appropriate.
- Gleason score ≥7, higher PSA and younger age associated with higher morbidity and mortality; best treatment strategy (surgery, radiation, androgen suppression, etc) is not known.

Treatment of Early Prostate Cancer

- Radical prostatectomy (reduced overall and disease-specific mortality, metastasis, and local progression compared with watchful waiting in men <75 yr with early disease, well or moderately well differentiated histology, and PSA <50 ng/mL)
- Radiation therapy
  ○ External beam
  ○ Brachytherapy (radioactive seed implantation)
- Watchful waiting (avoid if life expectancy >15 yr or Gleason score ≥7)
- Hormonal therapy is generally reserved for locally advanced or metastatic disease.

Pharmacotherapy for Locally Advanced and Metastatic Disease

- Use hormonal therapy (**Table 77**) in ≥Stage III or T3 (tumor extension beyond prostate capsule); treatment of earlier stage disease is controversial.
- In case of relapse:
  ○ Withdrawal of antiandrogen may induce remission.
  ○ Patients often respond when changed to a second antiandrogen.
  ○ When antiandrogens no longer control disease, adrenal suppression with aminoglutethimide or ketoconazole and hydrocortisone replacement may be effective.

Therapy for Metastatic Bone Disease

In hormone-therapy cancer and bone metastasis, zoledronic acid reduces the proportion of patients with skeletal-related events or fracture.

Table 77. Common Drugs for Prostate Cancer Therapy

Class, Agent	Dosage	Metabolism	Adverse Events
LH-RH Agonists			
Goserelin acetate implant (*Zoladex*)	3.6 mg SC q 28 d or 10.8 mg q 3 mo	Rapid urinary and hepatic excretion, no dosage adjustment in renal impairment	Hot flushes (60%), breast swelling, libido change, impotence, nausea
Leuprolide acetate (*Lupron Depot*)	7.5 mg IM q mo or 22.5 mg q 3 mo or 30 mg q 4 mo	Unknown; active metabolites for 4–12 wk, dose-dependent	Certain symptoms (urinary obstruction, spinal cord compression, bone pain) may be exacerbated early in treatment; adverse events: hot flushes (60%), edema (12%), pain (7%), nausea, vomiting, impotence, dyspnea, asthenia (all 5%), thrombosis, PE, MI (all 1%); headache as high as 32%
Triptorelin (*Trelstar Depot, Trelstar LA*)	Depot: 37.5 mg q 28 d IM LA: 11.25 mg q 84 d	Hepatic metabolism and renal excretion (42% as intact peptide)	Hot flushes, ↑ glucose, ↓ Hb, ↓ RBC, ↑ alk phos, ↑ ALT or AST, skeletal pain, ↑ BUN
Histrelin acetate (*Vantas*)	50-mg SC implant q 12 mo	Hepatic metabolism	Hot flushes, fatigue, headaches, nausea, mild renal impairment
Antiandrogens			Class adverse events: nausea, hot flushes, breast pain, gynecomastia, hematuria, diarrhea, liver enzyme elevations, galactorrhea
Bicalutamide (*Casodex*)	50 mg po qd [T: 50]	Metabolized in liver, excreted in urine; half-life 10 d at steady state	
Flutamide (*Eulexin*)	250 mg po q 8 h [C: 125]	Renally excreted; half-life 5–6 h	Greatest GI toxicity in the class; severe liver dysfunction reported
Nilutamide (*Nilandron*)	300 mg for 30 d, then 150 mg po qd [T: 50]	80% protein bound; liver metabolism, renal excretion; half-life 40–60 h	Delayed light adaptation
GnRH Antagonist			
Abarelix (*Plenaxis*)	100 mg IM q 28 d	Liver metabolism, 13% renal excretion; half-life 13 d	Hypersensitivity 4%, prolonged QT interval; use limited to initial treatment of advanced cancer

PSYCHOTIC DISORDERS

DIAGNOSIS
Differential Diagnosis
- Bipolar affective disorder
- Delirium
- Dementia
- Drugs: eg, antiparkinsonian agents, anticholinergics, benzodiazepines or alcohol (including withdrawal), stimulants, corticosteroids, cardiac drugs (eg, digitalis), opioid analgesics
- Late-life delusional (paranoid) disorder
- Major depression
- Physical disorders: hypo- or hyperglycemia, hypo- or hyperthyroidism, sodium or potassium imbalance, Cushing's syndrome, Parkinson's disease, B_{12} deficiency, sleep deprivation, AIDS
- Pain, untreated
- Schizophrenia
- Structural brain lesions: tumor or stroke
- Seizure disorder: eg, temporal lobe

Risk Factors for Psychotic Symptoms in Older Adults
Chronic bed rest, cognitive impairment, female gender, sensory impairment, social isolation

MANAGEMENT
- Alleviate underlying physical causes.
- Address identifiable psychosocial triggers.
- If psychotic symptoms are severe, frightening, or may affect safety, use antipsychotic.
- Olanzapine, quetiapine, risperidone first choice because of fewer adverse events (TD extremely high in older adults taking typical antipsychotics).

Table 78. Representative Medications for Treatment of Psychosis

Class, Agent	Dosage*	Formulations	Comments (Metabolism)
Atypical Antipsychotics			
Aripiprazole (*Abilify*)	10–15 (1) initially; max 30/d	T: 10, 15, 20, 30	Sedation; wait 2 wk between dosage changes (CYP2D6, 3A4) (L)
Clozapine (*Clozaril*)	25–150 (1)	T: 25, 100	May be useful for parkinsonism and TD; sedation, orthostasis, anticholinergic effects, agranulocytosis, weight gain; high risk of diabetes mellitus and dyslipidemia (L)
✒Olanzapine (*Zyprexa*)	2.5–10 (1)	T: 2.5, 5, 7.5, 10, 15, 20; disintegrating tab: 5, 10, 15, 20	Sedation, anticholinergic effects at high doses, high risk of weight gain, hyperglycemia, diabetes mellitus, risk of cerebrovascular adverse events; dose-related EPS (L)

(cont.)

Table 78. Representative Medications for Treatment of Psychosis (cont.)

Class, Agent	Dosage*	Formulations	Comments (Metabolism)
✔Quetiapine (*Seroquel*)	25–800 (1–2)	T: 25, 100, 200, 300	Sedation, orthostasis, no dose-related EPS; intermediate risk of diabetes mellitus and dyslipidemia; limited geriatric data (L, K)
✔Risperidone (*Risperdal*)	0.5–1 (1–2)	T: 0.25, 0.5, 1, 2, 3, 4 scored; S: 1 mg/mL; IM long-acting: 25, 37.5, and 50 mg/2 mL	Orthostasis, dose-related EPS; caution in patients at risk of stroke, risk of cerebrovascular adverse events, intermediate risk of diabetes mellitus and dyslipidemia; IM not for acute treatment; do not exceed 6 mg (L, K)
Ziprasidone (*Geodon*)	20–80 (1–2)	C: 20, 40, 60, 80; IM: 20 mg/mL	May increase QT$_c$; very limited geriatric data (L)
Low Potency			
Thioridazine (eg, *Mellaril*)	25–200 (1–3)	T: 10, 15, 25, 50, 100, 150, 200; S: 30 mg/mL	Anticholinergic effects, orthostasis, QT$_c$ prolongation, sedation, TD; for acute use only (L, K)
Intermediate Potency			
Loxapine (*Loxitane*)	2.5–20 (1–3)	C: 5, 10, 25, 50; S: 25 mg/mL	Anticholinergic effects, orthostasis, sedation, TD; for acute use only (L, K)
High Potency			
Haloperidol (*Haldol*)	0.5–2 (1–3); depot 100–200 mg IM q 4 wk	T: 0.5, 1, 2, 5, 10, 20; S: conc 2 mg/mL; Inj	EPS, TD; for acute use only (L, K)

✔ = preferred for treating older adults but does not imply lower risk; mortality may be increased in patients with dementia.
* Total mg/d (frequency/d).

Table 79. Management of Adverse Events of Antipsychotic Medications

Adverse Event	Treatment	Comment
Drug-induced parkinsonism	Lower dosage or switch to atypical antipsychotic	Often dose related; avoid anticholinergic agents
Akathisia (motor restlessness)	Switch to atypical antipsychotic, β-blocker (eg, propranolol [*Inderal*] 20–40 mg/d) or low-dose benzodiazepine (eg, lorazepam 0.5 mg bid)	Also seen with atypical antipsychotics; more likely with traditional agents
Hypotension	Slow titration; reduce dosage; change drug class	More common with low-potency agents
Sedation	Reduce dosage; give at bedtime; change drug class	More common with low-potency agents
TD	Stop drug (if possible); change to atypical antipsychotic	Increased risk in elderly; may be irreversible

Note: Periodic (q 4 mo) reevaluation of antipsychotic dosage and ongoing need is important (see OBRA Regulations, p 232). Older adults are particularly sensitive to adverse events of antipsychotic drugs. They are also at higher risk of developing TD. Periodic use of an adverse-event scale such as the AIMS (p 223) is highly recommended.

ALLERGIC RHINITIS

Definition
- The most common atopic disorder.
- Symptoms include rhinorrhea; sneezing; and irritated eyes, nose, and mucous membranes.
- May be seasonal, but in older adults is more often perennial.
- Postnasal drip, mainly from chronic rhinitis, is the most common cause of chronic cough.

Therapy

Nonpharmacologic: Saline and sodium bicarbonate nasal irrigation may be helpful (eg, Sinu*Cleanse*); avoid allergens, eliminate pets and their dander, dehumidify to reduce molds; reduce outdoor exposures during pollen season; reduce house dust mites by encasing pillows and mattresses. Arachnocides reduce mites.

Pharmacologic: Target therapy to symptoms and on whether symptoms are seasonal or perennial; see **Table 80** and **Table 81**.

Table 80. Choosing Drug Therapy for Allergic Rhinitis or Conjunctivitis

Agent or Class	Rhinitis	Sneezing	Pruritus	Congestion	Eye Symptoms
Nasal steroids*	+++	+++	++	++	++
Ipratropium, nasal*	++	0	0	0	0
Antihistamines**†	++	++	++	+	++
Pseudoephedrine, nasal‡	0	0	0	++++	0
Cromolyn, nasal†	+	+	+	+	0
Leukotriene modifiers	+	0	0	++	++

Note: 0 = drug is not effective; the number of "+'s" grades the drug's effectiveness.

* Effective in seasonal, perennial, and vasomotor rhinitis.

** Better in seasonal than in perennial rhinitis; nasal, ocular, and oral forms; ocular form effective only for eye symptoms, and nasal form only for nasal symptoms.

† Start before allergy season.

‡ Topical therapy rapid in onset but results in rebound if used for more than a few days; enhances effectiveness of nasal steroids and sleep during severe attacks.

Table 81. Drug Therapy for Allergic Rhinitis or Conjunctivitis

Type, Drug	Geriatric Dosage	Formulations	Geriatric Half-life	Adverse Events/Comments
H₁-Receptor Antagonists or Antihistamines				Class adverse events: bitter taste, nasal burning, sneezing (nasal preparations), eye burning, stinging (ocular preparations)
✒Azelastine (*Astelin*)	2 spr bid*	topical spr 0.1% (100 spr)	22–25 h	
(*Optivar*)	1 gtt OU qid	ophthalmic 0.05%		
✒Cetirizine (*Zyrtec*)	5 mg/d (max)	T: 5, 10; syr 5 mg/5 mL	Prolonged	
✒Desloratadine (*Clarinex*)	5 mg/d	T: 5	27 h	

(cont.)

Table 81. Drug Therapy for Allergic Rhinitis or Conjunctivitis (cont.)

Type, Drug	Geriatric Dosage	Formulations	Geriatric Half-life	Adverse Events/Comments
Emedastine (*Emadine*)	1 gtt OU qid	0.05%		
Fexofenadine (✔*Allegra, Allegra-D***)	60 mg po bid; once a day if CrCl <40	T: 30, 60, 180; C: 60	14 h	Least sedating in the class
Levocabastine (*Livostin*)	1 gtt OU qid	0.05%		
Loratadine (✔*Claritin, Claritin-D,*** generic, OTC)	5–10 mg qd	T: 10; rapid-disintegrating tab 10 mg; syr 1 mg/mL	Metabolites >12 d; wide variation	
Chlorpheniramine (eg, *ChlorTrimeton,* OTC)	8–12 mg bid	T: 4, 8, 12; ChT: 2; CR: 8, 12; S: 2 mg/5 mL	20 h, longer with kidney dysfunction	Sedation, dry mouth, confusion, urinary retention; dries lung secretions
Diphenhydramine (eg, *Benadryl,* OTC)	25–50 mg bid	T: 25, 50; S: elixir 12.5 mg/mL	13.5 h	Same as chlorpheniramine
Hydroxyzine (eg, *Atarax*)	25–30 mg bid	T: 10, 25, 50	30 h	Same as chlorpheniramine
Decongestants				
Pseudoephedrine (eg, *Sudafed,* combinations, OTC)	60 mg po q 4–6 h	T: 30, 60; SR: 120; S: elixir 30 mg/5 mL	2–16 h; varies with urine pH	Arrhythmia, insomnia, anxiety, restlessness, elevated BP, urinary retention in men
Nasal Steroids				
Beclomethasone (eg, *Beconase, Vancenase*)	1 spr bid–qid*	topical spr 16 g (80 spr)	Rapid absorption, hepatic metabolism	Class adverse events: nasal burning, sneezing, bleeding; septal perforation (rare); fungal overgrowth (rare); no significant systemic effects
Budesonide (eg, *Rhinocort*)	2 spr bid or 4 qd*	7 g (200 spr)		
Dexamethasone (eg, *Dexacort*)	2 spr bid or tid*	25 mL (200 spr)		
Flunisolide (eg, *Nasalide, Nasarel*)	2–4 spr bid or tid*	25 mL (200 spr)		
Fluticasone (eg, *Flonase*)	2 spr qd*	16 g (120 spr)		
Mometasone (*Nasonex*)	2 spr qd*	17 g (120 spr)		
Triamcinolone (eg, *Nasacort*)	2–4 spr qd*	10 g (100 spr)		

(cont.)

Table 81. Drug Therapy for Allergic Rhinitis or Conjunctivitis (cont.)

Type, Drug	Geriatric Dosage	Formulations	Geriatric Half-life	Adverse Events/Comments
Mast Cell Stabilizers				
Cromolyn (*NasalCrom*)	1 spr tid–qid;* begin 1–2 wk before exposure to allergen	2%, 4%		Nasal irritation, headache, itching of throat
Lodoxamide (*Alomide*)	1–2 gtt OU qid	0.1%		Ocular irritation, burning, stinging
Nedocromil (*Alocril*)	1–2 gtt OU bid	2%		Headache, ocular irritation, burning, stinging
Pemirolast (*Alamast*)	1–2 gtt OU qid	0.1%		Headache, rhinitis, flu-like symptoms, ocular irritation, burning, stinging
Mast Cell Stabilizers and H₁ antagonists				
Ketotifen (*Zaditor*)	1 gtt OU q 8–12 h	0.025%		Conjunctival injection, headache, rhinitis, ocular irritation
Olopatadine (*Patanol*)	1 gtt OU bid	0.1%		Cold syndrome, dysgeusia, headache, keratitis, ocular irritation
NSAID				
Ketorolac (*Acular*)	1 gtt OU qid	0.5%		Ocular irritation, burning, stinging
Other				
Ipratropium (*Atrovent NS*)	2 spr bid–qid*	0.03, 0.06%† sol	1.6 h	Epistaxis, nasal irritation, upper respiratory infection; sore throat, nausea. Caution: Do not spray in eyes.
Montelukast (*Singulair*)	10 mg po qd	T: 10 mg; gran 4 mg/packet		Less effective than nasal steroids

✔ = preferred for treating older adults.
* Spr per nares.
** *Allegra-D* and *Claritin-D*, also available as *Allegra-D 24 Hour* and *Claritin-D 24 Hour*, are not recommended; all contain pseudoephedrine. Contraindicated in narrow angle glaucoma, urinary retention, MAOI use within 14 d, severe HTN, or CAD. May cause headache, nausea, insomnia.
† Use 0.06% for treatment of viral upper respiratory infection.

CHRONIC OBSTRUCTIVE PULMONARY DISEASE
Definition
A spectrum of chronic respiratory diseases characterized by:
- Airflow limitation
- Cough
- Dyspnea
- Frequent pulmonary infection
- Impaired gas exchange
- Sputum production

Therapy

Smoking Cessation: Essential at any age. See p 16.

Nebulizers: Consider for patients with disabling or distressing breathlessness on maximal therapy with inhalers.

Mucolytic Therapy: (See **Table 83**.) Consider for patients with chronic productive cough; continue if reduced cough and sputum during a trial. Treatment with mucolytics is associated with a small reduction in acute exacerbations and a greater reduction in total number of days of disability.

Rehabilitation: Patients at all stages benefit from exercise training, ie, increased exercise tolerance results in decreased dyspnea and fatigue.

Long-term Oxygen Therapy: For indications, see **Table 87**. Assess patients with FEV_1 <30%, cyanosis, edema, HF, resting O_2 sats ≤92%

MDIs and Dry Powder Inhalers: Educate patients on use; dry powder inhalers should be used with an AeroChamber (requires separate prescription). Use a separate AeroChamber for inhaled steroids; wash AeroChamber monthly.

Stepped Approach: Add steps when symptoms inadequately controlled; D/C agent if no improvement. Assess improvement in symptoms, ADLs, exercise capacity, rapidity of symptom relief. See **Table 82** and **Table 86**.

Table 82. **COPD Therapy**

Stage	Treatment	
Mild COPD		
FEV_1 ≥80%	Short-acting β_2-agonist when needed	
Moderate COPD		
50% ≤FEV_1 <80%	Regular treatment with one or more bronchodilators* Rehabilitation	Long-acting bronchodilator if needed for added benefit or if ≥2 exacerbations/yr
30% ≤FEV_1 <50%	Regular treatment with one or more bronchodilators* Rehabilitation	Inhaled steroids[†] if significant symptoms and lung function response or if ≥2 exacerbations/yr
Severe COPD		
FEV_1 <30% or respiratory or right HF	Regular treatment with one or more bronchodilators* Inhaled steroids[†] if significant symptoms and lung function response or if repeated exacerbations Treatment of complications Long-term O_2 therapy if respiratory failure	
COPD Exacerbation		
(increased breathlessness, wheezing, cough, sputum)	Increase dose and/or frequency of bronchodilators* Consider IV methylxanthine Add steroid (eg, methylprednisolone 30–40 mg po qd × 10–14 d) Add antibiotics if ↑ sputum with ↑ purulence (cover *Streptococcus pneumoniae, Haemophilus influenzae, Moraxella catarrhalis*) CXR, ECG, ABG; titrate O_2 to 90% sat and recheck ABG If 2 or more of severe dyspnea, respiratory rate ≥25, or Pco_2 45–60, then noninvasive positive pressure ventilation reduces risk of ventilator use and mortality and length of hospital stay	

* β_2-agonists, ipratropium, slow-release theophylline (caution in older adults with other conditions and taking other medications).

† Consider osteoporosis prophylaxis.

Source: Chronic obstructive pulmonary disease. National Clinical Guideline on Management of Chronic Obstructive Pulmonary Disease in Adults in Primary and Secondary Care. *Thorax* 2004;59(Suppl 1):1–232.

Table 83. Mucolytic Agents for Use in COPD with Chronic Productive Cough and Frequent Exacerbation

Drug	Formulation	Dosage	Adverse Events (Metabolism)
Acetylcysteine (Mucomyst)	10% sol 20% sol 200 mg/mL	6–10 mL 3–5 mL by nebulizer tid–qid 600 mg po qd	Inhaled: occasional bronchospasm; oral form: nausea, vomiting, diarrhea, dyspepsia (unknown, K excretion)
Iodinated glycerol (Iocen)	T: 30 S: 60 mg/5 mL	60 mg qid	Long-term use may cause thyroid suppression, other symptoms of iodism, eg, rash (unknown)
Guiafenesin (Robitussin, Hytuss, Humabid LA)	T: 100, 200 LA: 600 S: 100, 200 mg/mL	200–400 po qid LA: 600 bid	Nausea, vomiting (unknown)

ASTHMA
Definition
Chronic inflammatory disorder of the airways; may be triggered by:
- Air pollution
- Allergens
- Chemicals
- Emotional distress
- Exercise
- Tobacco smoke
- Viruses

Characteristics
- Can present at any age, but in old age **cough** is a common presentation, it is less variable and episodic, presents more fixed obstruction, and is more difficult to classify.
- Symptoms include chest tightness, cough, reversible and variable PEF, shortness of breath, and wheezing.
- Symptoms may be confused with those of HF, COPD; PEF not reliable.

Therapy
Nonpharmacologic
Avoid triggers; educate patients on disease management, use of MDIs and dry powder inhalers, and peak flow meters (document severity and response to therapy).
Pharmacologic
Stepped approach:
- Based on severity of symptoms (see **Table 84**).
- When symptoms controlled for 3 mo, try stepwise reduction.
- If control not achieved, step up, but first review medication technique, adherence, and avoidance of triggers (see **Table 85** and **Table 86**).

MDIs should be used with an AeroChamber (requires separate prescription), and patients should be educated on their use. Use separate AeroChamber for steroids; wash AeroChamber monthly.

Table 84. Classification of Asthma Severity

	Symptoms During Day	Symptoms at Night	PEF or FEV$_1$	PEF Variability
Intermittent	<1/wk; asymptomatic between attacks	<2/mo	≥80%	<20%
Mild, persistent	>2/wk; attacks may affect activity	>2/mo	≥80%	20%–30%
Moderate, persistent	Daily, attacks affect activity	>1/wk	60%–80%	>30%
Severe, persistent	Continual; limited physical activity	Frequent	≤60%	>30%

Source: Adapted from Global Initiative for Asthma, *Global Strategy for Asthma Prevention and Management.* Bethesda, MD: National Heart, Lung, and Blood Institute, April 2002. NIH Publication No. 02-3659. http://www.ginasthma.com

Table 85. Asthma Therapy for Older Adults

	Daily Medications	Other Options	Geriatric Notes
Step 1 Intermittent	None	Inhaled β_2-agonist prn	
Step 2 Mild, persistent	Low-dose inhaled steroid	Long-acting β_2-agonist, SR-theophylline, or cromone or leukotriene inhibitor	Many drug interactions with theophylline; leukotrienes have not been studied in older adults
Step 3 Moderate, persistent	Low- to medium-dose inhaled steroid plus long-acting inhaled β_2-agonist	Medium-dose inhaled steroid plus SR-theophylline, or medium-dose inhaled steroid plus either oral β_2-agonist or leukotriene inhibitor, or high-dose inhaled steroid	Oral β_2-agonists cause tremors, tachycardia, angina; many older adults have fixed obstruction, and ipratropium is helpful and well tolerated
Step 4 Severe, persistent	High-dose inhaled steroid plus long-acting inhaled β_2-agonist plus one or more of SR-theophylline, leukotriene inhibitor, oral long-acting β_2-agonist, oral steroid		

Sources: Adapted from National Asthma Education and Prevention Program, *NAEPP Working Group Report: Considerations for Diagnosing and Managing Asthma in the Elderly.* Bethesda, MD: National Heart, Lung, and Blood Institute; Feb. 1996. NIH Publication No. 96-3662; and Global Initiative for Asthma, *Global Strategy for Asthma Management and Prevention.* Bethesda, MD: National Heart, Lung, and Blood Institute, April 2004. NIH Publication No. 02-3659. http://www.ginasthma.com

Table 86. Asthma and COPD Medications

Drug Packaging Color (Body/Cap)*	Dosage	Adverse Events (Metabolism, Excretion)
Anticholinergics		
✔ Ipratropium (*Atrovent*, generic) (silver/green)	2–6 puffs qid or 0.5 mg by nebulizer qid	Dry mouth, bitter taste (lung, poorly absorbed; F)
Tiotropium (*Spiriva*) (gray/green)	1 inhalation cap (18 mcg) qd	Same as ipratropium (14% K, 86% F)

(cont.)

Table 86. Asthma and COPD Medications (cont.)

Drug Packaging Color (Body/Cap)*	Dosage	Adverse Events (Metabolism, Excretion)
Short-acting β₂-Agonists**		Class adverse events: tremor, nervousness, headache, palpitations, tachycardia, cough, hypokalemia. Caution: use half-doses in patients with known or suspected coronary disease (L)
✔ Albuterol (*Proventil, Ventolin*) (yellow/orange)	2–6 puffs q 4–6 h or 2.5 mg by nebulizer qid; 1.5–3.5 mg bid–qid by nebulizer; ER tablets 4–8 mg po q 12 h	Adverse events more common with oral formulation
(*Ventolin Rotacaps*) (light blue/dark blue)	1–2 caps q 4–6 h; dry powder inhaler 200 mcg/inhalation	
✔ Bitolterol (*Tornalate*)	1–3 puffs q 4–6 h	
Isoetharine (eg, *Bronkometer, Bronkosol,* generic)	0.25–0.5 mL of 1% sol; 2 mL NS by nebulizer q 1–4 h; inhaler 1–2 puffs q 4 h	Use limited by short duration of action; not widely used for this reason (lung, L)
Levalbuterol (*Xopenex*)	0.31, 0.63, 1.25 mg q 6–8 h by nebulizer	Expensive; no advantage over racemic albuterol (intestine, L)
Pirbuterol (*Maxair*) (blue/white)	2–3 puffs q 4–6 h	Mechanism may be difficult for older patients to trigger (L, K)
Long-acting β-Agonists ✔ Salmeterol (*Serevent Diskus*) (teal/light teal)	1 cap bid; dry powdered inhaler 50 mcg/inhalation	Class adverse events: tremor, nervousness, headache, palpitations, tachycardia, cough, hypokalemia. Caution: use half-doses in patients with known or suspected coronary disease; not for acute exacerbation (L)
✔ Formoterol (*Foradil*) (white/light blue)	1 puff q 12 h	Onset of action 1–3 min (L, K)
Corticosteroids: Inhaled ✔ Beclomethasone (*Beclovent*) (white/brown) (*Vanceril*) (pink/dark pink)	2–4 puffs bid–qid [42, 84 mcg/puff, max 840 mcg/d]	Class adverse events: nausea, vomiting, diarrhea, abdominal pain; oropharyngeal thrush; dosages >1.0 mg/d may cause adrenal suppression, reduce calcium absorption and bone density, and cause bruising (L)
✔ Budesonide (eg, *Pulmicort*) (white/brown)	1–2 puffs bid–qid [100, 200, 400 mcg/puff]	
✔ Dexamethasone (eg, *Dexacort*)	3 puffs tid–qid [100 mcg/puff]	
✔ Flunisolide (eg, *AeroBid*) (gray/purple or green)	2–4 puffs bid [250 mcg/puff]	
✔ Fluticasone (eg, *Flovent*) (orange/light orange)	1 puff bid [44, 110, 220 mcg/puff]	
Mometasone (*Asmanex*)	1 inhalation/d [220 mcg]	
✔ Triamcinolone (eg, *Azmacort*) (white/white)	2 puffs tid–qid or 4 puffs bid [100 mcg/puff]	

(cont.)

Table 86. Asthma and COPD Medications (cont.)

Drug Packaging Color (Body/Cap)*	Dosage	Adverse Events (Metabolism, Excretion)
Corticosteroids: Oral		
Prednisone (eg, *Deltasone, Orasone*)	20 mg po bid [T: 1, 2.5, 5, 10, 20, 50; elixir 5 mg/5 mL]	Leukocytosis, thrombocytosis, sodium retention, euphoria, depression, hallucination, cognitive dysfunction; other effects with long-term use (L)
Methylxanthines		
Long-acting Theophyllines (eg, *Quibron-T/SR*)	300–400 mg/d [T: 300 bisect, trisect tabs]	Class adverse events: atrial arrhythmias, seizures, increased gastric acid secretion, ulcer, reflux, diuresis; clearance ↓ by 30% after 65 yr; initial dose ≤400 mg/d, titrate using blood levels (L)
(eg, *Theo-Dur, Slo-Bid*)	100–200 mg po bid [T: 100, 200, 300, 450]	
(eg, *Uniphyl, Theo-24*)	400 mg po qd [T: 100, 200, 300, 400]	
Leukotriene Modifiers		
Montelukast (*Singulair*)	10 mg po in AM [T: 10; ChT: 4, 5]	Headache, drowsiness, fatigue, dyspepsia; minimal data in older adults; leukotriene-receptor antagonist (L)
Zafirlukast (*Accolate*)	20 mg po bid 1 h before or 2 h after meals [T: 10, 20]	Headache, somnolence, dizziness, nausea, diarrhea, abdominal pain, fever; monitor LFTs; monitor coumarin anticoagulants; leukotriene-receptor antagonist (L, reduced by 50% >65 yr)
Zileuton (*Zyflo*)	600 mg po qid [T: 600]	Dizziness, insomnia, nausea, abdominal pain, abnormal LFTs, myalgia; monitor coumarin anticoagulants; other drug interactions; inhibits synthesis of leukotrienes (L)
Other Medications		
✔ Albuterol-Ipratropium (*Combivent*) (silver/orange)	0.09/0.018 mg/puff, 2–3 puffs qid; 3 mg/0.5 mg by nebulizer qid	Same as individual agents (L, K)
Cromolyn sodium (eg, *Intal*) (white/blue)	2–4 puffs or 20-mg caps qid	Because of propellant, use MDI with caution in coronary disease or arrhythmia (L, K)
Nedocromil (*Tilade*) (white/white)	2 puffs qid	Bitter taste, headache, dizziness, sore throat, cough, chest tightness (K, F)
✔ Salmeterol-Fluticasone combination (*Advair Diskus*) (purple/light purple)	1 puff bid (50 mcg/100, 250, or 500 mcg/inhalation)	

✔ = preferred for treating older adults.
 * Generics may have different color on body and cap.
** Older nonselective β_2-agonists such as isoproterenol, metoproterenol, or epinephrine are not recommended and are more toxic.

Table 87. Indications for Long-term Oxygen Therapy*

Pao₂ Level	Sao₂ Level	Other
$\leq$55 mm Hg	$\leq$88%	>15 h/d for benefit[†], greater if 20 h/d
55–59 mm Hg	$\geq$89%	Signs of tissue hypoxia (ie, cor pulmonale by ECG, HF, hematocrit >55%); or nocturnal desaturation, sats <90% for >30% of the time
$\geq$60 mm Hg	$\geq$90%	Desaturation with exercise
		Desaturation with sleep apnea not corrected by CPAP

* Titrate O₂ saturation to approximately 90%.
† Improves survival, hemodynamics, polycythemia, exercise capacity, lung mechanics, and cognition.
Source: Adapted from Global Strategy for the Diagnosis, Management, and Prevention of Chronic Obstructive Pulmonary Disease, Global Initiative for Chronic Obstructive Lung Disease (GOLD). NHLBI/WHO Workshop Report, Executive Summary. National Institutes of Health, National Heart, Lung, and Blood Institute. March 2001. NIH Publication No. 2701A (for full report, see http://www.goldcopd.com).

COUGH
• Symptom of acute and chronic respiratory and cardiac illnesses.
• Chronic rhinitis is most common cause in older adults (see **Table 81**).

Management
• Identify cause, then treat underlying problem.
• Do not suppress cough in stable COPD.
• For symptomatic relief, see **Table 88**.
• Evaluate for adverse events from other medications, eg, ACE inhibitors.

Table 88. Antitussives and Expectorants

Drug	Dosage	Formulations	Adverse Events (Metabolism)
Benzonatate* (*Tessalon Perles*)	100 mg po tid (max: 600 mg/d)	C: 100, 200	CNS stimulation or depression, headache, dizziness, hallucination, constipation (L)
Dextromethorphan** (eg, *Robitussin DM*)	10–30 mL po q 4–8 h	C: 30 S: 10 mg/5 mL	Mild drowsiness, fatigue; interacts with fluoxetine, paroxetine; combination may cause serotonin syndrome (L)
Guaifenesin** (eg, *Robitussin*)	5–20 mL po q 4 h	S: 100 mg/5 mL	None at low dosages; high dosages cause nausea, vomiting, diarrhea, drowsiness, abdominal pain (L)
*Histussin HC***	10 mL q 4 h up to 40 mL/d	S: hydrocodone 2.5 mg + phenylephrine 5 mg + chlorpheniramine 2 mg/mL	Sedation, constipation, nervousness, tachycardia, hypertension, urinary retention (L)
Hydrocodone** (*Hycodan*)	5 mL po q 4–6 h	S: 5 mg/5 mL	Sedation, constipation, confusion (L)

* Antitussive and expectorant
** Antitussive

PULMONARY EMBOLISM (PE)
Symptoms
Classic triad—dyspnea, chest pain, hemoptysis—seen in ≤20% of cases.
Consider PE with any of the following:
- Chest pain
- Hemoptysis
- Hypotension
- Hypoxia
- Shortness of breath
- Syncope
- Tachycardia

Diagnosis

Figure 10. Evaluation of Suspected Pulmonary Embolism

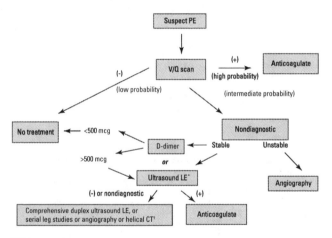

* LE = lower extremity
† Helical CT may not detect peripheral emboli.

Pharmacologic Therapy
- Low-molecular-weight heparin (LMWH) (see **Table 12**) is preferred to unfractionated heparin (UFH) in most patients due to lower risk of hemorrage and mortality. UFH should be used when CrCl <25 mL/min.
- UFH: mix infusion 100 U/mL in D5W; cleared through the reticuloendothelial system, half-life of anticoagulation effect 1.5 h
- Warfarin may be started on the same day as heparin (see p 18 and **Table 10**)
- Acute massive PE (filling defects in 2 or more lobar arteries, or the equivalent, by angiogram) associated with hypotension or severe hypoxia or high pulmonary pressures on echocardiogram should usually be treated with thrombolytic therapy within 48 h of onset (see **Table 12**).

IMPOTENCE (ERECTILE DYSFUNCTION)
Definition
Inability to achieve sufficient erection for intercourse. Prevalence nearly 70% by age 70.

Causes
Often multifactorial; >50% of cases arterial, venous, or mixed vascular cause. Also:

- Diabetes mellitus
- Drug adverse events
- Hyperprolactinemia
- Hypogonadism
- Neurologic: eg, disorders of the CNS, spinal cord, or PNS; autonomic neuropathy; temporal lobe epilepsy
- Psychologic: eg, depression, anxiety, bereavement
- Thyroid or adrenal disorders

Decreased bioavailable testosterone is associated more with decreased libido than with erectile dysfunction.

Evaluation
History: Type and duration of problem; relation to surgery, trauma, medication. Problems with orgasm, libido, or penile detumescence are not erectile dysfunction.

Physical Findings:
- Neuropathy: orthostatic hypotension, impaired response to Valsalva's maneuver, absent bulbocavernosus or cremasteric reflexes
- Peyronie's disease: penile bands, plaques
- Hypogonadism: diminished male pattern hair, gynecomastia, small (<20–25 mm long) testes

Assessment:
- Reduced penile-to-brachial pressure index suggests vascular disease.
- Cavernosometry used for diagnosing venous leak syndrome; reserved for surgical candidates.
- Test dose of prostaglandin E or papaverine can exclude vascular disease or confirm venous leak syndrome.
- For libido problems check total and bioavailable testosterone, luteinizing hormone, TSH, and prolactin. Most late-life hypogonadism is hypothalamic failure.
- Total testosterone <200 ng/dL is clearly hypogonadal. Levels 200–500 ng/dL are questionable hypogonadism. If symptoms are troublesome, a replacement trial can be given.
- Because sex hormone binding globulin increases with age, bioavailable testosterone should be a better test in older men. Currently, data are insufficient to set treatment thresholds for bioavailable testosterone for men of different ages.

Therapy

Table 89. **Management of Male Sexual Dysfunction**

Cause	Therapy	Comments
Hypogonadism, poor libido	Testosterone: scrotal transdermal (*Testoderm*) [4, 5, 6] 4–6 mg qd; *or* skin transdermal (*Androderm*) [2.5, 5] 5 mg/d;	

(cont.)

Table 89. Management of Male Sexual Dysfunction (cont.)		
Cause	Therapy	Comments
	or testosterone cypionate or enanthate 200 mg IM q 2–4 wk	When given IM, can cause polycythemia, fluid retention, gynecomastia, liver dysfunction, but IM testosterone is inexpensive and generally well tolerated
	or testosterone gel 1% (*AndroGel*) [5 g (50 mg/24 h), 7.5 g (75 mg), 10 g (100 mg)] begin with 5 g pk qam; (*Testim*) [5 g (50 mg/24 h)] begin with 5 g pk qam	Squeeze pk contents into palm of hand and apply, let dry; wash hands immediately. Check serum testosterone after 14 d and adjust dose; do not use in women
Neuropathic, vascular, or mixed	Vacuum tumescence devices (*Osbon-Erec Aid, Catalyst Vacuum Device, Pos-T-Vac, Rejoyn*)	Rare: Ecchymosis, reduced ejaculation, coolness of penile tip. Good acceptance in older population; intercourse successful in 70%–90% of cases
	Intracavernosal [5, 10, 20, 40 mcg] *or* intraurethral [125, 250, 500, 1000 mcg] prostaglandin E (*Alprostadil*)	Risks: hypotension, bruising, bleeding, priapism; erection >4 h requires emergency treatment; intraurethral safer and more acceptable
	Penile prosthesis	Complications: infection, mechanical failure, penile fibrosis
Organic, psychogenic, or mixed	PDE5 Inhibitors	All agents: Contraindicated with use of nitrates; caution in vascular disease, least effective in vascular impotence. Metabolism reduced in liver, kidney disease. Adverse events: headache, flushing, dyspepsia, dizziness, rhinitis. Nonarteritic ischemic optic neuropathy has been reported with sildenafil and tadalafil; may be a class effect, but cause and effect has not been proved.
	Sildenafil (*Viagra*) [25, 50, 100] Start 25 mg 1 h before sexual activity	Precaution: 50 or 100 mg should not be taken within 4 h of an α-blocker; 25 mg may be taken any time. Other adverse events: color tinge in vision, increased sensitivity to light, blurred vision
	Vardenafil (*LEVITRA*) [2.5, 5, 10, 20] Start 2.5 mg 1 h before sexual activity	Contraindicated with use of any α-blocker; caution with CYP3A4 inhibitors.
	Tadalafil (*Cialis*) [5, 10, 20] Start 5 mg 30 min–1 h before sexual activity; lasts 24 h	Caution with use of any α-blocker; both agents may lower BP; patients should be on stable dose of α-blocker before starting lowest dose of *Cialis*. Caution with CYP3A4 inhibitors. Other adverse events: back pain, myalgia, pain in limb.

DYSPAREUNIA

Definition

Pain with intercourse.

Aggravating Factors

- Gynecologic tumors
- Interstitial cystitis
- Myalgia from overexertion during Kegel's exercises
- Osteoarthritis
- Pelvic fractures
- Retroverted uterus
- Sacral nerve root compression
- Vaginal atrophy from estrogen deprivation
- Vulvar or vaginal infection

Evaluation
- Ask about sexual problems (eg, changes in libido, partner's function, and health issues).
- Screen for depression.
- Perform pelvic examination for vulvovaginitis, vaginal atrophy, conization (decreased distensibility and narrowing of the vaginal canal), scarring, pelvic inflammatory disease, cystocele, and rectocele.

Management
- Identify and treat clinical pathology.
- Educate and counsel patients.
- Discuss hormone therapy (see pp 212–214).
- Water-soluble lubricants (eg, *Replens*) are highly effective as monotherapy for those who cannot or will not use hormones, or as a supplement to estrogen.
- For vaginismus (vaginal muscle spasm), trial cessation of intercourse and gradual vaginal dilation may help.
- For diminished libido, short-term use of androgens (which used long-term adversely affect health) may help; refer for counseling or sex therapy.
- Topical estrogens (**Table 90**) treat symptoms and complications of estrogen deficiency such as dyspareunia and recurrent urinary tract infections with minimal systemic absorption.

Table 90. Topical Estrogens Without Systemic Effects

Estrogen	Dosage
Estrogen cream (*Premarin, Ogen, Estrace*)	Use min dose (0.5 g for *Premarin*, 2 g for *Ogen* and *Estrace*) daily × 2 wk, then 1–3 times/wk thereafter
Estradiol vaginal ring (*Estring*)	Insert intravaginally and change q 90 d
Estradiol vaginal tablets (*Vagifem*)	Insert 25 mcg intravaginally daily × 2 wk, then twice/wk

SSRI-INDUCED SEXUAL DYSFUNCTION
- Incidence varies widely, from 1% to 20% of patients making spontaneous reports to 75% when patients are systematically questioned.
- Symptoms include anorgasmia, decreased libido, and ejaculatory dysfunction.
- Wait for tolerance to develop (12 wk of treatment may be needed).
- Pharmacologic management:
  ○ For sertraline and citalopram (not other SSRIs), reducing dose or "drug holidays" (skip or reduce weekend dose) may help.
  ○ Adjuvant medications reported as effective in case reports include sildenafil (*Viagra*) 25–100 mg 1 h before intercourse
  ○ Controlled trials of mirtazapine, yohimbine, olanzapine, and bupropion did not show a benefit different from that of placebo, although most trials were small.
  ○ Change from sertraline to netazadone was found to be associated with significantly less re-emergence of sexual dysfunction than restarting sertraline and was not associated with any worsening of depression.

SKIN ULCERS

CHRONIC WOUND ASSESSMENT AND TREATMENT
Wound Assessment
Evaluation of chronic wounds should include the following (see **Table 91** for wound characteristics specific to ulcer type):
- Location
- Wound size and shape: length, width, depth, stage (pressure ulcer), grade (diabetic foot ulcer)
- Wound bed: color, presence of slough, necrotic tissue, granulation tissue, epithelial tissue, undermining or tunneling
- Exudate: purulent versus nonpurulent (serous, serosanguineous)
- Wound edges: distinct, diffuse, rolled under
- Periwound surface: erythema, edema, induration, temperature
- Presence of pain
- Signs of wound infection
  - Increased necrotic tissue
  - Foul odor of exudates
  - Purulent exudates
  - Faint halo of erythema at wound edges
  - Wound breakdown
  - Increasing pain
  - Edema
  - Granulation tissue that bleeds easily
  - Serous exudates with inflammation
  - Nonhealing or enlarging wound
- Swab culture is of limited value in diagnosing infection due to contaminated wound bed.

Wound Treatment
- Remove devitalized tissues and surface contaminants
  - Sharp debridement
  - Autolytic enzymatic preparations (eg, moisture-retaining dressings or hydrogels)
  - Mechanical (eg, wet-to-dry dressings)
  - Chemical (eg, topical enzymes such as *Accuzyme, Santyl*)
  - Cleanse with irrigation or whirlpool using normal saline or lactated Ringer's solution
  - Avoid antiseptics because of cytotoxicity
- Control bacterial burden of wound
  - Monitor for signs of infection
  - Debride all necrotic tissue (*except* when wound is ischemic)
  - Use silver product (topical such as *Silvadene* or silver dressing) if critical bacteria load is suspected
  - Limit use of topical antibiotics because of risk of developing resistant organisms
  - Use systemic antibiotics only in presence of spreading cellulitis, sepsis, or osteomyelitis
- Provide moist wound environment and control exudates (see **Table 92** and **Table 93**)
  - Dressings
  - Negative-pressure wound therapy (ie, vacuum-assisted closure [*VAC*])
    - Indications: Stage III and IV pressure ulcers, neuropathic ulcers, venous ulcers, dehisced incisions with trapping of third-space fluid around wound
    - Contraindications: Presence of *any* nonviable, necrotic tissue in wound; untreated osteomyelitis; malignancy in or surrounding wound
    - Precautions: unstable hemostasis, anticoagulant therapy

- Guidelines for use:
  - □ Negative pressure = 75–125 mm Hg depending on wound characteristics
  - □ Dressing change regimen: 48 hr after placement, then every other day
  - □ Cycle: continuous for initial 48 hr, then intermittent (5 min negative pressure followed by 2 min of no pressure) for remainder of treatment
  - □ Specialized training in application and monitoring of therapy essential to successful outcome
- Prevent further injury; position to avoid any pressure on the wound
- Support repair process
  - ○ Protein (1.25–1.5 g/kg/d) and calories (30–35/kg/d)
  - ○ Vitamin and mineral supplements if deficiencies suspected
  - ○ Avoid exposure to cold; vasoconstriction reduces blood flow to wound

Table 91. Wound Characteristics by Ulcer Type

	Arterial	Diabetic	Pressure	Venous
Location	Tips of toes or between toes, on pressure points of foot (eg, heel or lateral foot), or in areas of trauma	Plantar surface of foot, especially over metatarsal heads, toes, and heel	Over bony prominences (eg, trochanter, coccyx, ankle)	Gaiter area, particularly medial malleolus
Size and shape	Small craters with well-defined borders	Even wound margins with callus	Variable length, width, depth depending on stage (see staging system, p 195–196)	Edges may be irregular with depth limited to dermis or shallow subcutaneous tissue
Wound bed	Pale or necrotic	Granular tissue unless PAD present	Varies from bright red, shallow crater to deeper crater with slough and necrotic tissue; tunneling and undermining	Ruddy red; yellow slough may be present; undermining or tunneling uncommon
Exudate	Minimal amount due to poor blood flow	Variable amount; serous unless infection present	Purulent, becoming serous as healing progresses; foul odor with infection	Copious; serous unless infection present
Surrounding skin	Halo of erythema or slight fluctuance indicates infection	Normal	May be distinct, diffuse, rolled under; erythema, edema, induration if infected	May appear macerated, crusted, or scaly
Pain	Cramping or constant deep aching	None, because of neuropathy	Painful, unless sensory function impaired	Variable; may be severe, dull, aching, or bursting in character

ARTERIAL ULCERS
Definition
Any lesion caused by severe tissue ischemia secondary to atherosclerosis.

Causes
• Progressive occlusion
• Minor trauma (eg, footwear)

Intrinsic Risk Factors
• PAD
• Diabetes mellitus
• Systolic HTN
• Smoking
• Advanced age

Evaluation
In addition to evaluation under Chronic Wound Assessment (see p 189):
• Determine severity of PAD (see **Table 24**)
  ○ Venous filling time: Prolonged venous filling (>20 sec) predictive of severe PAD
  ○ Pedal pulses: Absence of both a dorsalis pedis and a posterior tibialis pulse indicative of PAD
  ○ Skin temperature: Unilateral coolness and sudden, marked change from proximal to distal
  ○ Ankle-brachial index (ABI): If ABI value <0.5, wound healing unlikely without revascularization
• Assess wound characteristics (see **Table 91**)
• Assess pain characteristics (see Pain, p 148)

Prevention and Management
Protective Skin Care:
• Inspect feet and legs daily
• Use emollients after bathing to prevent cracking and fissures
• Dry skin between toes to prevent maceration
• Avoid friction and pressure by using lamb's wool or foam between toes
• Use positioning devices to avoid pressure on feet (eg, heel protectors)
Protection from Mechanical Trauma:
• Wear proper fitting, protective footwear consistently
• Seek professional foot and nail care
Protection from Thermal Trauma:
• Wear warm socks to prevent vasoconstriction
• Avoid exposure of feet and legs to heat-producing devices and hot bathing water
Local Wound Care
Treatment dictated by adequacy of perfusion and status of wound bed:
• Avoid debridement of necrotic tissue until perfusion status is determined.
• If wound is infected, revascularization procedures, surgical removal of necrotic tissue, and systemic antibiotics are treatments of choice.

- Topical antibiotics should not be used solely to treat infected ischemic wounds and may cause sensitivity reactions.
- If wound is uninfected and dry eschar is present, maintain dry intact eschar as a barrier to bacteria. Application of an antiseptic may decrease bacterial burden on wound surface.
- If wound is uninfected and soft slough and necrotic tissue are present, apply moisture-retaining dressings that allow frequent inspection of wound for signs of infection.
- Assess vascular perfusion and refer for surgical intervention if consistent with overall goals of care.

DIABETIC FOOT ULCERS
Definition
Any lesion on the plantar surface of the foot caused by neuropathy.

Causes
Repetitive stress, unrelieved pressure, and trauma in an insensate foot

Intrinsic Risk Factors
- Peripheral neuropathy
- Structural foot deformity
- Limited joint mobility
- History of previous ulcers
- History of amputation
- Retinopathy
- Nephropathy
- History of uncontrolled or poorly controlled diabetes
- Advanced age
- Vascular insufficiency
- Poorly fitting footwear

Evaluation
In addition to evaluation under Chronic Wound Assessment (see p 189):
- Assess the feet in patients with one or more risk factors:
  ○ Visual inspection for rubor, pallor, callus, dry skin, ingrown toenails, and fissures
  ○ Vascular assessment for pulses, dorsal vein distention, temperature
  ○ Sensory assessment for pressure, touch, vibration
  ○ Motor assessment for joint rigidity, muscle wasting, gait disturbance
- Assess wound characteristics (see **Table 91**)
- Assess for presence of infection:
  ○ Sudden increase in blood glucose
  ○ Wound can be probed to the bone—highly sensitive indicator of osteomyelitis
- Determine grade of ulcer (Wagner Classification)
  ○ Grade 0: Preulcerative lesions; healed ulcers present; bony deformity present
  ○ Grade 1: Superficial ulcer without subcutaneous tissue involvement
  ○ Grade 2: Penetration through subcutaneous tissue
  ○ Grade 3: Osteitis, abscess, or osteomyelitis
  ○ Grade 4: Gangrene of digit
  ○ Grade 5: Gangrene of foot requiring disarticulation

Prevention and Management
- Inspect feet daily
- Use emollients after bathing to prevent cracking and fissures
- Wear proper fitting, protective footwear consistently
- Seek professional foot and nail care
- Avoid exposure to heat-producing devices (eg, heating pads) and hot bathing water

Local Wound Care
In addition to recommendations under Chronic Wound Treatment (see p 189):
- Debride devitalized tissue and callus: surgical debridement is method of choice for effective, rapid removal of nonviable tissue
- Avoid occlusive dressings due to risk of wound infection
- Offload pressure and stress from foot
  - Avoidance of pressure on foot essential to management of diabetic foot ulcer
  - Use orthotic that redistributes weight on plantar surface of foot when ambulating (eg, total contact cast, *DH Pressure Relief Walker*)
- Infected diabetic foot ulcers should be treated with systemic antibiotics because of development of resistant organisms with topical antibiotics.

Pharmacologic Therapy
Regranex, a recombinant platelet-derived growth factor, applied topically in thin layer to a clean wound bed for 12 h followed by 12 h of saline-moistened gauze dressing:
- Must be used in conjunction with offloading of pressure on foot, regular sharp debridement, and maintenance of uninfected status.
- If wound closure is not ≥30% in 10 wk or complete in 20 wk, reevaluate treatment plan and consider surgical intervention (especially if osteomyelitis is present).
- Monitor healing progress; if no signs of healing over 2-wk period, reevaluate factors affecting healing and wound management strategies.

Surgical Intervention
If ulceration is resistant to more conservative therapies or if osteomyelitis is suspected, referral for surgical evaluation is warranted.

PRESSURE ULCERS
Definition
Any lesion caused by unrelieved pressure resulting in damage of underlying tissue; usually develops over bony prominence.

Causes
- Pressure
- Shear
- Friction

Intrinsic Risk Factors
- Immobility (eg, chairbound)
- Increased age
- Malnutrition
- Moisture (eg, incontinence)
- Decreased sensory perception

Table 92. Wound and Pressure Ulcer Products, by Drainage and Stage

Product	Drainage			Wound Stage			
	Light	Moderate	Heavy	I	II	III	IV
Transparent film	•			•	•		
Foam island	•	•				•	
Hydrocolloids	•	•			•	•	
Petroleum-based nonadherent	•				•	•	
Alginate		•	•			•	•
Hydrogel	•				•	•	•
Gauze packing (moistened with saline)		•	•			•	•

Table 93. Common Dressings for Pressure Ulcer Treatment

Dressing	Indications/Use	Contraindications
Transparent film (eg, *Bioclusive, Tegaderm, Op-site*)	Stage I, II Protection from friction Superficial scrape Autolytic debridement of slough Apply skin prep to intact skin to protect from adhesive	Draining ulcers Suspicion of skin infection or fungus
Foam island (eg, *Allevyn, Lyofoam*)	Stage II, III Low to moderate exudate Can apply as window to secure transparent film	Excessive exudate Dry, crusted wound
Hydrocolloids (eg, *DuoDERM, Extra thin film DuoDERM, Tegasorb, RepliCare, Comfeel, Nu-derm*)	Stage II, III Low to moderate drainage Good periwound skin integrity Autolytic debridement of slough Left in place 3–5 d Can apply as window to secure transparent film Can apply over alginate to control drainage Must control maceration Apply skin prep to intact skin to protect from adhesive	Poor skin integrity Infected ulcers Wound needs packing
Alginate (eg, *Sorbsan, Kaltostat, Algosteril, AlgiDERM*)	Stage III, IV Excessive drainage Apply dressing within wound borders Requires secondary dressing Must use skin prep Must control maceration	Dry or minimally draining wound Superficial wounds with maceration

(cont.)

Table 93. **Common Dressings for Pressure Ulcer Treatment (cont.)**

Dressing	Indications/Use	Contraindications
Hydrogel (amorphous gels) (eg, *IntraSite gel, SoloSite gel, Restore gel*)	Stage II, III, IV Needs to be combined with gauze dressing Stays moist longer than saline gauze Changed 1–2 times/d Used as alternative to saline gauze for packing deep wounds with tunnels, undermining Reduces adherence of gauze to wound Must control for maceration	Macerated areas Wounds with excess exudate
(gel sheet) (eg, *Vigilon, Restore Impregnated Gauze*)	Stage II Needs to be held in place with topper dressing	Macerated areas Wounds with moderate to heavy exudate
Gauze packing (moistened with saline) (eg, square 2 × 2s/ 4 × 4s, *Fluffed Kerlix, Plain NuGauze*)	Stage III, IV Wounds with depth, especially those with tunnels, undermining Must be remoistened often to maintain moist wound environment	
Silver dressings (silver with alginates, gels, charcoal) (eg, *Silvercel, Silvadene, Aquacel Ag, Acticoat*)	Malodorous wounds High level of exudates Wound highly suspicious for critical bacterial load Periwound with signs of inflammation Slow-healing wound	Systemic infection Cellulitis Signs of systemic side effects, especially erythema multiforme Fungal proliferation Sensitivity of skin to sun Interstitial nephritis Leukopenia Skin necrosis Concurrent use with proteolytic enzymes

Source: Copyright © 2006 by Rita Frantz. Used with permission.

Evaluation

In addition to evaluation under Chronic Wound Assessment (see p 189):
- Determine intensity of risk status using validated tool, eg, Braden Scale. See Braden BJ, Bergstrom N. Clinical utility of the Braden Scale for predicting pressure sore risk. *Decubitus* 1989;2(3):44–51; for an online version of the scale: http://www.bradenscale.com/bradenscale.htm (for a downloadable PDF file) http://www.ncbi.nlm.nih.gov/books/bv.fcgi?rid=hstat2.section.4947 (in AHRQ pressure ulcer practice guideline).
- Assess wound characteristics (see **Table 91** and below)
- Determine level of tissue injury by using Pressure Ulcer Staging System:
  ○ **Stage I:** An observable pressure-related alteration of intact skin that, as compared with an adjacent or opposite area on the body, may include changes in one or more of the following: skin temperature (warmth or coolness), tissue consistency (firm or boggy feel), and/or sensation (pain, itching). The ulcer appears as a defined area of persistent redness in lightly pigmented skin, whereas in darker skin tones, it may appear with persistent red, blue, or purple hues.

- **Stage II:** Partial-thickness skin loss involving epidermis and/or dermis; presents as abrasion, blister, or shallow crater.
- **Stage III:** Full-thickness skin loss involving damage or necrosis of subcutaneous tissue that may extend down to, but not through, underlying fascia; presents as deep crater with or without undermining of adjacent tissue.
- **Stage IV:** Full-thickness skin loss with extensive destruction; tissue necrosis; or damage to muscle, bone, or supporting structures. May have associated undermining of sinus tracts. Note: eschar-covered ulcers cannot be staged until eschar is removed.

Prevention and Management
In addition to recommendations under Chronic Wound Treatment (see p 189):
Protect Wound and Surrounding Skin from Further Trauma
- Avoid positioning directly on the ulcer.
- Use pressure-reduction strategies:
  - Reposition q 2 h.
  - Use pressure-reducing cushions, mattresses, and heel protectors.
  - Avoid massaging reddened bony prominences.
  - Avoid positioning directly on the trochanter.
- Reduce friction and shear:
  - Maintain head of bed elevation <30 degrees.
  - Use lift sheet to reposition.
Promote Clean Wound Bed, Prevent Infection
- Debride necrotic tissue, eschar.
- Consider use of autolytic methods or topical enzymes in conjunction with sharp debridement to facilitate more rapid removal of necrotic tissue.
- Cleanse with each dressing change using normal saline. Irrigate using 8 mm Hg pressure (19-gauge IV catheter and 35-mL syringe) when wound is deep, tunneled, or undermined.
Maintain Moist Wound Environment (see **Table 92** and **Table 93**)
Control Exudate (see **Table 92** and **Table 93**)
Eliminate Dead Space: Pack dead space (tunnels, undermining) with moistened gauze dressings or strips of calcium alginate.
Diagnose and Treat Infection
- Ensure that necrotic tissue has been debrided completely from wound bed.
- Consider 2-wk trial of topical antibiotic for clean ulcers that are not healing after 2–4 wk optimal care; antibiotic spectrum should include gram-negative, gram-positive, and anaerobic organisms.
- Avoid using systemic antibiotics in the absence of advancing cellulitis or systemic infection.
Support Healing Systemically
- Provide nutritional support (see p 118).
- Provide adequate hydration with oral or parenteral fluids.
Surgical Repair
- Consider surgical referral for Stage IV pressure ulcers and for severely undermined or tunneled wounds.
- Monitor healing progress; in absence of signs of healing over 2-wk period, reevaluate factors affecting healing and wound management strategies.

VENOUS ULCERS
Definition
Any lesion caused by venous insufficiency precipitated by venous hypertension

Cause
Venous insufficiency

Intrinsic Risk Factors
- DVT
- Multiple pregnancies
- Edema
- Ascites
- Congenital anomalies
- Severe trauma to legs
- Tumors
- Sedentary lifestyle or job

Evaluation
In addition to evaluation under Chronic Wound Assessment (see p 189):
- Assess status of venous insufficiency
  ○ Lower-extremity edema
  ○ Lipodermatosclerosis (hyperpigmentation and induration around gaiter area)
  ○ Varicosities
  ○ Hemosiderosis
  ○ Venous dermatitis
- Diagnostic studies: Doppler ultrasonograpy, duplex imaging
- Assess wound characteristics (see **Table 91**)

Prevention and Management
Compression Therapy
- Essential component of venous ulcer treatment
- Provides externally applied pressure or static support to lower extremity to facilitate normal venous return
- Therapeutic level of compression is 30–40 mm Hg at ankle, decreasing toward knee
- Contraindicated in arterial insufficiency, uncompensated HF, and active thrombus
- Avoid compression therapy when ABI <0.8
- Types of compression therapy:
  ○ Static compression
    ■ Therapeutic stockings: Use with stable venous insufficiency to prevent ulceration or with an existing ulcer once edema has been controlled.
    ■ Compression wraps
      □ Combination short- and long-stretch elastic wraps (eg, *Dynaflex, Profore*) provide sustained compression for ambulatory or sedentary patient
      □ Avoid long-stretch elastic wraps (eg, *Ace* bandages, antiembolism hose) that provide subtherapeutic levels of compression
      □ Inelastic devices (paste bandages) and orthotic devices (eg, *Unna's boot, Circ-Aid Thera-Boot*) work by compressing calf during ambulation; most effective for ambulatory patients
    ■ Compression stockings: Stocking system containing light compression understocking and medium compression overstocking that provides high-compression therapy *(SurePress Comfort)*

○ Dynamic compression: Powered devices that propel venous blood upward when applied to lower extremity (eg, intermittent pneumatic pumps, sequential gradient compression devices, A-V impulse device)

Local Wound Care
In addition to recommendations under Chronic Wound Treatment (see p 189):
• Use exudate-absorbing dressings (eg, calcium alginate dressings, foam dressings)
• Use skin sealant to protect skin around wound from exudates
• Infected venous ulcers should be treated with systemic antibiotics because of development of resistant organisms with topical antibiotics.

Pharmacologic Therapy
Pentoxifylline (*Trental*) 400–800 mg tid has been shown to accelerate healing by decreasing blood viscosity and WBC adhesion while increasing fibrinolysis.

Surgical Intervention
• If manifestations of chronic venous insufficiency and ulceration are resistant to more conservative therapies or if venous obstruction is present, surgical repair (eg, skin graft) is treatment of choice.
• Monitor healing progress; if no signs of healing over 2-wk period, reevaluate factors affecting healing and wound management strategies.

SLEEP DISORDERS

CLASSIFICATION
- Disturbance of the sleep-wake cycle
- Hypersomnolence
- Insomnia (difficulty initiating or maintaining sleep)
- Parasomnias (disorders of arousal, partial arousal, and sleep stage transition)
- Sleep apnea

SLEEP DISORDERS OTHER THAN SLEEP APNEA
Risk Factors and Aggravating Factors
Treatable Associated Medical and Psychiatric Conditions: Adjustment disorders, anxiety, bereavement, cough, depression, dyspnea (cardiac or pulmonary), GERD, nocturia, pain, paresthesias, stress

Medications That Cause or Aggravate Sleep Problems: Alcohol, antidepressants, β-blockers, bronchodilators, caffeine, clonidine, cortisone, diuretics, levodopa, methyldopa, nicotine, phenytoin, progesterone, quinidine, reserpine, sedatives, sympathomimetics including decongestants

Management
Sleep improvements are better sustained over time with behavioral treatment.
Nonpharmacologic—Measures Recommended to Improve Sleep Hygiene:
- During the daytime:
  - Get out of bed at the same time each morning regardless of how much you slept the night before.
  - Exercise daily but not immediately before bedtime.
  - Get adequate exposure to bright light during the day.
  - Decrease or eliminate naps, unless necessary part of sleeping schedule.
  - Limit or eliminate alcohol, caffeine, and nicotine, especially before bedtime.
- At bedtime:
  - Maintain a regular sleeping time, but don't go to bed unless sleepy.
  - If hungry, have a light snack before bed (unless there are symptoms of GERD or it is otherwise medically contraindicated), but avoid heavy meals at bedtime.
  - Don't read or watch television in bed.
  - Relax mentally before going to sleep; don't use bedtime as worry time.
  - Relax before bedtime, and maintain a routine period of preparation for bed (eg, washing up and going to the bathroom).
  - Control nighttime environment, ie, comfortable temperature, quiet, dark.
  - Wear comfortable bedclothes.
  - If it helps, use soothing noise, eg, a fan or other appliance or a "white noise" machine.
  - If unable to fall asleep within 15–20 min, get out of bed and perform soothing activity, such as listening to soft music or reading (but avoid exposure to bright light).

Pharmacologic—Principles of Prescribing Medications for Sleep Disorders:
- Use lowest effective dose.
- Use intermittent dosing (2–4 times/wk).
- Prescribe medications for short-term use (no more than 3–4 wk).

- Discontinue medication gradually.
- Be alert for rebound insomnia after discontinuation.

Table 94. Useful Medications for Sleep Disorders in Older Adults

Class, Drug	Usual Dose	Formulations	Half-life	Comments (Metabolism, Excretion)
Antidepressant, sedating				
✔ Trazodone (*Desyrel*)	25–150 mg	T: 50, 100, 150, 300	12 h	Moderate orthostatic effects; effective for insomnia with or without depression (L)
Benzodiazepine, intermediate-acting				
Estazolam (*ProSom*)	0.5–1.0 mg	T: 1, 2	12–18 h	Rapidly absorbed, effective in initiating sleep; slightly active metabolites that may accumulate (K)
Lorazepam (*Ativan*)	0.25–2 mg	T: 0.5, 1, 2	8–12 h	Effective in initiating and maintaining sleep; associated with falls, memory loss, rebound insomnia (K)
Temazepam (*Restoril*)	7.5–15 mg	C: 7.5, 15, 30	8–10 h*	Daytime drowsiness may occur with repeated use; effective for sleep maintenance; delayed onset of effect (K)
Nonbenzodiazepine, short-acting				
Eszopiclone (*Lunesta*)	1–2 mg	T: 1, 2, 3	5–6 h	CYP3A4 interactions; avoid administration with high-fat meal; not for treatment of anxiety (L)
Zaleplon (*Sonata*)	5 mg	C: 5, 10	1 h	Avoid taking with alcohol or food (L)
Zolpidem (*Ambien*)	5 mg	T: 5, 10	1.5–4.5 h**	Confusion and agitation may occur but are rare (L)
(*Ambien CR*)	6.25 mg	T: 6.25, 12.5	1.6–5.5 h	Do not divide, crush or chew.
CNS depressant, nonbarbiturate and nonbenzodiazepine				
Chloral hydrate (*Aquachloral, Supprettes*)	500–1000 mg (not to exceed 2 g as single dose or total daily dose)	C: 500; syr 500 mg/5 mL; Sp: 324, 500, 648	8 h (active metabolite)	Hypnotic effect lost after 2 wk of continual use; contraindicated in marked cardiac, hepatic, or renal impairment (K, L)
Hormone and Hormone Receptor Agonist				
Melatonin	0.3–5 mg	various	1 h	Not regulated by FDA
Ramelteon (*Rozerem*)	8 mg within 30 min of bedtime	T: 8	Ramelteon: 1–2.6 h; active metabolite: 2–5 h	Do not administer with or immediately after high-fat meal (L, K)

✔ = preferred for treating older adults.
* Can be as long as 30 h in older adults.
** 3 h in older adults; 10 h in those with hepatic cirrhosis.

SLEEP APNEA
Definition
Repeated episodes of apnea (cessation of airflow for ≥10 sec) or hypopnea (transient reduction [≥30% decrease in thoracoabdominal movement or airflow and with ≥4% oxygen desaturation, or an arousal] of airflow for ≥10 sec) during sleep with excessive daytime sleepiness or altered cardiopulmonary function.

Classification
Obstructive (90% of cases): Airflow cessation as a result of upper airway closure in spite of adequate respiratory muscle effort
Central: Cessation of respiratory effort
Mixed: Features of both obstructive and central

Associated Risk Factors, Clinical Features
Family hx, HTN, increased neck circumference, male gender, obesity, smoking, snoring, upper airway structural abnormalities (eg, soft palate, tonsils)

Evaluation
• Full night's sleep study (polysomnography) in sleep laboratory is indicated for those who habitually snore and either report daytime sleepiness or have observed apnea.
• Results are reported as the apnea-hypopnea index (AHI), which is the number of episodes of apneas and hypopneas per hour of sleep.
• Medicare reimbursement threshold for CPAP based on a min of 2 h sleep by polysomnography is AHI (1) ≥15 or (2) ≥5 and ≤14 with documented symptoms of excessive daytime sleepiness, impaired cognition, mood disorders, or insomnia, or documented HTN, ischemic heart disease, or hx of stroke.

Management
Nonpharmacologic:
• Use CPAP by nasal mask, nasal prongs, or mask that covers the nose and mouth (considered initial treatment for clinically important sleep apnea).
• Avoid use of alcohol or sedatives.
• Lie in lateral rather than supine position; may be facilitated by soft foam ball in a backpack.
• Lose weight (obese patients).
• Use oral appliances that keep the tongue in an anterior position during sleep or keep the mandible forward.
Pharmacologic:
• Modafinil (*Provigil*) 200 mg qam for excessive daytime sleepiness (CYP3A4 inducer and CYP2C19 inhibitor) [T: 100, 200]; use in addition to (not instead of) CPAP
• Protriptyline (*Vivactil*) 10–20 mg/d [T: 5, 10] (men commonly experience urinary hesitancy or frequency and impotence)
• Fluoxetine (*Prozac*) 10–20 mg [T: 10, 20, 40; S: 20 mg/5 mL]
Surgical:
• Tracheostomy (indicated for patients with severe apnea who cannot tolerate positive pressure or when other interventions are ineffective)
• Uvulopalatopharyngoplasty (curative in fewer than 50% of cases)
• Maxillofacial surgery (rare cases)

OTHER CONDITIONS ASSOCIATED WITH SLEEP DISORDERS

Nocturnal Leg Cramps

Stretching exercises or use of heating pad 10 min before bedtime may be helpful. Quinine, 200–300 mg po hs [T: 200, 260, 300, 325] may reduce the frequency though not the severity of leg cramps. Cinchonism, hemolysis, thrombocytopenia, and visual disturbances are notable adverse events.

Restless Legs Syndrome

Diagnostic Criteria:

- A compelling urge to move the limbs, usually associated with paresthesias or dysesthesias
- Motor restlessness (eg, floor pacing, tossing and turning in bed, rubbing legs)
- Vague discomfort, usually bilateral, most commonly in calves
- Symptoms exacerbated by rest, especially at night
- Symptoms relieved by movement—jerking, stretching, or shaking of limbs; pacing

Secondary Causes: Iron deficiency, spinal cord and peripheral nerve lesions, uremia, drugs (eg, TCAs, SSRIs, lithium, dopamine antagonists, caffeine)

Nonpharmacologic Treatment:

- Sleep hygiene measures (see p 199).
- Avoid alcohol, caffeine, nicotine.
- Rub limbs.
- Use hot or cold baths, whirlpools.

Pharmacologic Treatment

- Exclude or treat iron deficiency, peripheral neuropathy.
- If possible, avoid SSRIs, TCAs, lithium, and dopamine antagonists. Start at low dose, increase as needed:
- First line: dopamine agonists (see **Table 62**) or carbidopa-levodopa (*Sinemet*) 25/100 mg, 1–2 h before bedtime. Symptom augmentation may develop earlier in the day (eg, afternoon instead of evening) and may be more severe; treatment may require reducing dose or switching to dopamine agonist.
- Second-line agents include carbamazepine and gabapentin (see **Table 63**).
- For refractory cases, benzodiazepines or opioids can be tried.

Periodic Limb Movement Disorder

Diagnostic Criteria:

- Insomnia or excessive sleepiness
- Repetitive, highly stereotyped limb muscle movements (eg, extension of big toes with partial flexion of ankle, knee, and sometimes hip)
- Polysomnographic monitoring showing repetitive episodes of muscle contractions and associated arousals or awakenings
- No evidence of a medical, mental, or other sleep disorder that can account for symptoms

Treatment: Indicated for clinically significant sleep disruption or frequent arousals documented on a sleep study.

- Nonpharmacologic: sleep hygiene measures (see p 199).
- Pharmacologic: See restless legs syndrome, above.

DEFINITION
Visual acuity 20/40 or worse; severe visual impairment (legal blindness) 20/200 or worse

EVALUATION
Acuity Testing
Near Vision: Check each eye independently with glasses using handheld Rosenbaum card at 14" or Lighthouse Near Acuity Test at 16".
Far Vision: Snellen wall chart at 20'

Visual Fields: By confrontation

Ophthalmoscopy

Tonometry: Using Tono-pen (portable)

Causes of Visual Impairment in Decreasing Order of Frequency
Refractive Error: Most common cause of impairment
Cataracts: Lens opacity on ophthalmoscopic examination. Risk factors: Age, sun exposure, smoking, corticosteroids, diabetes mellitus.
Age-related Macular Degeneration (AMD): Atrophy of cells in the central macular region of retinal pigmented epithelium; on ophthalmoscopic examination, white-yellow patches (drusen) or hemorrhage and scars in advanced stages. Risk factors: Age, smoking, sun exposure, family hx, white race.
Diabetic Retinopathy: Microaneurysms, dot and blot hemorrhages on ophthalmoscopy with proliferative retinopathy ischemia and vitreous hemorrhage. Risk factors: Chronic hyperglycemia, smoking.
Glaucoma: Intraocular pressure >21 mm Hg, optic cupping and nerve head atrophy, and loss of peripheral visual fields. Risk factors: Black race, age, family hx, elevated ocular pressures.

MANAGEMENT
Prevention
Biennial full eye examinations for persons >65 yr old, annually for people with diabetes.

Nonpharmacologic Treatment
AMD: Photodynamic therapy for some wet forms: monitor for conversion to wet form using Amsler grid daily.
Cataract:
- Reduce UV light exposure.
- Surgery (AHRQ guidelines [AHCPR Publication No. 93-0542]):
  ○ if acuity 20/50 or worse with symptoms of poor functional acuity
  ○ if 20/40 or better with disabling glare or frequent exposure to low light situations, diplopia, disparity between eyes, or occupational need
  ○ when cataract removal will treat another lens-induced disease (eg, glaucoma)

○ when cataract coexists with retinal disease requiring unrestricted monitoring (eg, diabetic retinopathy)

Diabetic Retinopathy: Laser treatment of proliferative retinopathy or macular edema

Glaucoma Surgery:
• Open angle—laser trabeculoplasty or surgical trabeculectomy
• Angle closure—laser iridotomy
• Used primarily when pressures are poorly controlled by topical agents or when visual loss progresses.

Pharmacologic Treatment

AMD: For intermediate or more advanced stages: Zinc oxide 80 mg, cupric oxide 2 mg, β-carotene 15 mg, vitamin C 500 mg, and vitamin E 400 IU taken in divided doses bid reduces risk of progression (eg, *Ocuvite PreserVision* 2 tabs po bid). Not recommended for smokers (β-carotene) or for people with CAD (vitamin E). Pagaptanib *(Macugen),* a vascular endothelial growth factor antagonist, at 0.3 mg intravitreous q 6 wk for up to 2 yr, slows vision loss in wet AMD.

Diabetic Retinopathy: Glycemic control HbA$_{1c}$ 7%–9%; BP <130/80; lipid control not well studied (see p 62)

Glaucoma: Treat when pressures are >25 mm Hg or with optic nerve damage or visual field loss (see **Table 95**). Instill drops under lower lid, close eye for at least 1 min to reduce systemic absorption; wait 5 min before instilling a second type of drop.

Table 95. Agents for Treating Glaucoma			
Drug	**Strength**	**Dosage**	**Comments (Metabolism)**
Adrenergic Agonists (bottles with purple caps)			
Apraclonidine (*Iopidine*)	0.5%, 1%	1–2 drops tid	Low BP, fatigue, drowsiness, dry mouth, dry nose (unknown)
Brimonidine (*Alphagan*)	0.2%	1 drop tid	Low BP, fatigue, drowsiness, dry mouth, dry nose (L)
(*Alphagan P*)	0.15%	1 drop tid	Benzalkonium-chloride free (L)
Dipivefrin (*AKPro, Propine*)	0.1%	1 drop bid	HTN, headache, tachycardia, arrhythmia (eye, L)
Epinephrine (*Epifrin, Glaucon*)	0.1%–2%	1 drop qd–bid	HTN, headache, tachycardia, arrhythmia (L)
Epinephrine borate (*Epinal*)	0.25%–0.5%	1 drop bid	HTN, headache, tachycardia, arrhythmia (L)
β-Blockers (bottles with blue or yellow caps)			Class adverse events: hypotension, bradycardia, HF, bronchospasm, anxiety, confusion, hallucination, diarrhea, nausea, cramps, lethargy, weakness, masking of hypoglycemia, impotence (L)
✔Betaxolol (*Betoptic, Betoptic-S*)	0.25%, 0.5%	1–2 drops bid	
✔Carteolol (*Ocupress*)	1%	1 drop bid	
✔Levobunolol (*AKBeta, Betagan*)	0.25%, 0.5%	1 drop bid	
✔Metipranolol (*OptiPranolol*)	0.3%	1 drop bid	

(cont.)

Table 95. Agents for Treating Glaucoma (cont.)

Drug	Strength	Dosage	Comments (Metabolism)
✔Timolol drops (*Betimol, Timoptic*)	0.25%, 0.5%	1 drop bid	
Miotics, Direct-acting (bottles with green caps)			
Pilocarpine gel (*Pilopine HS*) (*Ocusert*)	4% 20, 40 mcg/h	1/2" qhs weekly	Systemic cholinergic effects (tissues, K)
Pilocarpine (*Adsorbocarpine, Akarpine, Isopto Carpine, Pilagan, Pilocar, Piloptic, Pilostat*)	0.25%–10%	1 drop qid	Systemic cholinergic effects are rare (K)
Miotics, Cholinesterase Inhibitors (bottles with green caps)			Class adverse events: cholinomimetic effects (sweating, tremor, headache, salivation), confusion, high or low BP, bradycardia, bronchoconstriction, urinary frequency, cramps, diarrhea, nausea, deterioration of mental status in people with AD
Demecarium (*Humorsol*)	0.125%, 0.25%	1–2 drops bid	
Echothiophate (*Phospholine*)	0.03%–0.25%	1 drop bid	
Isoflurophate (*Floropryl*)	0.025% oint	0.25" strip 8–72 h	
Physostigmine (*Eserine, Fisostin, Isopto Eserine*)	0.25% oint	1" tid	(L)
Carbonic Anhydrase Inhibitors (bottles with orange caps)			
Topical			Caution in kidney failure (K)
✔Brinzolamide (*Azopt*)	1%	1 drop tid	
✔Dorzolamide (*Trusopt*)	2%	1 drop tid	
Oral			Class adverse events: fatigue, weight loss, paresthesias, depression, COPD exacerbation, cramps, diarrhea, kidney failure, blood dyscrasias, hypokalemia, acidosis; not recommended in kidney failure (K)
Acetazolamide (eg, *Diamox*)	125–500 mg, SR 500 mg	250–500 mg bid–qid, SR 500 mg bid	
Dichlorphenamide (*Daranide*)	50 mg	25–50 mg qd–tid	
Methazolamide (eg, *Neptazane*)	25–50 mg	50–100 mg bid–tid	(L, K)
Prostaglandin Analogs			Class adverse events: change in eye color and periorbital tissues, hyperemia, itching; expensive
✔Bimatoprost (*Lumigan*)	0.03%	1 drop hs	(L, K, F)
✔Latanoprost (*Xalatan*)	0.005%	1 drop hs	(L)

(cont.)

Table 95. Agents for Treating Glaucoma (cont.)			
Drug	Strength	Dosage	Comments (Metabolism)
✔Travoprost (*Travatan*)	0.004%	1 drop hs	(L)
✔Unoprostone (*Rescula*)	0.15%	1 drop hs	(L)
Other Topical			
Dorzolamide/timolol (*Cosopt*)	0.05%, 0.2%	1 drop bid	Unusual taste, ocular itching, burning (K, L)

✔ = preferred for treating older adults.
Note: Patients may not know names of drugs but instead refer to them by the color of the bottle cap. The usual colors are listed above.

Low-vision Services
• Address the full range of functional visual impairment from blindness to partial sight. Refer patients with uncompensated visual loss that reduces function.
• Recommend optical aids:
  ○ Magnifiers with lights
  ○ Wearable telescopes for distance vision
  ○ Closed-circuit television to enlarge text
  ○ A variety of high-technology devices are available and under development (see products at http://www.lighthouse.org).
  ○ Optical aids (like the above) may improve mood unlike traditional aids such as talking books, Braille watches, etc, which do not.
• Strategies include magnification, improved illumination, increased contrast, and auditory and tactile feedback.
• Environmental modifications that improve function include color contrast, floor lamps to reduce glare, and motion sensors to turn on lights.
• Many states have "Services for the Visually Impaired" through the state health department.

Dry Eye Syndrome
Symptoms: Itchy or sandy (foreign body sensation)
Etiology: Many; consider autoimmune (Sjögren's syndrome), drug-induced, refer to ophthalmology for diagnostic assistance.
Therapy:
• Artificial tear formulations (eg, *HypoTears*)
• Viscoelastic tear formulations containing either chondroitin sulfate or hyaluronic acid are not better than artificial tears.
• Cyclosporine ophthalmic emulsion 0.05% (*Restasis*) 1 gtt OU q 12 h. Indicated when tear production is suppressed by inflammation. Does not increase tears in people using topical anti-inflammatories or punctal plugs. Adverse events: burning, hyperemia, discharge, pain, blurring.

Acute Conjunctivitis
Symptoms: Red eye, foreign body sensation, discharge, photophobia

Signs: Conjunctival hyperemia and discharge. Visual acuity, pupillary light reflexes, and visual fields are normal. If eye functions are abnormal, refer to ophthalmology for urgent diagnosis.

Differential Diagnosis: Acute iritis, acute glaucoma, episcleritis, or scleritis.

Etiology: Viral, bacterial, chlamydial, chemical, foreign body

Viral Versus Bacterial:

Viral—profuse tearing, minimal exudation, preauricular adenopathy common, monocytes in stained scrapings and exudates.

Bacterial—moderate tearing, profuse exudation, preauricular adenopathy uncommon, bacteria and polymorphonuclear cells in stained scrapings and exudates.

Both—minimal itching, generalized hyperemia, occasional sore throat and fever.

Treatment: Majority are viral; treat symptoms with artificial tears and cool compresses. If purulent discharge, suspect bacterial; start broad-spectrum topical antibiotics (see **Table 96**). If severe, obtain culture and Gram's stain, then start treatment. If signs and symptoms do not improve in 24–48 h, refer to ophthalmologist. If vision decreased or severe pain, refer to ophthalmologist immediately.

Other: Wash hands frequently and use separate towels to avoid spread.

Table 96. Treatment for Acute Bacterial Conjunctivitis*

Agent	Formulations**	Comments
Ciprofloxacin (*Ciloxan Ophthalmic*)	0.3% sol, 0.3% oint	Very broad spectrum, well tolerated, a first choice in severe cases, expensive
Erythromycin ophthalmic (*AK-Mycin, Ilotycin*)	5 mg/g oint	Good if staphylococcal blepharitis is present
Gatifloxacin (*Tequin*)	0.3% sol	Very broad spectrum, well tolerated, a first choice in severe cases, expensive
Moxifloxacin (*Avelox*)	0.5% sol	Very broad spectrum, well tolerated, a first choice in severe cases, expensive
Norfloxacin (*Chibroxin*)	0.3% sol	Very broad spectrum, well tolerated, a first choice in severe cases, expensive
Ofloxacin (*Floxin, Ocuflox Ophthalmic*)	0.3% sol, 0.3% oint	Very broad spectrum, well tolerated, a first choice in severe cases, expensive
Sulfacetamide sodium (*Sodium Sulamyd*)	10%, 30% drops, 10% oint	Well tolerated
Tobramycin (*AKTob, Tobrex*)	3 mg/g oint, 3 mg/mL sol	Well tolerated, but more corneal toxicity
Trimethoprim and polymyxin (*Polytrim*)	1 mg/mL, 10,000 IU/mL sol	Well tolerated but some gaps in coverage

* Do not use steroid or steroid-antibiotic preparations in initial treatment.

** In mild cases, solution is applied qid and gel or ointment bid for 5–7 d. In more severe cases, solution is applied q 2–3 h and ointment qid; as the eye improves, solution is applied qid and ointment bid.

Allergic Conjunctivitis

For therapy, see **Table 81**.

Systemic Medications with Ocular Adverse Events (symptoms, signs)
• Amiodarone: halos, blurred vision, corneal changes, optic neuropathy
• Anticholinergics: blurry near vision, angle-closure glaucoma (rare)
• Cisplatin: decreased central and color vision, optic disk edema, neuritis, corneal blindness
• Corticosteroids: cataracts, glaucoma
• Digoxin: yellowish orange vision; snowy, flickering vision
• Ethambutol or INH: loss of color vision, visual acuity, visual field
• Hydroxychloroquine or chloroquine: loss of color vision, visual acuity, visual field
• Niacin: decreased visual field, maculopathy
• Sildenafil: color tinge in vision (often blue haze), increased sensitivity to light, blurred vision; nonarteritic ischemic optic neuropathy has been reported in association with sildenafil and tadalafil (may be class effect of PDE5 inhibitors), but cause and effect has not been proved.

PREVENTION
(See also **Table 75**.)
- Annual breast and pelvic and perineal examination
- Annual mammography if life expectancy >4 yr
- Discuss HRT risks and benefits with patients on and considering treatment.
- Only one negative Pap smear needed after 65 yr if low risk (ie, one established sexual partner, good prior screening, no hx of abnormal Pap smear)
- Osteoporosis evaluation (see p 145)
- Heart disease
  ○ The leading cause of death in older women.
  ○ Assess risk based on Framingham criteria using the online calculator that uses age, smoking, systolic BP, total and HDL cholesterol at http://www.nhlbi.nih.gov/guidelines/cholesterol/index.htm.
  ○ Encourage all women to make lifestyle changes, including smoking cessation, regular exercise, weight management, and heart-healthy diet. Other recommendations are based on whether patient is at high, intermediate, or low risk. See **Table 18** for cholesterol treatment recommendations.
  ○ ASA (75–162 mg/d) is recommended in older women.

COMMON DISORDERS
Breast Cancer
Prevention: See also **Table 75**. Tamoxifen 20 mg po qd reduces breast cancer risk by 49% in women at high risk. For risk assessment, see prevention section of http://www.cancer.gov/cancerinfo/pdq/prevention/breast/healthprofessional
Monitoring:
- History, physical
- LFTs, calcium q 4–6 mo for 5 yr, then yearly
- Annual mammography, pelvic, and FOBT
Oral Hormone Adjuvant Therapy: Postmenopausal women with estrogen-receptor- or progesterone-receptor-positive tumors at high risk of recurrence (tumors >1 cm, or positive nodes) should be treated with oral adjuvant therapy. Therapy should include an aromatase inhibitor, which may be the initial treatment. Options include an aromatase inhibitor for 5 yr, or sequential treatment with tamoxifen (for 2–5 yr) followed by an aromatase inhibitor for 2–5 yr. See **Table 97**.
Adjuvant Chemotherapy: Reduces risk of recurrence for receptor-negative tumors. Recurrence is reduced by an additional 5%–10% in estrogen-receptor- or progesterone-receptor-positive tumors treated with both oral hormone adjuvant and chemotherapy.
Therapy for Metastatic Bone Disease: Pamidronate or zoledronic acid reduces morbidity and delays time to onset of bone symptoms. Consult oncology.

Table 97. Oral Agents for Breast Cancer Treatment

Class, Agent	Dosage	Formulations	Monitoring	Adverse Events (Metabolism)
Anti-estrogen Drugs				
Fulvestrant (*Faslodex*)	250 mg IM 1/mo in 1 or 2 injections	Inj	Blood chemistry, lipids	Has potent CYP3A4 inhibitors; GI reactions, anesthesia, pain (back, pelvic, headache), hot flushes (L)
Tamoxifen* (*Nolvadex*)	20 mg po qd	T: 10, 20	Annual eye examination; endometrial cancer screening	Drug interactions: erythromycin, calcium channel blockers; ↑ risk of thrombosis (L)
Toremifene (*Fareston*)	60 mg po qd	T: 60	CBC, Ca, LFTs, BUN, Cr	Drug interactions with CYP3A4–6 inhibitors and inducers (see **Table 7**); ↑ warfarin effect (L)
Aromatase Inhibitors				
Anastrozole (*Arimidex*)	1 mg po qd	T: 1	Periodic CBC, lipids, serum chemistry profile	Common: arthritis, arthralgia, bone pain, asthenia, cough, dyspnea, pharyngitis, depression, headache, nausea, rash, edema. Less common: anemia, leukopenia, thromboembolism, thrombophlebitis, hypercholesterolemia, fractures, vaginal hemorrhage. (L)
Exemestane (*Aromasin*)	25 mg po qd	T: 25	Periodic WBC count with differential, lipids, serum chemistry profile	Common: anxiety, depression, fatigue, insomnia, dyspnea, hot flushes, weight gain, nausea, pain at tumor site. Rare: myocardial infarction (L)
Letrozole (*Femara*)	2.5 mg po qd	T: 2.5	Periodic CBC, LFTs, TSH	Common: arthralgia, back pain, bone pain, dyspnea, hot flushes, nausea. Less common: fracture, myocardial infarction or ischemia, pancytopenia, thromboembolism, pleural effusion, pulmonary embolism. Metabolized by CYP3A4, CYP2A6; strongly inhibits CYP2A6 and moderately inhibits CYP2C19. (L)

* Reduce dosage if CrCl <10 mL/min.

Vulvar Diseases
Non-neoplastic:
- Lichen sclerosus—Common on vulva of middle-aged and older women; causes 1/3 of benign vulvar lesions, extends to perirectal areas (classic hourglass appearance); lesions are white to pink macules or papules, may coalesce; asymptomatic or itching, soreness, or dyspareunia. Must biopsy for diagnosis: Associated with squamous cell cancer in 4%–5%. Treatment: Clobetasol propionate 0.05% qd–bid for 8–12 wk; then taper gradually to zero. Long-term follow-up advised.
- Squamous hyperplasia—Raised white keratinized lesions difficult to distinguish from VIN; must biopsy to exclude malignancy. Treatment: Betamethasone dipropionate 0.05% for 6–8 wk, then 1% hydrocortisone if symptoms persist. Long-term follow-up advised.

Neoplastic:
- VIN—Most often seen in postmenopausal women; asymptomatic or may cause pruritus; hypo- or hyperpigmented keratinized lesions; often multifocal; inspection ± colposcopy of the entire vulva with biopsy of most worrisome lesions; lesions graded on degree of atypia. Treatment: surgical or other ablative therapy.
- Vulvar malignancy—Half of cases are in women >70 yr old; 80% are squamous cell, with melanoma, sarcoma, basal cell, and adenocarcinoma <20%; biopsy any suspicious lesion. Treatment: radical surgery is preferred treatment.

Postmenopausal Bleeding
Bleeding after 1 yr of amenorrhea:
- Exclude malignancy, identify source, treat symptoms.
- Examine genitalia, perineum, rectum.
- If endometrial source, use endometrial biopsy or vaginal probe ultrasound to assess endometrial thickness (<5 mm virtually excludes malignancy).
- D&C when endometrium not otherwise adequately assessed.
- Evaluation is needed for:
  ○ Women on combination continual estrogen and progesterone who bleed after 12 mo.
  ○ Women on cyclic replacement with bleeding at unexpected times (ie, bleeding other than during the second week of progesterone therapy).
  ○ Women on unopposed estrogen who bleed at any time.

Symptoms Associated with the Postmenopausal State
- Hot flushes and night sweats
- Vaginal dryness and dyspareunia
- Sleep disturbances
- Insufficient evidence exists to link the following commonly reported symptoms to the postmenopausal state: mood symptoms, cognitive disturbances, somatic symptoms, sexual dysfunction.

Therapy for Menopausal Symptoms
- Vasomotor and vaginal symptoms respond to estrogen (see **Table 99**) in dose-response fashion; start at low dosage, titrate to effect. Dyspareunia and vaginal dryness respond to topical estrogen (see **Table 90**).
- If estrogen cannot be taken or if patient feels risks exceed benefits, try one of the less effective alternatives for vasomotor symptoms:
  ○ Megestrol (*Megace*): [T: 20, 40] 20 mg qd–bid

○ Venlafaxine (*Effexor*) 75–150 mg/d
○ Fluoxetine (*Prozac*) 20 mg/d
○ Paroxetine (*Paxil*) 12.5–25 mg/d
○ Gabapentin (*Neurontin*) [C: 100, 300, 400; T: 600, 800; S: 250/5 mL] usually 300–600 tid
○ Clonidine (*Catapres, Duraclon*): [T: 0.1, 0.2, 0.3] 0.1–0.3 mg/d; use lowest effective dosage, watch for orthostatic hypotension and rebound increase in BP if used intermittently.

Vaginal Prolapse
- Child-bearing and other causes of increased intra-abdominal pressure weaken connective tissue and muscles supporting the genital organs, leading to prolapse.
- Symptoms include pelvic pressure, back pain, fecal or urinary incontinence, difficulty evacuating the rectum. Symptoms may be present even with mild prolapse.
- The degree of prolapse and organs involved dictate therapy; no therapy if asymptomatic.
- Estrogen and Kegel's exercises may help in mild cases.
- Pessary or surgery indicated with increase in symptoms. Surgery needed for 4th-degree symptomatic prolapse.
- Precise anatomic defect(s) dictates the surgical approach. Surgical closure of the vagina is a simple option for frail patients who are not sexually active.
- A common classification (ACOG) for degrees of prolapse:
  ○ First degree—extension to mid-vagina
  ○ Second degree—approaching hymenal ring
  ○ Third degree—at hymenal ring
  ○ Fourth degree—beyond hymenal ring

HORMONE THERAPY
Estrogen Therapy
- For current understanding of risks for women >65 yr old on estrogen replacement, see **Table 98**.
- If the woman has a uterus, estrogen can be combined with progesterone to reduce risk of endometrial cancer.
- Some women prefer unopposed estrogen and annual endometrial biopsy.
- For common regimens, see **Table 99**.
- Older women can get hot flushes if estrogen is discontinued suddenly. Tapering (eg, qod for 1–2 mo and then q 3 d for a few months) is better tolerated.

Table 98. Hormone Therapy Risks and Benefits After Age 65

Outcome	Estrogen	Estrogen/Progesterone
MI	none	↑
Thromboembolic disease	↑ DVT	↑ DVT, PE
Stroke	↑	↑
Breast cancer	possibly ↓	↑
Hip fracture	↓	↓
Colon cancer	none	↓

(cont.)

Table 98. **Hormone Therapy Risks and Benefits After Age 65 (cont.)**

Outcome	Estrogen	Estrogen/Progesterone
Endometrial cancer	↑	no change or ↓
Gallbladder disease	↑	↑
Urogenital disease*	↓	↓
Dementia	unknown	↑
Ovarian cancer	↑	unknown

* Dyspareunia, UTI, vaginal dryness, and possibly incontinence

Contraindications:
- Undiagnosed vaginal bleeding
- Thromboembolic disease
- Breast cancer
- Endometrial cancer more advanced than Stage 1
- Possibly gallbladder disease
- CHD

Table 99. **Common Regimens for Systemic Hormone Therapy**

Preparation	Starting Dosage (mg/d)	Cyclic Dosing	Continual Dosing	Formulations
Oral				
Conjugated equine estrogen (*Premarin*)*	0.3–0.625	—	Daily	T: 0.3, 0.625, 0.9, 1.25, 2.5
Conjugated synthetic estrogen (*Cenestin*)	0.625	—	Daily	T: 0.625, 0.9, 1.25
Esterified estrogen (eg, *Estratab*, *Menest*)*	0.3–0.625	—	Daily	T: 0.3, 0.625, 1.25, 2.5
Estradiol acetate (*Femtrace*)	0.45	—	Daily	T: 0.45, 0.9, 1.8
Estropipate (*Ogen, Ortho-Est*)*	0.625	—	Daily	T: 0.625, 1.25, 2.5
Micronized 17-β estradiol (*Estrace*)*	0.5–1	—	Daily	T: 0.5, 1, 2
Synthetic conjugated estrogens, B (*Enjuvia*)	0.625	—	Daily	T: 0.625, 1.25
Oral Combinations				
Conjugated estrogen *and* medroxyprogesterone (*Prempro*)	0.625, 0.45 1.5, 2.5, 5	—	Daily	Fixed dose 0.625/2.5 or 0.625/5 or 0.45/1.5
Conjugated estrogen *and* medroxyprogesterone (*Premphase*)	0.625 5	Days 1–28 Days 15–28	—	Fixed dose 0.625 days 1–14, 0.625/5 days 15–28
Estradiol *and* norethindrone (*FEMHRT 1/5*)	1 5	—	Daily	Fixed dose 1/5
Transdermal				
Transdermal estrogen (*Alora*)	0.05–0.75	—	Biweekly	0.05, 0.075, 0.1

(cont.)

Table 99. Common Regimens for Systemic Hormone Therapy (cont.)

Preparation	Starting Dosage (mg/d)	Cyclic Dosing	Continual Dosing	Formulations
(Bio-E-Gel)	0.75	—	Apply 1 packet topically daily	Gel (0.06%), 1.25 g/packet
(Estrasorb)	0.05	—	Apply 2 packets topically daily	Emulsion, 1.74 g/packet
(Estraderm)*	0.05–0.75		Biweekly	0.05, 0.1
(Vivelle)*	0.0375–0.05		Biweekly	0.025, 0.0375, 0.05, 0.075, 0.1
(Climara)*	0.025–0.05	—	Weekly	0.025, 0.05, 0.075, 0.1
(FemPatch)	0.025–0.05	—	Weekly	0.025
(EstroGel)	0.75	—	Daily	Metered-dose pump: 1.25 g/pump (0.75 mg estradiol)
Estradiol and norethindrone (CombiPatch)	0.05/0.14	Biweekly for 3 wk, 1 wk off	—	0.05/0.14, 0.05/0.25
Other				
Femring	0.05	—	Intravaginal ring, change q 90 d	0.05, 0.10
Medroxyprogesterone (Cycrin, Provera)	2.5–10	5–10 mg, days 1–14	2.5–5 mg/d	T: 2.5, 5, 10

Note: See also **Table 90** for topical estrogens without systemic effects.
* FDA approved for long-term use to prevent osteoporosis.

MINI-COG ASSESSMENT INSTRUMENT FOR DEMENTIA

The Mini-Cog assessment instrument combines an uncued 3-item recall test with a clock-drawing test (CDT) that serves as a recall distractor. The Mini-Cog can be administered in about 3 min, requires no special equipment, and is relatively uninfluenced by level of education or language differences.

Administration

The test is administered as follows:

1. Make sure you have the patient's attention. Instruct the patient to listen carefully to and remember 3 unrelated words and then to repeat the words back to you (to be sure the patient heard them).
2. Instruct the patient to draw the face of a clock, either on a blank sheet of paper, or on a sheet with the clock circle already drawn on the page. After the patient puts the numbers on the clock face, ask him or her to draw the hands of the clock to read a specific time (11:10 or 8:20 are most commonly used and more sensitive than some others). These instructions can be repeated, but no additional instructions should be given. If the patient cannot complete the CDT in ≤3 min, move on to the next step.
3. Ask the patient to repeat the 3 previously presented words.

Scoring

Give 1 point for each recalled word after the CDT distractor. Score 0–3 for recall. Give 2 points for a normal CDT, and 0 points for an abnormal CDT. The CDT is considered normal if all numbers are depicted, once each, in the correct sequence and position, and the hands readably display the requested time. Add the recall and CDT scores together to get the Mini-Cog score:

• 0–2 indicates positive screen for dementia.
• 3–5 indicates negative screen for dementia.

Source: Adapted from Borson S, Scanlan J, Brush M, Vitaliano P, Dokmak A. The Mini-Cog: a cognitive "vital signs" measure for dementia screening in multi-lingual elderly. *Int J Geriatr Psychiatry* 2000; 15(11):1021–1027, and Borson S, Scanlan JM, Watanabe J, Tu SP, Lessig M. Improving identification of cognitive impairment in primary care. *Int J Geriatr Psychiatry*, in press.

PHYSICAL SELF-MAINTENANCE SCALE (ACTIVITIES OF DAILY LIVING, OR ADLs)

In each category, circle the item that most closely describes the person's highest level of functioning and record the score assigned to that level (either 1 or 0) in the blank at the beginning of the category.

A. Toilet _____
1. Care for self at toilet completely; no incontinence 1
2. Needs to be reminded, or needs help in cleaning self, or has rare (weekly at most) accidents. 0
3. Soiling or wetting while asleep more than once a week. 0
4. Soiling or wetting while awake more than once a week. 0
5. No control of bowels or bladder 0

B. Feeding ____

1. Eats without assistance. 1
2. Eats with minor assistance at meal times and/or with special preparation of food, or help in cleaning up after meals. 0
3. Feeds self with moderate assistance and is untidy. 0
4. Requires extensive assistance for all meals. 0
5. Does not feed self at all and resists efforts of others to feed him or her. 0

C. Dressing ____

1. Dresses, undresses, and selects clothes from own wardrobe 1
2. Dresses and undresses self with minor assistance 0
3. Needs moderate assistance in dressing and selection of clothes. 0
4. Needs major assistance in dressing but cooperates with efforts of others to help. 0
5. Completely unable to dress self and resists efforts of others to help 0

D. Grooming (neatness, hair, nails, hands, face, clothing) ____

1. Always neatly dressed and well-groomed without assistance 1
2. Grooms self adequately with occasional minor assistance, eg, with shaving. 0
3. Needs moderate and regular assistance or supervision with grooming 0
4. Needs total grooming care but can remain well-groomed after help from others. 0
5. Actively negates all efforts of others to maintain grooming .0

E. Physical Ambulation ____

1. Goes about grounds or city 1
2. Ambulates within residence on or about one block distant. 0
3. Ambulates with assistance of (check one)
   a ( ) another person, b ( ) railing, c ( ) cane, d ( ) walker, e ( ) wheelchair 0
   1.__Gets in and out without help. 2.__Needs help getting in and out
4. Sits unsupported in chair or wheelchair but cannot propel self without help 0
5. Bedridden more than half the time 0

F. Bathing ____

1. Bathes self (tub, shower, sponge bath) without help. 1
2. Bathes self with help getting in and out of tub. 0
3. Washes face and hands only but cannot bathe rest of body. .0
4. Does not wash self but is cooperative with those who bathe him or her. 0
5. Does not try to wash self and resists efforts to keep him or her clean. 0

For scoring interpretation and source, see note after the next instrument.

INSTRUMENTAL ACTIVITIES OF DAILY LIVING SCALE (IADLs)

In each category, circle the item that most closely describes the person's highest level of functioning and record the score assigned to that level (either 1 or 0) in the blank at the beginning of the category.

A. Ability to Use Telephone ____

1. Operates telephone on own initiative; looks up and dials numbers. 1
2. Dials a few well-known numbers. 1
3. Answers telephone but does not dial. 1
4. Does not use telephone at all. 0

B. Shopping ____

1. Takes care of all shopping needs independently. 1
2. Shops independently for small purchases. 0
3. Needs to be accompanied on any shopping trip. 0
4. Completely unable to shop. 0

C. Food Preparation _____

1. Plans, prepares, and serves adequate meals independently. 1
2. Prepares adequate meals if supplied with ingredients. 0
3. Heats and serves prepared meals or prepares meals but does not maintain
   adequate diet. 0
4. Needs to have meals prepared and served. 0

D. Housekeeping _____

1. Maintains house alone or with occasional assistance (eg, domestic help for
   heavy work). 1
2. Performs light daily tasks such as dishwashing, bedmaking. 1
3. Performs light daily tasks but cannot maintain acceptable level of cleanliness. 1
4. Needs help with all home maintenance tasks. 1
5. Does not participate in any housekeeping tasks. 0

E. Laundry _____

1. Does personal laundry completely. 1
2. Launders small items; rinses socks, stockings, etc. 1
3. All laundry must be done by others. 0

F. Mode of Transportation _____

1. Travels independently on public transportation or drives own car. .1
2. Arranges own travel via taxi but does not otherwise use public transportation. 1
3. Travels on public transportation when assisted or accompanied by another. 1
4. Travel limited to taxi or automobile with assistance of another. 0
5. Does not travel at all. 0

G. Responsibility for Own Medications _____

1. Is responsible for taking medication in correct dosages at correct time. 1
2. Takes responsibility if medication is prepared in advance in separate dosages. 0
3. Is not capable of dispensing own medication. 0

H. Ability to Handle Finances _____

1. Manages financial matters independently (budgets, writes checks, pays rent
   and bills, goes to bank); collects and keeps track of income. 1
2. Manages day-to-day purchases but needs help with banking, major
   purchases, etc. 1
3. Incapable of handling money. 0

Scoring Interpretation: For ADLs, the total score ranges from 0 to 6, and for IADLs, from 0 to 8. In some categories, only the highest level of function receives a 1; in others, two or more levels have scores of 1 because each describes competence at some minimal level of function. These screens are useful for indicating specifically how a person is performing at the present time. When they are also used over time, they serve as documentation of a person's functional improvement or deterioration.

Source: Lawton MP, Brody EM. Assessment of older people: self-maintaining and instrumental activities of daily living. _Gerontologist_ 1969, 9:179–186. Copyright by the Gerontological Society of America. Reproduced by permission of the publisher.

PHQ-9 QUICK DEPRESSION ASSESSMENT
INSTRUCTIONS FOR USE (_for doctor or healthcare professional use only_)
For initial diagnosis:

1. Patient completes PHQ-9 Quick Depression Assessment.
2. If there are at least 4 ✔s in the shaded section (including Questions #1 and #2),
   consider a depressive disorder. Add score to determine severity.

3. *Consider Major Depressive Disorder*
—if there are at least 5 ✔s in the shaded section (one of which corresponds to Question #1 or #2)
Consider Other Depressive Disorder
—if there are 2 to 4 ✔s in the shaded section (one of which corresponds to Question #1 or #2)
Note: Since the questionnaire relies on patient self-report, all responses should be verified by the clinician and a definitive diagnosis made on clinical grounds, taking into account how well the patient understood the questionnaire, as well as other relevant information from the patient. Diagnoses of Major Depressive Disorder or Other Depressive Disorder also require impairment of social, occupational, or other important areas of functioning (Question #10) and ruling out normal bereavement, a history of a Manic Episode (Bipolar Disorder), and a physical disorder, medication, or other drug as the biological cause of the depressive symptoms.

To monitor severity over time for newly diagnosed patients or patients in current treatment for depression:
1. Patients may complete questionnaires at baseline and at regular intervals (eg, every 2 wk) at home and bring them in at their next appointment for scoring, or they may complete the questionnaire during each scheduled appointment.
2. Add up ✔s by column. For every ✔:
   Several days = 1
   More than half the days = 2
   Nearly every day = 3
3. Add together column scores to get a TOTAL score.
4. Refer to the PHQ-9 Scoring Card to interpret the TOTAL score.
5. Results may be included in patients' files to assist in setting up a treatment goal, determining degree of response, as well as guiding treatment intervention.

PHQ-9 SCORING CARD FOR SEVERITY DETERMINATION
(for healthcare professional use only)
Scoring—add up all checked boxes on PHQ-9
For every ✔:
Not at all = 0; Several days= 1; More than half the days = 2; Nearly every day = 3

Interpretation of Total Score	
Total Score	**Depression Severity**
1–4	Minimal depression
5–9	Mild depression
10–14	Moderate depression
15–19	Moderately severe depression
20–27	Severe depression

PATIENT HEALTH QUESTIONNAIRE (PHQ-9)
NAME: _____   DATE: _____

Over the last 2 weeks, how often have you been bothered by any of the following problems? (use "✔" to indicate your answer)	Not at all	Several days	More than half the days	Nearly every day
1. Little interest or pleasure in doing things	0	1	2	3
2. Feeling down, depressed, or hopeless	0	1	2	3
3. Trouble falling or staying asleep, or sleeping too much	0	1	2	3
4. Feeling tired or having little energy	0	1	2	3
5. Poor appetite or overeating	0	1	2	3
6. Feeling bad about yourself—or that you are a failure or have let yourself or your family down	0	1	2	3
7. Trouble concentrating on things, such as reading the newspaper or watching television	0	1	2	3
8. Moving or speaking so slowly that other people could have noticed. Or the opposite—being so fidgety or restless that you have been moving around a lot more than usual	0	1	2	3
9. Thoughts that you would be better off dead, or of hurting yourself in some way	0	1	2	3

add columns: _____ + _____ + _____

(Healthcare professional: For interpretation of TOTAL, please refer to scoring card.)   **TOTAL:** _____

10. If you checked off *any* problems, how difficult have these problems made it for you to do your work, take care of things at home, or get along with other people?

Not difficult at all _____
Somewhat difficult _____
Very difficult _____
Extremely difficult _____

GERIATRIC DEPRESSION SCALE (GDS, SHORT FORM)

Choose the best answer for how you felt over the past week.

1. Are you basically satisfied with your life?   yes/**no**
2. Have you dropped many of your activities and interests?   **yes**/no
3. Do you feel that your life is empty?   **yes**/no
4. Do you often get bored?   **yes**/no

5. Are you in good spirits most of the time? yes/**no**
6. Are you afraid that something bad is going to happen to you? **yes**/no
7. Do you feel happy most of the time? yes/**no**
8. Do you often feel helpless? **yes**/no
9. Do you prefer to stay at home, rather than going out and doing new things? **yes**/no
10. Do you feel you have more problems with memory than most? **yes**/no
11. Do you think it is wonderful to be alive now? yes/**no**
12. Do you feel pretty worthless the way you are now? **yes**/no
13. Do you feel full of energy? yes/**no**
14. Do you feel that your situation is hopeless? **yes**/no
15. Do you think that most people are better off than you are? **yes**/no

Score 1 point for each bolded answer. Cut-off: normal 0–5; above 5 suggests depression.

Source: Courtesy of Jerome A. Yesavage, MD. For 30 translations of the GDS, see
http://www.stanford.edu/~yesavage/GDS.html
For additional information on administration and scoring, refer to the following references:
Sheikh JI, Yesavage JA. Geriatric Depression Scale: recent evidence and development of a shorter version. *Clin Gerontol.* 1986;5:165–172.
Feher EP, Larrabee GJ, Crook TH 3rd. Factors attenuating the validity of the Geriatric Depression Scale in a dementia population. *J Am Geriatr Soc.* 1992;40:906–909.
Yesavage JA, Brink TL, Rose TL et al. Development and validation of a geriatric depression rating scale: a preliminary report. *J Psychiatr Res.* 1983;17:27.

BRIEF HEARING LOSS SCREENER

	Points
1. Age:_____	_____

If age >70 years = 1 point

2. Sex: Male_____ Female_____ _____
If male = 1 point

3. Highest grade attended: _____
12th grade or less_____
higher than 12th grade_____
If ≤12th grade = 1 point

4. Have you ever had deafness or trouble hearing with one or both ears? __0__
Yes_____, go to Question #5.
No_____, go to Question #6.
No points assigned to this question.

5. Did you ever see a doctor about it? _____
Yes_____ No_____
If "Yes" = 2 points

6. Without a hearing aid, can you usually hear and understand what a person says _____
without seeing his or her face if that person whispers to you from across the room?
Yes_____ No_____
If "No" = 1 point

7. Without a hearing aid, can you usually hear and understand what a person says _____
without seeing his or her face if that person talks to you in a normal voice from
across the room?
Yes_____ No_____
If "No" = 2 points

TOTAL _____
3 or more points is a positive score indicating the need for further evaluation.

Test Characteristics of This Screener With Established Hearing Loss Criteria

	Sensitivity	Specificity	Pos Predictive Value	Neg Predictive Value
Ventry-Weinstein criteria	80%	80%	45%	95%
High-frequency pure-tone average	59%	88%	76%	77%

Source: Reuben DB, Walsh K, Moore AA, et al. Hearing loss in community-dwelling older persons: national prevalence data and identification using simple questions. *J Am Geriatr Soc.* 1998;46:1011. Reprinted with permission.

PERFORMANCE-ORIENTED MOBILITY ASSESSMENT (POMA)
Balance

Chair: Instructions: Place a hard armless chair against a wall. The following maneuvers are tested.

1. Sitting down
   0 = unable without help or collapses (plops) into chair or lands off center of chair
   1 = able and does not meet criteria for 0 or 2
   2 = sits in a smooth, safe motion *and* ends with buttocks against back of chair and thighs centered on chair

2. Sitting balance
   0 = unable to maintain position (marked slide forward or leans forward or to side)
   1 = leans in chair slightly or slight increased distance from buttocks to back of chair
   2 = steady, safe, upright

3. Arising
   0 = unable without help or loses balance or requires >3 attempts
   1 = able but requires 3 attempts
   2 = able in 1 or 2 attempts

4. Immediate standing balance (first 5 sec)
   0 = unsteady, marked staggering, moves feet, marked trunk sway, or grabs object for support
   1 = steady but uses walker or cane, or mild staggering but catches self without grabbing object
   2 = steady without walker or cane or other support

Stand

5a. Side-by-side standing balance
   0 = unable or unsteady *or* holds ≤3 sec
   1 = able but uses cane, walker, or other support or holds for 4–9 sec
   2 = narrow stance without support for 10 sec

5b. Timing __ __.__ seconds

6. Pull test (person at max position attained in #5, examiner stands behind and exerts mild pull back at waist)
   0 = begins to fall
   1 = takes more than 2 steps back
   2 = fewer than 2 steps backward and steady

7a. Able to stand on right leg unsupported
   0 = unable or holds onto any objects or able for <3 sec
   1 = able for 3 or 4 sec
   2 = able for 5 sec

7b. Timing __ __.__ seconds

8a. Able to stand on left leg unsupported
   0 = unable or holds onto any object or able for <3 sec
   1 = able for 3 or 4 sec
   2 = able for 5 sec

8b. Timing __ __.__ seconds

9a. Semitandem stand
   0 = unable to stand with one foot half in front of other with feet touching *or* begins to fall *or* holds for ≤3 sec
   1 = able for 4–9 sec
   2 = able to semitandem stand for 10 sec

9b. Timing __ __.__ seconds

10a. Tandem stand
   0 = unable to stand with one foot in front of other or begins to fall or holds for ≤3 sec
   1 = able for 4–9 sec
   2 = able to tandem stand for 10 sec

10b. Timing __ __.__ seconds

11. Bending over (to pick up a pen off floor)
   0 = unable or is unsteady
   1 = able but requires more than one attempt to get up
   2 = able and is steady

12. Toe stand
   0 = unable
   1 = able but for <3 sec
   2 = able for 3 sec

13. Heel stand
   0 = unable
   1 = able but for <3 sec
   2 = able for 3 sec

Gait

Bare Floor (flat, even surface): Instructions: Person stands with examiner, walks down 10-ft walkway (measured). Ask the person to walk down walkway, turn, and walk back. The person should use customary walking aid.

1. Type of surface: 1 = linoleum or tile; 2 = wood; 3 = cement or concrete; 4 = other____ (not included in scoring)

2. Initiation of gait (immediately after told to "go")
   0 = any hesitancy or multiple attempts to start
   1 = no hesitancy

3. Path (estimated in relation to tape measure). Observe excursion of foot closest to tape measure over middle 8 feet of course.
   0 = marked deviation
   1 = mild or moderate deviation or uses walking aid
   2 = straight without walking aid

4. Missed step (trip or loss of balance)
   0 = yes, and would have fallen or more than 2 missed steps
   1 = yes, but appropriate attempt to recover and no more than 2 missed steps
   2 = none

5. Turning (while walking)
   0 = almost falls
   1 = mild staggering but catches self, uses walker or cane
   2 = steady without walking aid

6.   Step over obstacles (to be assessed in a separate walk with 2 shoes placed on course 4 feet apart)

0 = begins to fall at any obstacle or unable or walks around any obstacle or >2 missed steps

1 = able to step over all obstacles but some staggering and catches self or 1–2 missed steps

2 = able and steady at stepping over all obstacles with no missed steps

Source: Courtesy of Mary E. Tinetti, MD. Adapted with permission.

ABNORMAL INVOLUNTARY MOVEMENT SCALE (AIMS)

Examination Procedure

Either before or after completing the examination procedure, observe the patient unobtrusively, at rest (eg, in waiting room). The chair to be used in this examination should be a hard, firm one without arms.

1. Ask patient to remove shoes and socks.
2. Ask patient whether there is anything in his or her mouth (ie, gum, candy, etc) and if there is, to remove it.
3. Ask patient about the **current** condition of his or her teeth. Ask patient if he or she wears dentures. Ask if teeth or dentures are bothering patient **now**.
4. Ask patient whether he or she notices any movements in mouth, face, hands, or feet. If yes, ask to describe and to what extent they **currently** bother patient or interfere with his or her activities.
5. Have patient sit in chair with hands on knees, legs slightly apart, and feet flat on floor. (Look at entire body for movements while patient is in this position.)
6. Ask patient to sit with hands hanging unsupported; if male, between legs, if female and wearing a dress, hanging over knees. (Observe hands and other body areas.)
7. Ask patient to open mouth. (Observe tongue at rest within mouth.) Do this twice.
8. Ask patient to protrude tongue. (Observe abnormalities of tongue movement.) Do this twice.
9. Ask patient to tap thumb with each finger as rapidly as possible for 10–15 sec; separately with right hand, then with left hand. (Observe facial and leg movements.)
10. Flex and extend patient's left and right arms (one at a time). (Note any rigidity.)
11. Ask patient to stand up. (Observe in profile. Observe all body areas again, hips included.)
12. Ask patient to extend both arms outstretched in front with palms down. (Observe trunk, legs, and mouth.)
13. Have patient walk a few paces, turn, and walk back to chair. (Observe hands and gait.) Do this twice.

Instructions: Complete examination procedure before making ratings. Rate highest severity observed.

Code:

1 None
2 Minimal, may be extreme normal
3 Mild
4 Moderate
5 Severe

Facial and Oral Movements

1. Muscles of facial expression (eg, movements of forehead, eyebrows, periorbital area, cheeks [including frowning, blinking, smiling, grimacing])

   1   2   3   4   5

2. Lips and perioral area (eg, puckering, pouting, smacking)

   1   2   3   4   5

3. Jaw (eg, biting, clenching, chewing, mouth opening, lateral movement)

   1   2   3   4   5

4. Tongue (rate only increase in movement both in and out of mouth, **not** inability to sustain movement)

   1   2   3   4   5

Extremity Movements

5. Upper—arms, wrists, hands, fingers: include choreic movements (ie, rapid, objectively purposeless, irregular, spontaneous), athetoid movements (ie, slow, irregular, complex, serpentine). Do **not** include tremor (ie, repetitive, regular, rhythmic).

   1   2   3   4   5

6. Lower—legs, knees, ankles, toes: eg, lateral knee movement, foot tapping, heel dropping, foot squirming, inversion and eversion of foot.

   1   2   3   4   5

Trunk Movements

7. Neck, shoulders, hips (eg, rocking, twisting, squirming, pelvic gyrations)

   1   2   3   4   5

Global Judgments

8. Severity of abnormal movements
   1. None, normal
   2. Minimal
   3. Mild
   4. Moderate
   5. Severe
9. Incapacitation due to abnormal movements
   1. None, normal
   2. Minimal
   3. Mild
   4. Moderate
   5. Severe
10. Patient's awareness of abnormal movements (rate only patient's report)
    1. No awareness
    2. Aware, no distress
    3. Aware, mild distress
    4. Aware, moderate distress
    5. Aware, severe distress

Dental Status

11. Current problems with teeth and/or dentures
    1. No
    2. Yes
12. Does patient usually wear dentures?
    1. No
    2. Yes

Source: Adapted from Department of Health and Human Services, Public Health Service, Alcohol, Drug Abuse and Mental Health Administration, National Institute of Mental Health. *Treatment Strategies in Schizophrenia Study.* ADM-117. Revised 1985.

PAIN SCALES FOR ASSESSING PAIN INTENSITY
Use copies of pain scales that are large enough for older adults to see comfortably (14-point font or larger).

Faces Pain Scale
Place an X under the face that best represents the severity or intensity of your pain right now.

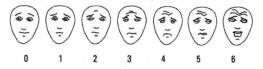

Source: Reprinted from *Pain*, 41(2), Bien D, Reeve R, Champion G, et al. The Faces Pain Scale for the self-assessment of the severity of pain experienced by children: development and initial validation, and preliminary investigation for ratio scale properties. 139–150, Copyright 1990, with permission from the International Association for the Study of Pain.

0–10 Numeric Rating Scales
Verbal: On a scale of 0–10, with 0 being no pain and 10 being the most intense pain imaginable, what would you rate the severity or intensity of your pain right now? _____

Source: Keela Herr, 2006.

Visual: Circle the number that best represents the severity or intensity of your pain right now.

0	1	2	3	4	5	6	7	8	9	10
No pain					Moderate pain					Worst possible pain

Source: Carr DB, Jacox AK, Chapman CR, et al. *Acute Pain Management: Operative Medical Procedures and Trauma.* Clinical Practice Guideline No. 1. Rockville, MD: AHCPR, Public Health Service, US Dept of Health and Human Services; February 1992. AHCPR Publication No. 92-0032.

Verbal Descriptor Scale

Place an X beside the words that best describe the severity or intensity of your pain right now. Mark one set of words.

—— Most intense pain imaginable
—— Very severe pain
—— Severe pain
—— Moderate pain
—— Mild pain
—— Slight pain
—— No pain

Source: Keela Herr, 2006.

Reference

AGS Panel on Persistent Pain in Older Persons. The management of persistent pain in older persons. *J Am Geriatr Soc.* 2002;50(6, Suppl):S205–S224.

BRIEF PAIN INVENTORY (Short Form)

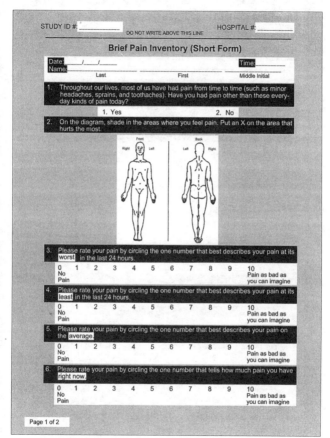

STUDY ID #: _____   HOSPITAL #: _____
DO NOT WRITE ABOVE THIS LINE

Date: ___/___/___   Time: _____
Name: _____
            Last   First   Middle Initial

7. What treatments or medications are you receiving for your pain?

_____
_____

8. In the last 24 hours, how much relief have pain treatments or medications provided? Please circle the one percentage that most shows how much relief you have received.

0%	10%	20%	30%	40%	50%	60%	70%	80%	90%	100%
No Relief										Complete Relief

9. Circle the one number that describes how, during the past 24 hours, pain has interfered with your:

A. General Activity

0	1	2	3	4	5	6	7	8	9	10
Does not Interfere										Completely Interferes

B. Mood

0	1	2	3	4	5	6	7	8	9	10
Does not Interfere										Completely Interferes

C. Walking Ability

0	1	2	3	4	5	6	7	8	9	10
Does not Interfere										Completely Interferes

D. Normal Work (includes both work outside the home and housework)

0	1	2	3	4	5	6	7	8	9	10
Does not Interfere										Completely Interferes

E. Relations with other people

0	1	2	3	4	5	6	7	8	9	10
Does not Interfere										Completely Interferes

F. Sleep

0	1	2	3	4	5	6	7	8	9	10
Does not Interfere										Completely Interferes

G. Enjoyment of life

0	1	2	3	4	5	6	7	8	9	10
Does not Interfere										Completely Interferes

Worst pain, or the arithmetic mean of the 4 severity items (items 3, 4, 5, and 6), can be used as measures of pain severity. The arithmetic mean of the 7 interference item (items 9A-G) can be used as a measure of pain interference. Scores on the BPI pain severity items are defined as mild (1–4), moderate (5–6), and severe (7–10). The tool can be used to follow the course of pain and response to interventions.

KARNOFSKY SCALE

This 10-point scale is a quick and easy way to indicate how a patient is feeling on a given day, without going through several multiple-choice questions or symptom surveys.

Score	Description
100	Able to work; normal, no complaints, no evidence of disease
90	Able to work; able to carry on normal activity, minor symptoms
80	Able to work; normal activity with effort, some symptoms
70	Unable to work or carry on normal activity, cares for self independently
60	Mildly disabled, dependent; requires occasional assistance, cares for most needs
50	Moderately disabled, dependent; requires considerable assistance and frequent care
40	Severely disabled, dependent; requires special care and assistance
30	Severely disabled; hospitalized, death not imminent
20	Very sick; active supportive treatment needed
10	Moribund; fatal processes rapidly progressing

Source: Karnofsky DA, Burchenal JH. The clinical evaluation of chemotherapeutic agents in cancer. In: MacLeon CM, ed. *Evaluation of Chemotherapeutic Agents*. Columbia University Press; 1949:196.

PALLIATIVE PERFORMANCE SCALE, VERSION 2 (PPSv2)

%	Ambulation	Activity and Evidence of Disease	Self-care	Intake	Conscious Level
100	Full	Normal activity and work, no evidence of disease	Full	Normal	Full
90	Full	Normal activity and work, some evidence of disease	Full	Normal	Full
80	Full	Normal activity with effort, some evidence of disease	Full	Normal or reduced	Full
70	Reduced	Unable to do normal job or work, significant disease	Full	Normal or reduced	Full
60	Reduced	Unable to do hobby or housework, significant disease	Occasional assistance required	Normal or reduced	Full or confusion
50	Mainly sit/lie	Unable to do any work, extensive disease	Considerable assistance required	Normal or reduced	Full or confusion
40	Mainly in bed	Unable to do most activity, extensive disease	Mainly assistance	Normal or reduced	Full or drowsy, ± confusion
30	Totally bed bound	Unable to do any activity, extensive disease	Total care	Normal or reduced	Full or drowsy, ± confusion
20	Totally bed bound	Unable to do any activity, extensive disease	Total care	Minimal to sips	Full or drowsy, ± confusion
10	Totally bed bound	Unable to do any activity, extensive disease	Total care	Mouth care only	Drowsy or coma ± confusion
0	Death	—	—	—	—

The Palliative Performance Scale, version 2 (PPSv2), copyright 2001, Victoria Hospice Society. Reprinted with permission. Instructions for use of PPSv2 can be found at: http://www.victoriahospice.org/pdfs/PPSv2.pdf
The PPSv2 replaces the first PPS published in Anderson F et al., Palliative performance scale (PPS): A new tool. *J Pall Care* 1996;(9)4:26-32.

REISBERG FUNCTIONAL ASSESSMENT STAGING (FAST) SCALE

This 16-item scale is designed to parallel the progressive activity limitations associated with AD. Stage 7 identifies the threshold of activity limitation that would support a prognosis of ≤6 mo life expectancy.

FAST Scale Item	Activity Limitation Associated with AD
Stage 1	No difficulty, either subjectively or objectively
Stage 2	Complains of forgetting location of objects; subjective work difficulties
Stage 3	Decreased job functioning evident to coworkers; difficulty in traveling to new locations
Stage 4	Decreased ability to perform complex tasks (eg, planning dinner for guests, handling finances)
Stage 5	Requires assistance in choosing proper clothing
Stage 6	Decreased ability to dress, bathe, and toilet independently
Substage 6a	Difficulty putting clothing on properly
Substage 6b	Unable to bathe properly, may develop fear of bathing
Substage 6c	Inability to handle mechanics of toileting (ie, forgets to flush, does not wipe properly)
Substage 6d	Urinary incontinence
Substage 6e	Fecal incontinence
Stage 7	Loss of speech, locomotion, and consciousness
Substage 7a	Ability to speak limited (1–5 words a day)
Substage 7b	All intelligible vocabulary lost
Substage 7c	Nonambulatory
Substage 7d	Unable to smile
Substage 7e	Unable to hold head up

Source: Reisberg, B. Functional assessment staging (FAST), *Psychopharmacol Bull.* 1988;24(4):653–659. Copyright MedWorks Media LLC. Reprinted with permission.

AUA SYMPTOM INDEX FOR BPH

Questions to be answered (circle one number on each line)	Not at all	Less than 1 time in 5	Less than half the time	About half the time	More than half the time	Almost always
1. Over the past month or so, how often have you had a sensation of not emptying your bladder completely after you finished urinating?	0	1	2	3	4	5
2. Over the past month or so, how often have you had to urinate again less than 2 hours after you finished urinating?	0	1	2	3	4	5

(cont.)

Questions to be answered (circle one number on each line)	Not at all	Less than 1 time in 5	Less than half the time	About half the time	More than half the time	Almost always
3. Over the past month or so, how often have you found you stopped and started again several times when you urinated?	0	1	2	3	4	5
4. Over the past month or so, how often have you found it difficult to postpone urination?	0	1	2	3	4	5
5. Over the past month or so, how often have you had a weak urinary stream?	0	1	2	3	4	5
6. Over the past month or so, how often have you had to push or strain to begin urination?	0	1	2	3	4	5
7. Over the last month, how many times did you most typically get up to urinate from the time you went to bed at night until the time you got up in the morning?	none	1 time	2 times	3 times	4 times	5 or more times

AUA Symptom Score = sum of responses to questions 1–7 =_____. For interpretation, see p 171.

Source: Barry MJ, Fowler FJ Jr, O'Leary MP et al. The American Urological Association symptom index for benign prostatic hyperplasia. *J Urol.* 1992;148(5):1549–1557. Reprinted with permission.

MEDICATION APPROPRIATENESS ASSESSMENT

To assess the appropriateness of a drug, the following questions should be considered in view of the patient's medical problems and current medications. For combination drugs, the questions should be considered for each drug. See also p 9.
• Is there an indication for the drug?
• Is the medication effective for the condition?
• Is the dosage correct?
• Are the directions correct?
• Are the directions practical?
• Are there clinically significant drug-drug interactions?
• Are there clinically significant drug-disease or drug-condition interactions?
• Is there unnecessary duplication with other drug(s)?
• Is the duration of therapy acceptable?
• Is this drug the least expensive alternative compared with others for the same use?

Source: Adapted from Hanlon JT, Schmader KE, Samsa GP, et al. A method for assessing drug therapy appropriateness. *J Clin Epidemiol* 1992; 45(10):1045–51, copyright (1992) with permission from Elsevier.

OBRA REGULATIONS

Centers for Medicare and Medicaid Services (CMS [formerly US Health Care Financing Administration]) regulations regarding the use of certain medications in nursing homes are contained in the Omnibus Budget Reconciliation Act (OBRA) of 1987.

ANTIDEPRESSANT MEDICATIONS

	Table 100. Recommended Maximum Doses of Antidepressants	
Drug	Usual Max Daily Dose (mg) for Age ≥65	Usual Max Daily Dose (mg)
Amitriptyline (*Elavil*)	150	300
Amoxapine (*Asendin*)	200	400
Desipramine (*Norpramin*)	150	300
Doxepin (*Adapin, Sinequan*)	150	300
Imipramine (*Tofranil*)	150	300
Maprotiline (*Ludiomil*)	150	300
Nortriptyline (*Aventyl, Pamelor*)	75	150
Protriptyline (*Vivactil*)	30	60
Trazodone (*Desyrel*)	300	600
Trimipramine (*Surmontil*)	150	300

ANTIPSYCHOTIC MEDICATIONS

Indications for appropriate use of antipsychotic medications are outlined in OBRA. In addition to psychotic disorders, these indications include specific nonpsychotic behavior associated with organic mental syndromes:

• Agitated psychotic symptoms (biting, kicking, scratching, assertive and belligerent behavior, sexual aggressiveness) that present a danger to patients themselves or to others or that interfere with family's and/or staff's ability to provide care (ADLs)
• Psychotic symptoms (hallucinations, delusions, paranoia)
• Continual (24-h) crying out and screaming

Behaviors less responsive to antipsychotic therapy include:

• Repetitive, bothersome behavior (ie, pacing, wandering, repeated statements or words, calling out, fidgeting)
• Poor self-care
• Unsociability
• Indifference to surroundings
• Uncooperative behavior
• Restlessness
• Impaired memory
• Anxiety
• Depression
• Insomnia

Use of antipsychotic agents only for one or more of these symptoms is inappropriate. Because of their anticholinergic properties, antipsychotic agents may worsen these symptoms, as well as symptoms of sedation, lethargy, and "confusion."

Selection of an antipsychotic agent should be based on the adverse-event profile because all antipsychotic agents are equally effective at equivalent doses. Coadministration of two or more antipsychotics does not have any pharmacologic basis or clinical advantage. Coadministration of two or more antipsychotic agents does not improve clinical response and increases the potential for adverse events.

Once behavior is under control, assess patient to determine if precipitating event (eg, stress from drugs, fluid or electrolyte changes, infection, changes in environment) has been resolved or if patient has accommodated to the environment or situation. Determine whether the dosage can be decreased or tapered off completely by monitoring selected target symptoms for which the antipsychotic therapy was initiated. OBRA 1987 requires attempts to reduce dosage within a 6-mo period or documentation as to why this cannot be done. Identifying target symptoms is essential for adequate monitoring. Because of adverse events, intermittent use (not prn) is preferable (ie, only when patient exhibits behavior warranting use of these agents). For the recommended doses of antipsychotics, see **Table 101**.

Drug	Usual Max Daily Dose (mg) for Age ≥65	Usual Max Daily Dose (mg)	Daily Oral Dose (mg) for Patients with Organic Mental Syndromes
Acetophenazine (*Tindal*)	150	300	20
Chlorpromazine (*Thorazine*)	800	1600	75
Chlorprothixene (*Taractan*)	800	1600	75
Clozapine (*Clozaril*)	25	450	50
Fluphenazine (*Prolixin*)	20	40	4
Haloperidol (*Haldol*)	50	100	4
Loxapine (*Loxitane*)	125	250	10
Mesoridazine (*Serentil*)	250	500	25
Molindone (*Moban*)	112	225	10
Olanzapine (*Zyprexa*)	—	20	10
Quetiapine (*Seroquel*)	—	800	200
Perphenazine (*Trilafon*)	32	64	8
Promazine (*Sparine*)	50	500	150
Risperidone (*Risperdal*)	1	16	2
Thioridazine (*Mellaril*)	400	800	75
Thiothixene (*Navane*)	30	60	7
Trifluoperazine (*Stelazine*)	40	80	8
Triflupromazine (*Vesprin*)	100	200	—

Table 101. Recommended Maximum Doses of Antipsychotics

ANXIOLYTIC MEDICATIONS
Use of anxiolytics is acceptable as long as other disease processes that could explain anxious behavior have been excluded. Daily use, at any dose, should be limited to <4 consecutive months, unless an attempt at dosage reduction is unsuccessful. Proper indications include:

- Generalized anxiety disorder
- Organic mental syndrome (including dementia associated with agitation)
- Panic disorders
- Anxiety associated with other psychiatric disorder (eg, depression, adjustment disorder)

Table 102. Recommended Maximum Doses of Anxiolytics*

Drug	Usual Daily Dose (mg) for Age ≥65	Usual Daily Dose (mg) for Age <65
Alprazolam (*Xanax*)	2	4
Clorazepate (*Tranxene*)	30	60
Chlordiazepoxide (*Librium*)	40	100
Diazepam (*Valium*)	20	60
Halazepam (*Paxipam*)	80	160
Lorazepam (*Ativan*)	3	6
Meprobamate (*Miltown*)	600	1600
Oxazepam (*Serax*)	60	90
Prazepam (*Centrax*)	30	60

* CMS-OBRA guidelines strongly urge clinicians not to use barbiturates, glutethimide, and ethchlorvynol because of their adverse events, pharmacokinetics, and addiction potential in older adults. Also, CMS discourages use of long-acting benzodiazepines in treating older adults.

HYPNOTIC MEDICATIONS

Hypnotics can be used for 10 consecutive days. If attempts to reduce the dosage have been unsuccessful three times, then dosage reduction is clinically contraindicated.

Table 103. Recommended Maximum Doses of Hypnotics*

Drug	Usual Max Single Dose (mg) for Age ≥65	Usual Max Single Dose (mg)
Alprazolam (*Xanax*)	0.25	1.5
Amobarbital (*Amytal*)	150	300
Butabarbital (*Butisol*)	100	200
Chloral hydrate (*Noctec*)	750	1500
Chloral hydrate (various)	500	1000
Diphenhydramine (*Benadryl*)	25	50
Ethchlorvynol (*Placidyl*)	500	1000
Flurazepam (*Dalmane*)	15	30
Glutethimide (*Doriden*)	500	1000
Halazepam (*Paxipam*)	20	40
Hydroxyzine (*Atarax*)	50	100
Lorazepam (*Ativan*)	1	2
Methyprylon (*Noludar*)	200	400
Oxazepam (*Serax*)	15	30
Phenobarbital (*Nembutal*)	100	200
Secobarbital (*Seconal*)	100	200

(cont.)

Table 103. Recommended Maximum Doses of Hypnotics* (cont.)		
Drug	Usual Max Single Dose (mg) for Age ≥65	Usual Max Single Dose (mg)
Temazepam (*Restoril*)	15	30
Triazolam (*Halcion*)	0.125	0.5

* CMS-OBRA guidelines strongly urge clinicians not to use barbiturates, glutethimide, and ethchlorvynol because of their adverse effects, pharmacokinetics, and addiction potential in older adults. Also, CMS discourages use of long-acting benzodiazepines in treating older adults.

CMS CRITERIA: INAPPROPRIATE DRUG USE IN NURSING HOMES

On July 1, 1999, HCFA (the US Health Care Financing Administration, renamed in 2001 the Centers for Medicare and Medicaid Services, or CMS) modified its regulations regarding medication use by nursing home residents who are ≥65 yr old. As part of their review, surveyors determine if the resident is taking any medications considered to have a high potential ("high severity") for severe adverse drug reactions (ADRs) or medications with a high potential for less severe ("low severity") ADRs. Residents receiving any medications are monitored for ADRs. If an ADR is identified, the rationale for use of the medication must be justified and considered appropriate. If it is not, a deficiency is cited.

People wishing additional information are advised to contact the American Society of Consultant Pharmacists (http://www.ascp.com).

The medications in **Table 104** are considered "high severity" by CMS and should be considered potentially inappropriate for use in treating older adults.

Table 104. Drugs Considered "High Severity" by CMS	
Class or Drug	**Comments**
Amitriptyline (*Elavil*)	May be used for neurogenic pain if evaluation of risk vs. benefit of the drug is documented, including consideration of alternative therapies
Chlorpropamide (*Diabinese*)	
Digoxin, in dosages >0.125 mg/d	Unless an atrial arrhythmia is being treated; high severity is considered if started within the past month
Disopyramide (*Norpace*)	
GI antispasmodics (belladonna alkaloids, clidinium, dicyclomine, hyoscyamine, propantheline)	Use for short periods (≤7 d) on an intermittent basis (not more frequently than q 3 mo) does not require review by a surveyor.
Meperidine, oral	If started within past month
Methyldopa	If started within past month
Pentazocine	
Ticlopidine	Review by a surveyor is not necessary in individuals who receive ticlopidine because they have had a previous stroke or have evidence of stroke precursors (ie, TIAs) and cannot tolerate ASA.

The drug-diagnosis combinations in **Table 105** are considered "high severity" by CMS and should be considered potentially inappropriate for use in treating older adults.

Table 105. Diagnosis-Drug Combinations Considered "High Severity" by CMS		
Class or Drug	**Diagnosis**	**Comments**
Sedatives, hypnotics	COPD	Short-acting benzodiazepines are acceptable
NSAIDs	Active or recurrent gastritis, peptic ulcer disease, GERD	COX-2 inhibitors are not included on the list of NSAIDs

(cont.)

Table 105. Diagnosis-Drug Combinations Considered "High Severity" by CMS (cont.)

Class or Drug	Diagnosis	Comments
Metoclopramide	Seizures or epilepsy	
ASA, NSAIDs, dipyridamole, ticlopidine	Anticoagulation	
Anticholinergic drugs	BPH	
TCAs	Arrhythmias	If started within past month

The medications in **Table 106** are considered "low severity" by CMS and should be considered as potentially inappropriate in treating older adults.

Table 106. Drugs Considered "Low Severity" by CMS

Class or Drug	Comments
Antihistamines with anticholinergic properties	
Cyclandelate	
Digoxin, in dosages >0.125 mg/d	Unless an atrial arrhythmia is being treated; high severity is considered if started within the past month
Diphenhydramine	Review by a surveyor is not necessary if used for a short time (≤7 d) on an intermittent basis (not more frequently than q 3 mo) for allergies
Dipyridamole	
Ergot mesylates (eg, *Hydergine*)	
Indomethacin	Short-term use (eg, 1 wk) is considered acceptable for treatment of gouty arthritis
Meperidine, oral	If therapy longer than 1 mo
Muscle relaxants (eg, carisoprodol, chlorzoxazone, cyclobonzaprine, dantrolene, metaxalone, methocarbamol, orphenadrine)	Use for short periods (≤7 d) on an intermittent basis (not more frequently than q 3 mo) does not require review by a surveyor

The drug-diagnosis combinations in **Table 107** are considered "low severity" by the CMS and should be considered potentially inappropriate in treating older adults.

Table 107. Diagnosis-Drug Combinations Considered "Low Severity" by CMS

Class or Drug	Diagnosis	Comments
Corticosteroids	Diabetes mellitus	If started within past month
Potassium supplements or ASA at >325 mg/d	Active or recurrent gastritis, peptic ulcer disease, or GERD	Use of potassium supplements to treat low potassium concentrations until they return to the normal range is permissible if prescriber determines that intake of fresh fruits and vegetables or other dietary supplementation is not adequate or possible

(cont.)

Table 107. Diagnosis-Drug Combinations Considered "Low Severity" by CMS (cont.)

Class or Drug	Diagnosis	Comments
Antipsychotics	Seizures or epilepsy	Treatment of acute psychosis for ≤72 h is permissible
Narcotic drugs, including propoxyphene	BPH	Review by a surveyor is not necessary if use is for short duration (≤7 d) on an intermittent basis (once q 3 mo) for symptoms of an acute, self-limiting condition
Bladder relaxants (flavoxate, oxybutynin, bethanechol)	BPH	Review by a surveyor is not necessary if use is for short duration (≤7 d) on an intermittent basis (once q 3 mo) for symptoms of an acute, self-limiting condition
Anticholinergic antihistamines, GI antispasmodics, anticholinergic antidepressants, and narcotic drugs (including propoxyphene)	Constipation	Constipation can be worsened. Review by a surveyor is not necessary if use is for short duration (≤7 d) on an intermittent basis (once q 3 mo) for symptoms of an acute self-limiting condition
Antiparkinson medications	Constipation	Constipation can be worsened
Decongestants, theophylline, methylphenidate, SSRI antidepressants and desipramine, MAOIs, β-agonists	Insomnia	Insomnia can be worsened

MEDICARE PART D PRESCRIPTION DRUG PLAN

Dates and Events:
Oct 1, 2005: Prescription drug providers (PDP) release information on their individual plans.
Nov 15, 2005: Enrollment opens.
Jan 1, 2006: Part D prescription drug coverage begins.
May 15, 2006: Last day for Medicare-eligible individuals to enroll.
Nov 15-Dec 31, 2006: Next open enrollment period.

How it Works:
- Participants sign up with a PDP and pay a monthly premium (varies depending on plan). Those who sign up late may be charged a 1%/mo higher premium for every month late in signing up after May 15, 2006.
- Deductible: Once an individual has spent $250 for eligible drugs (monthly premium does not count toward the deductible), coinsurance begins.
- Coinsurance: The individual is responsible for 25% of the drug cost or a copay depending on the plan, and the plan pays 75% until the combined total equals $2000.
- The "gap" or "doughnut hole" is the time when there is no plan contribution once the $2000 annual threshold has been reached until a total of $3600 has been spent out-of-pocket for the year. Monthly premiums do not count toward the $3600.
- Catastrophic coverage begins once an individual has spent $3600 out-of-pocket for the year on medications. Once this threshold is crossed, participants pay a small percentage or flat copayment for each prescription and the plan pays the rest. There is no ceiling for this part of the program.
- A new cycle begins on January 1 of each year.

Drugs Excluded from Part D Plans
- Drugs for weight loss, weight gain, and anorexia
- Fertility agents
- Cosmetic agents (eg, for hair loss)
- Drugs intended for the symptomatic relief of cough or colds
- Vitamin and mineral products (excluding prenatal and fluoride preparations)
- Nonprescription drugs
- Inpatient drugs
- Barbiturates (including phenobarbital)
- Benzodiazepines

For more (and updated) information, contact Medicare at www.medicare.gov or 1-800-MEDICARE (1-800-633-4227).

IMPORTANT TELEPHONE NUMBERS AND WEB SITES

General Information on Aging

AGS Foundation for Health in Aging	www.healthinaging.org	800-563-4916
Administration on Aging	www.aoa.gov	202-619-0724
American Association of Retired Persons	www.aarp.org	888-OUR-AARP (888-687-2277)
American Geriatrics Society	www.americangeriatrics.org	800-247-4779
American Medical Directors Association	www.amda.com	800-876-2632
American Society of Consultant Pharmacists	www.ascp.com	800-355-2727
Assisted Living Federation of America	www.alfa.org	703-691-8100
Children of Aging Parents	www.caps4caregivers.org	800-227-7294
CDC National Prevention Information Network	www.cdcnpin.org	800-458-5231
Family Caregiver Alliance	www.caregiver.org	800-445-8106
Medicare Hotline	www.medicare.gov	800-MEDICARE (800-633-4227)
National Adult Day Services Association	www.nadsa.org	800-558-5301
National Council on the Aging	www.ncoa.org	202-479-1200
National Institute on Aging	www.nia.nih.gov	TTY: 800-222-4225 301-496-1752

Elder Mistreatment

National Center on Elder Abuse	www.elderabusecenter.org	202-898-2586

End-of-Life

National Hospice and Palliative Care Organization	www.nhpco.org	800-658-8898

Smoking Cessation

American Cancer Society	www.cancer.org	800-ACS-2345 (800-227-2345) TTY: 866-228-4327
American Lung Association	www.lungusa.org	800-LUNG-USA (800-586-4872)
CDC National Center for Chronic Disease Prevention and Health Promotion	www.cdc.gov/tobacco/how2quit.htm	800-311-3435
National Cancer Institute	www.smokefree.gov	877-448-7848 TTY: 800-332-8615

Specific Health Problems

Alzheimer's Association	www.alz.org	800-272-3900
American Cancer Society	www.cancer.org	800-ACS-2345 (800-227-2345)
Alzheimer's Disease Education and Referral Center	www.alzheimers.org	800-438-4380
American Academy of Ophthalmology	www.aao.org	800-222-3937

American Association for Geriatric Psychiatry	www.aagponline.org	301-654-7850
American College of Obstetricians and Gynecologists	www.acog.com	800-673-8444
American Diabetes Association	www.diabetes.org	800-DIABETES (800-342-2383)
American Foundation for the Blind	www.afb.org	800-AFB-LINE (800-232-5463)
American Heart Association	www.americanheart.org	800-AHA-USA1 (800-242-8721)
American Lung Association	www.lungusa.org	800-LUNG-USA (800-586-4872)
American Obesity Association	www.obesity.org	202-776-7711
American Pain Society	www.ampainsoc.org	847-375-4715
American Parkinson Disease Association	www.apdaparkinson.org	800-223-2732
American Urological Association	www.auanet.org	866-746-4282
Arthritis Foundation	www.arthritis.org	800-283-7800
Better Hearing Institute	www.betterhearing.org	800-EAR-WELL (800-327-9355)
Lighthouse International	www.lighthouse.org	800-829-0500
Meals On Wheels Association of America	www.mowaa.org	703-548-5558
National Association for Continence	www.nafc.org	800-BLADDER (800-252-3337)
National Diabetes Information Clearinghouse	www.diabetes.niddk.nih.gov	800-860-8747
National Digestive Disease Information Clearinghouse	www.digestive.niddk.nih.gov	800-891-5389
National Eye Institute	www.nei.nih.gov	301-496-5248
National Heart, Lung, and Blood Institute	www.nhlbi.nih.gov	301-592-8573
National Institute of Arthritis and Musculoskeletal and Skin Diseases	www.niams.nih.gov	877-22-NIAMS (877-226-4267)
National Institute of Mental Health	www.nimh.nih.gov	866-615-NIMH (866-615-6464)
National Institute of Neurological Disorders and Stroke	www.ninds.nih.gov	800-352-9424
National Institute on Deafness and Other Communication Disorders	www.nidcd.nih.gov	800-241-1044 TTY: 800-241-1055
National Kidney and Urologic Diseases Information Clearinghouse	www.kidney.niddk.nih.gov	800-891-5390
National Osteoporosis Foundation	www.nof.org	800-223-9994
National Parkinson Foundation	www.parkinson.org	800-327-4545
Self Help for Hard of Hearing People	www.hearingloss.org	301-657-2248 TTY: 301-657-2249
Sexuality Information and Education Council of the US	www.siecus.org	212-819-9770
The Simon Foundation for Continence	www.simonfoundation.org	800-23-SIMON (800-237-4666)

Page references followed by *t* and *f* indicate tables and figures, respectively.
Trade names are in *italics*.

INDEX (CONT.)

INDEX (CONT.)

INDEX (CONT.)

INDEX (CONT.)

INDEX (CONT.)

INDEX (CONT.)

INDEX (CONT.)

INDEX (CONT.)

INDEX (CONT.)

ABOUT THE AMERICAN GERIATRICS SOCIETY

Founded in 1942, the American Geriatrics Society (AGS) is the leading clinical society devoted to the care of older adults. The AGS promotes high quality, comprehensive, and accessible care for America's older population, including those who are chronically ill and disabled. The organization provides leadership to health care professionals, policy makers, and the public by developing, implementing, and advocating programs in patient care, research, professional and public education, and public policy.

Its members, who number just under 7000, include primary care physicians, geriatricians, geropsychiatrists, nurse practitioners, social workers, physician assistants, physical therapists, pharmacists, and others in the United States and around the world who are dedicated to improving the health, independence, and quality of life of the older population.

The AGS has long championed efforts to expand the national work force of clinicians with the specialized knowledge and skills to care for our aging population. Since the early 1990s, with funding from the John A. Hartford Foundation of New York City, the AGS has worked effectively to increase geriatrics expertise among subspecialists in internal medicine, practicing primary care physicians, and surgical and related medical specialists.

Current Major Publications and Programs of the AGS

Journal of the American Geriatrics Society—*JAGS* is rated in the top five of the ISI Science Citation Index for geriatrics and gerontology publications.

Annals of Long-Term Care: Clinical Care and Aging—This journal presents the highest quality clinical reviews, analysis, and opinions that impact the present and future of long-term care, and is the premier source of information for professionals in the long-term-care market.

Clinical Geriatrics—This journal focuses on both the clinical and practical issues related to the treatment and management of older adults.

Doorway Thoughts: Cross-Cultural Health Care for Older Adults—Developed by the AGS Ethnogeriatrics Committee, *Doorway Thoughts* uses illustrative case studies to discuss the unique cultural perspectives of seven different ethnic groups, focusing on issues such as preferred terms for cultural identity, nonverbal communication norms, differing expectations in the clinician-patient relationship, and views of end-of-life issues.

Geriatrics At Your Fingertips®—This annually updated, comprehensive pocket-sized reference to clinical geriatrics provides practical information on the evaluation and management of diseases and disorders most common to older adults. The complete content is available on the *GAYF* Web site, where versions for Pocket PC- and Palm-based PDAs are also available for download.

Geriatrics Review Syllabus: A Core Curriculum in Geriatric Medicine—The newly revised 6th (2006) edition of this ground-breaking self-assessment, continuing education program for primary care providers is a premier source of clinically relevant information in geriatric medicine.

Geriatrics Nursing Review Syllabus—This core curriculum in advanced practice geriatric nursing (GNRS) is a concise, up-to-date, and comprehensive text developed by the AGS in collaboration with the John A. Hartford Foundation Institute of Geriatric Nursing at New York University.

Geriatrics Review Syllabus Teaching Slides—This web-based subscription service can be found at http://www.frycomm.com/ags/teachingslides/. The series of one-hour PowerPoint® presentations on topics such as osteoporosis, delirium, palliative care, dementia, and preventive care is based on the *Geriatrics Review Syllabus* and works well for faculty, fellows, residents, students, and practicing clinicians. Each slide set includes case materials and can be modified to meet specific learning objectives for a session.

New Frontiers in Geriatrics Research: An Agenda for Surgical and Related Medical Specialties—www.frycomm.com/ags/rasp/ presents a research agenda specifically aimed at enhancing the quality of care for older adults who are cared for by specialists in surgical disciplines and related medical fields. This agenda and the accompanying Web site are useful to specialists who are interested in contributing to the evidence base in support of geriatrics practice in their respective disciplines.

AGS News and AGS Web site (http://www.americangeriatrics.org)—These excellent online sources provide information on AGS activities and programs, noteworthy news, public policy issues, career opportunities in geriatrics, and much more.

The AGS Annual Scientific Meeting—This is the premier forum on the latest information in clinical geriatrics, research on aging and health, health problems of older adults, and innovative models in health care delivery as well as teaching in geriatrics.

The Geriatrics Recognition Award—This award recognizes physicians and nurses who are committed to advancing their geriatrics knowledge to provide better care for older adults.

The AGS Awards Program—This program includes the Edward Henderson Award and State-of-the-Art Lecture, AGS Clinician of the Year, AGS/Merck New Investigator Awards, Dennis W. Jahnigen Memorial Award, the Dennis W. Jahnigen Career Development Scholars Awards, the Nascher/Manning Award, the Outstanding Scientific Clinical Investigator Award, and the Edward Henderson Student Award.

About the AGS Foundation for Health in Aging

In 1999, the AGS reached beyond its traditional role as a professional medical society and launched the **Foundation for Health in Aging (FHA)**. The FHA aims to build a bridge between the research and practice of geriatrics health care professionals and the public, and to advocate on behalf of older adults regarding issues of wellness and preventive care, self-responsibility and independence, and connections to family and community. For more information about FHA initiatives and its public education resources, please visit the Foundation Web site at www.healthinaging.org.

Current Major Publications and Programs of the FHA

Public Education Publications from the Foundation for Health in Aging—FHA publishes a variety of pamphlets and tools promoting disease prevention and healthy living, as well as describing the latest knowledge about age-associated chronic illness. All of these resources are available for free download on the FHA Web site at www.healthinaging.org.

Aging in the Know: Your Gateway to Health and Aging Resources on the Web—This new comprehensive Web site features information on over 50 health topics related to aging, a *What to Ask Series* designed to help older adults safely navigate the health care system, and topic-specific linkages to additional credible information on the Web. This free new resource can be found at www.healthinaging.org/agingintheknow/.

Eldercare at Home—Now in its 2nd edition, this is an extensive guide for families involved in providing care for older relatives who want to remain at home. In addition to the free online edition of *Eldercare at Home*, the FHA has created a fully illustrated workbook for individuals to use at home, and a PowerPoint® presentation package that can be used in community settings to teach family caregivers how to solve problems often faced when caring for an older adult at home. Information on these and other public education programs is available on the Foundation Web site.

FHA Awards Program—This program includes the Student Researcher Fund, the Hartford Geriatrics Health Outcomes Research Scholars Awards Program, and the T. Franklin Williams Research Scholars Award Program.

If you would like further information about the AGS or FHA, please visit our Web site at www.americangeriatrics.org

Or contact us at:
The American Geriatrics Society
The Empire State Building
350 5th Avenue, Suite 801
New York, NY 10118 USA

Call toll-free: (800) 247-4779

Outside the US, call: (212) 308-1414

E-mail: info.amger@americangeriatrics.org

GERIATRICS *At Your* FINGERTIPS®
2006–2007, 8th Edition
(ISBN 1-886775-18-4)
From the American Geriatrics Society

A guide to the evaluation and management of the diseases and disorders that most commonly affect older persons.

Portable, Practical, Fully Indexed, and Up-to-Date!

Send completed order form with payment to:

Fry Communications, Inc.
American Geriatrics Society
800 West Church Road
Mechanicsburg, PA 17055

For fast service
Call: 800-334-1429 x2529
Order online at www.geriatricsatyourfingertips.org

Please send me _____ copies of *Geriatrics At Your Fingertips*, 2006–2007, 8th Edition
@ $12.95 each
Subtotal _____

Shipping & Handling _____
North America: $2.50 + $1.00 ea additional
Overseas: $8.00 + $1.00 ea additional

TOTAL _____

To order quantities of 500 or greater please contact Elvy Ickowicz at 1-212-308-1414.

Method of Payment: _____ Check or money order payable to Fry Communications
_____ MasterCard   _____VISA
Card Number _____ Exp.Date _____
Signature _____

Shipping Instructions (must be complete)

Name: _____
Address: _____
City: _____ State: _____ Zip: _____
Phone: _____
E-mail Address: _____

GAYF2006–2007

Your request places you on the AGS e-alert electronic mailing list. You will be among the first in your discipline to find out about new releases, special offers, and program announcements from AGS. After you receive your first e-alert, you have the option of canceling the service at any time. Prices subject to change without notice.